CONSERVATIVE SURGERY FOR MENORRHAGIA

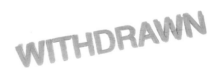

To my family, Katrina and Danny
P McG

To my parents, Patrick and Sheila, and my wife, Carmel
P O'D

To my wife Colleen
W P

CONSERVATIVE SURGERY FOR MENORRHAGIA

Peter O'Donovan
Consultant Obstetrician and Gynaecologist
Director, MERIT Centre
Bradford Royal Infirmary
UK

Paul McGurgan
Specialist Registrar
St Michael's Hospital
Bristol
UK

Walter Prendiville
Associate Professor
Coombe Women's Hospital
Dublin
Ireland

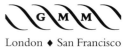

London ♦ San Francisco

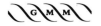

© 2003

GREENWICH MEDICAL MEDIA LTD
137 Euston Road
London
NW1 2AA

ISBN 1 84110097 8

First published 2003

Visit our website at:
www.greenwich–medical.co.uk

Distributed worldwide by Plymbridge Distributors Ltd

Typeset by Charon Tec Pvt. Ltd, Chennai, India
Printed by Bath Press Ltd, UK

CONTENTS

CHAPTER 7

CHAPTER 8

CHAPTER 9

CHAPTER 10

CHAPTER 11

CHAPTER 12

CHAPTER 13

CHAPTER 14

CHAPTER 15

CHAPTER 16

CHAPTER 17

CHAPTER 18

CHAPTER 19

CHAPTER 20

CHAPTER 21

CHAPTER 22

CHAPTER 23

CHAPTER 24

CONTRIBUTORS

J. Abbott
Research Fellow in MAS
Academic Department of Gynaecology
South Cleveland Hospital
Middlesbrough
UK

N. Amso
Senior Lecturer and
Honorary Consultant
University Hospital of Wales
Cardiff
UK

M.S. Baggish
Department of Obstetrics and
Gynaecology
Good Samaritan Hospital
Cincinnati
Ohio, USA

J.F. Bodle
Research Fellow
Department of Obstetrics and
Gynaecology
St James's University Hospital
Leeds
UK

T.H. Bourne
Gynaecological Ultra-sound and
Minimal Access Surgery Unit
St George's Hospital
London
UK

S.B. Brown
Department of Biochemistry and
Molecular Biology &

Centre for Photobiology and
Photodynamic Therapy
University of Leeds
UK

T.J. Clark
Department of Obstetrics and
Gynaecology
Education Resource Centre
Birmingham Women's Hospital
Birmingham
UK

J.D. Dobak
Chief Executive Officer
Innercool Ltd
San Diego
California, USA

J. Donnez
Professor and Head
Department of Gynaecology
University Catholique de Louvain
Brussels, Belgium

E.G.R. Downes
Consultant
Barnet and Chase Farm
Hospitals NHS Trust
Enfield
UK

S.R.G. Duffy
Senior Lecturer
Department of Obstetrics and
Gynaecology
St James's University Hospital
Leeds
UK

C.M. Farquhar
Associate Professor in
Obstetrics and Gynaecology
University of Auckland and
National Women's Hospital
Auckland
New Zealand

C.A. Fortin
Assistant Professor in
Obstetrics / Gynaecology
McGill University
Montreal
Canada

M.J. Gannon
Consultant in Obstetrics and
Gynaecology
General Hospital
Mullingar, Ireland &
Centre for Photobiology and
Photodynamic Therapy
University of Leeds
UK

R. Garry
Professor in Gynaecology
Academic Department of Gynaecology
South Cleveland Hospital
Middlesbrough
UK

M. Goldrath
5777 West Maple Road
Suite 2000
W. Bloomfield
Michegan
USA

D.A. Grainger
*Assistant Professor
Director, Division of
Reproductive Endocrinology
University of Kansas
School of Medicine
Wichita
Kansas, USA*

J. Hawe
*Consultant Obstetrician and
Gynaecologist
Countess of Chester Hospital
Liverpool Road
Chester
UK*

M.C.S. Heppard
*Innercool Ltd
San Diego
California, USA*

J. Higham
*Consultant
St Mary's Hospital
Praed Street
London
UK*

D. Hunter
*Research Fellow to
Professor Ray Garry
South Cleveland Hospital
Middlesbrough
UK*

K. Jermy
*Gynaecological Ultra-sound and
Minimal Access Surgery Unit
St George's Hospital
London
UK*

K. Johnson
*Specialist Registrar in Obstetrics and
Gynaecology
Bradford Royal Infirmary
UK*

N.P. Johnson
*Senior Lecturer in Obstetrics and
Gynaecology*

*National Women's Hospital
Auckland
New Zealand*

K.D. Jones
*Minimal Access Therapy Training Unit
The Royal Surrey County Hospital
Guildford
UK*

K.S. Khan
*Department of Obstetrics and
Gynaecology
Education Resource Centre
Birmingham Women's Hospital
Birmingham
West Midlands
UK*

C. Kremer
*Consultant
Pinderfields Hospital NHS Trust
Wakefield
UK*

A.E. Lethaby
*Cochrane Menstrual Disorders and
Subfertility Group
National Women's Hospital
Auckland
New Zealand*

T.C. Li
*Consultant Gynaecologist
Jessop Hospital for Women
Sheffield
UK*

A. Lower
*Consultant Gynaecologist
St Bartholomew's Hospital
London
UK*

A. Magos
*Minimally Invasive
Therapy Unit and
Endoscopy Training Centre
University Department of Obstetrics
and Gynaecology
The Royal Free Hospital
London
UK*

P. McGurgan
*Specialist Registrar in Obstetrics and
Gynaecology
St Michael's Hospital
Bristol
UK*

M. Nisolle
*Professor
Department of Gynaecology
Catholic University of Louvain
Brussels
Belgium*

K. Nakade
*Karl Storz Research Fellow
MERIT Centre
Bradford Royal Infirmary
Bradford
UK*

M.G. Okeahialam
*Department of Obstetrics amd
Gynaecology
Bradford Royal Infirmary
Duckworth Lane
Bradford
UK*

P.J. O'Donovan
*Department of Obstetrics and
Gynaecology
Bradford Royal Infirmary
Bradford
UK*

D.E. Parkin
*Consultant Gynaecologist
Aberdeen Royal Infirmary
Aberdeen
UK*

R. Polet
*Department of Gynaecology
Catholic University of Louvain
Brussels
Belgium*

W. Prendiville
*Associate Professor in Obstetrics and
Gynaecology
Coombe Womens Hospital*

Dolphins Barn, Dublin 8
Ireland

A. Prentice
Senior Lecturer
Rosie Maternity Hospital
Cambridge
UK

A. Rådestad
Karolinska Institutet Danderyd
Hospital
Division of Obstetrics and
Gynaecology
Danderyd
Sweden

L. Rogerson
Clinical Research Fellow
Department of Obstetrics and
Gynaecology
St James's University Hospital
Leeds
UK

P. Scott
Clinical Research Fellow
Minimally Invasive Therapy Unit and
Endoscopy Training Centre
University Department of Obstetrics
and Gynaecology
The Royal Free Hospital
Pond Street
Hampstead
London
UK

N. Sharp
Consultant

Obstetrics and Gynaecology
Royal United Hospital
Bath
UK

M. Smets
Department of Gynaecology
Catholic University of Louvain
Brussels, Belgium

L. Spangler
Valleylab
5920 Longbow Drive
Boulder CO 80301-3299
USA

J. Squifflet
Department of Gynaecology
Catholic University of Louvain
Brussels, Belgium

M.R. Stringer
Department of Medical Physics
Leeds General Infirmary
Centre for Photobiology and
Photodynamic Therapy
University of Leeds
UK

C.J.G. Sutton
Valleylab
5920 Longbow Drive
Boulder CO 80301-3299
USA

R. Teirney
Specialist Registrar
Rosie Hospital
Cambridge
UK

U. Ulmsten
Department of Obstetrics and
Gynaecology
University Hospital of Uppsala
Uppsala
Sweden

R.F. Valle
Department of Obstetrics and
Gynaecology
Northwestern University Medical
School
Chicago
Illinois, USA

G.A.Vilos
Professor of Obstetrics and
Gynecology
Director of Minimally Invasive
Surgery
University of Western Ontario
St Joseph's Health Centre
London, Ontario
Canada

W. Walker
Consultant Radiologist
Royal Surrey County Hospital
Guildford
Surrey, England

S.R. Watermeyer
Research Fellow
University Hospital of Wales
Cardiff
UK

FOREWORD

Menorrhagia is a major gynaecological problem which affects the health and quality of life of many women worldwide. In the first part of the last century, the options women had for management of this problem were limited. Dilatation and curettage was frequently used in spite of the fact there is no evidence that it has any therapeutic effect. For those women whose menorrhagia was a significantly debilitating problem, a hysterectomy was generally the only available solution. Occasionally, radiation therapy to obliterate the endometrium or to destroy ovarian function was used in those patients deemed unable to withstand a hysterectomy. Most women simply tolerated their bleeding problems until they became menopausal. With the availability of oral contraceptives in the latter half of the 20th century, medical therapy became an option for some women.

Although several techniques were attempted to destroy the lining of the endometrium in order to control menorrhagia, it was not until the early 1980s that a practical method was achieved. Endometrial ablation using the Nd:YAG laser was shown to be an effective, non-invasive, outpatient, method to control menorrhagia. It is interesting that this expensive and technologically sophisticated instrumentation became the first popular method of endometrial destruction. The resectoscope, a common piece of instrumentation found in all operating rooms was later shown to be equally as effective in endometrial destruction and to have the additional advantage of being able to resect many submucosal uterine fibroids and endometrial polyps. The resectoscopic methods and the Nd:YAG laser methods gave similar results.

The ready availability of resectoscopic equipment led most physicians entering the field to use either an ablation or resection technique for destroying the endometrial lining. Currently, the use of the Nd:YAG laser remains primarily in those original centres where the equipment is available and the surgical expertise exists for this technically more difficult procedure.

In spite of the ready availability, effectiveness and relative ease of resectoscopic techniques, destruction of the endometrial by either ablation or resection grew slowly and was commonly not offered to women as a method of managing menorrhagia. There were several reasons for this slow growth. In some countries, there was an economic dis-incentive for this type of treatment. More importantly, however, hysteroscopic endometrial destruction was far more skill dependent than many physicians realised. This led to poor results and not infrequently, complications.

During the last decade, global endometrial destruction techniques have been developed. Their goal was to provide a simple technique which required minimal training and would provide uniform and consistent good results while at the same time decreasing the risk of complications. In addition, these techniques lent themselves more readily to office procedures under local anesthesia than did the traditional hysteroscopic techniques. There are now over eight global procedures that are either under investigation or available to the practising gynaecologist. While some of the newer global procedures have improved results over the original ones they have become somewhat more skill dependent. It remains to be seen if this will translate into poorer results and more complications in the average users hands, as compared to the experts hands.

Drs O'Donovan, McGurgan and Prendiville have assembled a book, whose contents carefully cover the subject of menorrhagia and its conservative management. The chapters span from the epidemiology of menorrhagia to current techniques for treatment, and to future research and recommendations. They have logically divided the book into chapters which do not overlap but rather compliment each other. They have chosen as contributing authors experts whose knowledge of the subject material makes this book a unique publication and valuable resource.

Unfortunately, conservative surgery for menorrhagia is not yet available to all patients. This book provides understanding of the theory and practice necessary to provide this care. It challenges all gynaecological surgeons who seek to improve the health and life style of women to provide conservative care for this common problem.

Frankin Loffer
September 2002
USA

Introduction

Ellis G.R. Downes

Menorrhagia is now the commonest gynaecological complaint for women, leading them to seek the advice of both their family physicians and gynaecologists. Menorrhagia is increasingly going to have an even greater burden on our health care society due to the increasing numbers of menstrual cycles that women experience during their reproductive lifespan. On average today a woman will have 10 times more menstrual cycles than her predecessor did a hundred years ago.

Against such a background, the assessment of menorrhagia, its investigation and treatment, continues to be fraught with difficulties. We know there is a huge variation in a woman's perception of her menstrual symptoms compared to objective menstrual blood loss measurement. One woman's menorrhagia may be another woman's light period. It is not for the gynaecologist to dissuade a patient who does not have menorrhagia her symptoms are not worthy of treatment, it is for the gynaecologist to carefully assess her, counsel her and offer her the most appropriate treatment modality within the clinical armamentarium.

Over the coming years we must continue to strive for better ways of assessing menorrhagia in a way that will lead to easy and validated techniques to compare treatment modalities from both the acceptability point of view for the patient and the efficacy of treatment.

There must also continue to be challenges to the conventional medical model of care of menorrhagia — the cascade of intervention in which patients are offered medical treatment initially, and only if this 'fails' are patients offered surgical treatment. I believe increasingly that patients should be offered a range of options and ultimately the choice has to be the patients.

We are increasingly practising medicine in an age where patients are keen to look at alternatives to hysterectomy and while the safety and efficacy of hysteroscopic techniques such as endometrial resection (TCRE) and rollerball ablation are well documented, it is disappointing that few gynaecologists have the skills to offer these to their patients. There is thus a very real need for gynaecologists to be able to use alternative surgical methods to hysterectomy. We should not forget that even though hysterectomy is the most final surgical procedure, it is a major operation removing an organ, 95% of which (the myometrium) is unlikely

to be contributing to the patients menorrhagia (in dysfunctional uterine bleeding), and even in well-controlled randomised studies there is not, as one might expect, 100% patient satisfaction with the 'final solution' of hysterectomy.

Therefore, over the last 10 years there has been a proliferation of second-generation endometrial ablation techniques — balloon therapies, microwave endometrial ablation, hydrotherm ablation, cryotherapy, etc., all of which are trying to use different energy modalities to destroy the endometrium. The range of evidence supporting these views is varied from large prospective randomised control studies, to small retrospective data often with a disappointingly small follow-up period. The challenge between sharing new data allowing gynaecologists to evaluate new techniques and at the same time not publishing less robust data is a difficult balance which is all too often compromised by commercial pressures.

And so to the future, there are a number of intriguing questions that remain to be definitively answered:

1. How can we best assess a patient's symptoms of menstrual dysfunction, without needing to resort to objective menstrual blood loss measurement, but still having better than subjective 'history taking' idea of their severity?
2. What is the true long-term role of the Mirena Intrauterine System at reducing menstrual symptoms?
3. Which of the current second-generation endometrial ablation procedures are the best in terms of safety and efficacy?
4. If we are going to perform a hysterectomy for our patient, what is the best route hysterectomy should be performed?
5. Are there any other methods of destroying the endometrium that appear more promising than current techniques?
6. Before even offering intervention, what is the best method of investigating menorrhagia?

Over the next few years as scientists and clinicians work on these tantalising questions, we will strive towards a more effective, pragmatic and evidence-based approach to the commonest and most distressing symptom suffered by women — menorrhagia.

1

Epidemiology of menorrhagia

Raewyn Teirney and Andrew Prentice

Introduction

Menorraghia is a symptom synonymous with excessive heavy menstrual bleeding. It has become an increasingly common clinical problem for women, and their families in the western world, and is seen as a significant health burden on limited health resources. This may not be so surprising when one considers that the average woman today as a consequence of changing lifestyles and improved health, can expect up to 400 menstrual cycles, while historically her primitive counterpart would have experienced around only 40 menstrual cycles in her reproductive lifetime.[1]

This common gynaecological condition is often embarrassing and debilitating, and can have a significant adverse impact on the quality of women's lives as well as their health — causing disruption to work and daily routine, social life and physical health. Shaw and colleagues (1998) in a quality life survey asked women with perceived menorrhagia to list the effects and impact that the bleeding had on their health.[2] They found that the most important component was the effect on family life, followed by its impact on physical health. The effects on other areas such as work, psychological health, practical difficulties and social life were considered less important.

This chapter will give an overview on the epidemiological aspects of menorrhagia including its definitions, the prevalence, and the evidence for its aetiology and possible pathogenic mechanisms.

Definition

Menorrhagia is generally agreed to be excessive menstrual bleeding, but a variety of definitions exist in the literature relating to either objective or subjective assessment. The objective and 'gold standard' definition of menorrhagia is a measured menstrual blood loss (MBL) of greater than 80 ml per cycle. This cut-off point is based on population studies where menstrual blood loss greater than 80 ml lead to an increased likelihood of iron deficiency anaemia.[3] Several other definitions described for menorrhagia are based on a perceived or subjective change in a menstrual characteristic such as an increase in the frequency of bleeding or increased duration of bleeding (see Table 1.1). These include:

- *Polymenorrhoea*: frequent bleeding of intervals less than 21 days.

Table 1.1

	Normal	**Abnormal**
Cycle length	Regular 21–35 days	Irregular
Duration of bleeding	3–7 days	Greater than 7 days
Volume of blood loss	30–40 ml	Greater than 80 ml

- *Metrorrhagia*: irregular menstrual cycles with excessive flow and duration.
- *Hypermenorrhoea*: regular menstrual cycle with a menstrual flow lasting longer than 7 days duration. This is used commonly in the USA as a definition for menorrhagia.

Dysfunctional uterine bleeding (DUB) is another definition that is defined differently in different parts of the world. In most places it is defined as excessive bleeding (excessively heavy, prolonged or frequent) of uterine origin, where pathology has been excluded. In the USA, the usual definition of DUB appears to include solely causes of anovulation, but in other societies, menstrual cycles associated with DUB may be ovulatory or anovulatory.[4] However, menorrhagia is mainly a subjective complaint and to many women this means 'heavy periods'.

Prevalence of menorrhagia

Menorrhagia is a common complaint. In the United Kingdom it can account for about 5% of referrals to the GP, and 12% of all new gynaecological referrals.[5] Moreover, data shows that approximately 20% of women will have a hysterectomy before they reach the age of 60 years, and half of these will be for menorrhagia. In other words, 10% of women will have a hysterectomy for the problem of menorrhagia.[6]

However, determining the true prevalence of menorrhagia in the female population is difficult. Ideally one would require the objective measurement of MBL in a large population-based study of women, but this would be a difficult task to accomplish. Our knowledge and understanding of MBL is mainly based on subjective clinical data and results from early small population studies that objectively and semi-objectively measured MBL by a variety of methods. Based on these studies,

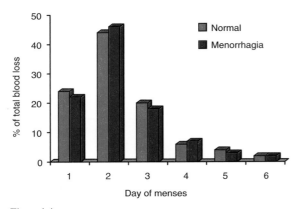

Figure 1.1

Table 1.2

Reference	n	Median (ml)	Range (ml)	Mean (ml)
7	100	35.9	6.6–178.8	50.6
3	476	30	1.6–200	43.4
8	348	27.5	0.1–280	37.5

it was determined that menstrual blood loss had a positive skewed distribution with the average or median blood loss to be about 35 ml per cycle, with the majority of this loss, in both normal cycles and those with excessive loss, occurring during the first 2–3 days of the menstrual period (Fig. 1.1). The 80 ml cut-off point which signifies menorrhagia represents the 90th centile of the distribution, where losses greater than this may cause iron deficiency anaemia, and therefore is regarded as pathological. They also showed that losses in excess of 80 ml are experienced by approximately 10% of all women[3,7,8] (see Table 1.2). Therefore, by definition menorrhagia should only be a clinical problem for 10% of the female population of reproductive age. However, subjective data suggests otherwise. One large subjective population survey on menstrual patterns by the World Health Organisation involving 5322 women from 14 countries reported a world-wide prevalence to be as high as 19% in women of reproductive age. While both Gath and colleagues[9] and Rees[10] reported that over one-third of women surveyed reported that their menstrual loss was heavy. Menorrhagia, therefore, is primarily a subjective complaint and will depend on how tolerant a woman is of her symptoms and her perception of what is normal. Furthermore, her ability to cope with her symptoms will in part be determined by her occupation or role in society.

In clinical practice, it is not generally feasible to measure MBL in women who present with the complaint of menorrhagia, rather, we rely on the history of the menstrual characteristics and the perception by the patient herself as to the heaviness and volume of blood loss. It is well known that subjective assessment of MBL is an unreliable indicator of menorrhagia, and that patients have a poor perception of what their actual blood loss may be at menstruation.[11] Furthermore, several studies have proven there to be a poor correlation between perceived and actual measured blood loss. Both Fraser[11] and Chimbria[12] have reported independently that only 40–50% of women who complained of excessive menstruation were in fact truly menorrhagic, with MBL greater than 80 ml. Conversely, Hallberg[3] found that a significant proportion of women with objective menstrual losses greater than 80 ml considered their periods to be either moderate or light. This highlights the problem that, either under- or over-reporting of the clinical problem could and probably does occur.

The physiology of menstruation

In order to understand the possible mechanisms involved in menorrhagia it is necessary first to review the physiology of menstruation during which two-thirds of the functioning endometrium is shed in a cyclical fashion leaving the basal endometrium, followed by regeneration. Our understanding of this complex process is still not clear. The majority of the knowledge is derived from studies by Markee et al (1940) who observed the transplanted endometrium of Rhesus monkeys in the anterior chamber of the eye of rabbits.

From Markee's study it was observed that with withdrawal of progesterone from an oestrogen primed endometrium, there was regression of the functional endometrium. The spiral arterioles thereafter underwent periods of vasoconstriction and vasodilation every 60 s, causing ischaemia, cell death and haemorrhage beneath the endometrium. Just prior to menstruation the spiral arterioles vasodilate. Blood passes into the ischaemic endometrium, white cells migrate through the capillary walls into the stroma, followed by shedding of the endometrium, with blood loss from rupture of the arterioles and damaged blood vessels. The majority of the bleeding during normal menstruation comes from the spiral arterioles and is actively limited in volume by vasoconstriction. Bleeding can also occur through capillaries or veins, from secondary haemorrhage via damaged vessels, and by diapedesis. Open-ended vessels become filled with fibrin and platelets in the first 20 h. By late menstruation, vessels ending on the shedding margin are constricted. Once shed, endometrial repair is achieved without scar tissue formation. Surface endometrium is regenerated by migration of epithelial cells from the basal portions of the endometrial glands. More recently, research has been concentrating on several local endometrial events that are thought to have a major role in controlling blood loss during menstruation.[13] To simplify, these endometrial events can be grouped into distinct mechanisms:

1. vascular control of the spiral arterioles in the endometrium by vaso-active prostaglandins, nitric oxide, and possibly endothelin;

2. local haemostasis involving mainly fibrinolysis; and

3. events involved in endometrial regeneration.[13]

Any aberration in these events could potentially lead to excessive heavy bleeding and will be discussed further on in the chapter under DUB.

Aetiology and pathophysiology of menorrhagia

Menorrhagia is associated with a variety of conditions. These include pelvic pathology such as fibroids, adenomyosis, endometrial disease, and polyps, as well as systemic diseases such as coagulopathies (see Fig. 1.2). However, objective evidence confirming the volume of menstrual blood loss in women with these diseases is limited. Furthermore, in over 50% of cases no pathology is found and is given the term DUB.

Pelvic pathology

Fibroids

Fibroids (leiomyomas) are smooth muscle tumours of the myometrium and have commonly been recognised as a cause of menorrhagia. They occur in approximately 20% of women of reproductive age and are divided into three groups according to their location in the uterus — submucus, intramural, and subserous.[14] The mechanisms as to how fibroids could cause excess bleeding are unclear but several explanations have

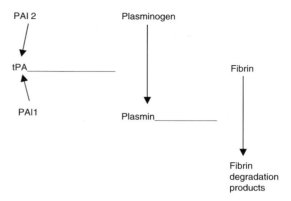

Figure 1.2 — *The fibrinolytic system:* This is the process whereby the haemostatic fibrin plug is broken down to form fibrin degradation products. This is mediated by the enzyme plasmin, which is formed from the cleavage of precursor plasminogen by tPA1 and tPA2. The tPAs are in turn inhibited by PAI1 and PAI2.

been hypothesised. The presence of fibroids, especially submucous ones increasing the surface area of the shedding endometrium, is one theory. Suggestions that they may act by affecting the contractility of the uterus or alter the production of local factors of prostaglandins and endothelins within the endometrium have also been put forward.[14,15] Certainly objective assessments of MBL confirm that the position of the fibroid in the uterus is correlated to the extent of menorrhagia. Fraser and colleagues (1990) demonstrated a decreasing order of MBL with submucous, intramural, and subserous fibroids.

It is unclear though what the proportion of association is, if any, that a fibroid has with excess menstrual loss. Results of objective MBL studies by Rybo and colleagues (1985) reported a 40% incidence of fibroids in women with MBL greater than 200 ml and a 10% incidence in those with a MBL of 80–100 ml. In women having a myomectomy, approximately 30% subjectively reported menorrhagia, while Fraser et al[16] found anaemia to be more common among those women with menorrhagia and fibroids. In his study of 18 women with fibroid uteri, 15 had menorrhagia defined by objective MBL measurements, while the remainder had a loss at the upper level of normal. Furthermore, there was a significant reduction in MBL (304–52 ml) after myomectomy suggesting that leiomyomas probably do have an association.

Adenomyosis

Adenomyosis is the presence of endometrial glands and stromal cells deep within the myometrium, causing smooth muscle proliferation. It has long been associated as a cause of dysmenorrhoea and menorrhagia. Evidence supporting this comes from several studies that have reported a high incidence of adenomyosis in the extirpated uteri of women with DUB who had symptoms of menorrhagia and dysmenorrhoea. Two groups, McCausland (1994) and Nishida,[17] found a significant correlation between the depth of invasion of adenomyotic lesions and severity of menorrhagia. A high incidence is also found in multiparous women, and those greater than 40 years.[18]

One of the problems is that diagnosis of adenomyosis is difficult. This is usually made retrospectively on uteri removed at hysterectomy. Consequently, the prevalence of adenomyosis and its contribution to menorrhagia is difficult to ascertain. The reported incidence can vary anywhere from 5% to 70% in the literature, depending on the thoroughness of uterine sampling and the many histological criteria used.[19]

The aetiology of this disease process and its pathogenic mechanisms in causing menorrhagia are not clear. Why this condition is present in some women and not others is a mystery and yet to be determined. Past classic opinions suggest that the development of adenomyosis arise from invagination of the basalis endometrius into the myometrium. Based on animal studies, one theory suggests that weakness in the myometrium caused by trauma such as curettage or myomectomy may predispose the uterus to its development. There is also some evidence to suggest the immune system may also have a role. Cameron (1987) showed that the potent vasodilator prostaglandins PGE_2 and PGI_2 are increased in the presence of adenomyosis and may act to affect menstruation and increase loss. This is also supported by results from studies demonstrating a reduced blood loss with mefanamic acid administration, also suggesting that prostaglandins may be involved.

Endometrial carcinoma

Endometrial carcinoma usually presents in the 5th to 6th decade as post-menopausal bleeding and is a rare but serious cause of menorrhagia in pre-menopausal women. Menorraghia has been reported to occur in 40% of pre-menopausal women with endometrial cancer in subjective studies[20] but Rybo[21] found only a 2% incidence of endometrial carcinoma in women with objective assessment of menorrhagia.

Endometrial hyperplasia is not as serious but, in the absence of treatment, 2% can progress to carcinoma. The incidence in pre-menopausal women with abnormal bleeding has been reported to be 4–10%.[20]

Farquahar and colleagues[22] have identified certain risk factors for endometrial disease in pre-menopausal women; these were women greater than 45 years, greater than 90 kg in weight, infertility, a family history of colonic cancer and nulliparity.

Endometrial cancers and hyperplasias are regarded as a consequence of excess oestrogen accompanied by inadequate cyclic exposure to progestogens. Oestrogen acting as a promoter of endometrial cancer development is plausible but the mechanisms involved in causing menorrhagia are unclear. It has been suggested that oestrogen may have a role in angiogenesis. Oestradiol appears to enhance vasodilation by stimulating nitric oxide synthesis and prostacyclin activity which then attenuates the vasoconstrictor activity of endothelin on vascular smooth muscle.[20]

Endometrial polyps

It is not known whether or how endometrial polyps cause menorrhagia. Often these small masses are seen at hysteroscopy during investigation for menstrual disturbances, with blood loss returning to normal in many cases following the removal. However, only a small percentage (4%) of women with objectively measured menorrhagia were found to have a polyp.[21]

Intra-uterine contraceptive device

Intra-uterine contraceptive devices (IUCDs) have been in use since the early 1960s as a contraceptive device for the prevention of pregnancy. The earlier inert devices used (Lippes loop) were shown to cause a marked increase in the measured volume of menstrual blood loss of up to 60% and, consequently, this was one of the main reasons for their poor continuation rate. The modern IUCDs, with the addition of copper, are much less likely to cause menorrhagia, although objective studies have demonstrated that blood loss is still greater than the pre-insertion loss. The underlying mechanism leading to this increased blood loss is thought to be a consequence of a change in the local endometrial environment. The devices are thought to play a role in increased bleeding by inducing a foreign body reaction within the endometrium, stimulating migration and infiltration of leucocytes and macrophages, leading to disturbances in the prostaglandin metabolism and fibrinolysis.[23,24] Others have suggested that movement of the device or uterine contractions against the device may cause damage to the superficial endometrial vessels.

The new hormone releasing devices, such as the levonorgestrel IUS (Mirena, Schering), significantly reduce the menstrual blood loss and are of great benefit to women with excess bleeding of unknown aetiology.

Systemic disorders

A number of systemic conditions can result in menorrhagia although these are rare. These include both hereditary and acquired disorders of coagulation factors and/or platelets. Endocrine disorders do not routinely cause menorrhagia with the exception of the endocrine consequences of an ovulation.[4]

Coagulation disorders

Disorders of primary haemostasis, including thrombocytopaenia and von Willebrand disease, are important when evaluating women with menorrhagia. These women usually present early at puberty. Von Willebrand disease is the most common of the hereditary disorders, affecting around 1% of the population world-wide. A prevalence study on these women reported menorrhagia as high as 90%.[25] The underlying abnormality is in the adhesive plasma protein — von Willebrand factor. Its function is to cause platelet adhesion by acting as a 'bridge' between platelet and injury sites in the vessel wall. Other hereditary disorders of coagulation that may be associated with menorrhagia are isolated deficiencies of factors VIII, IX, XI and in more rare disorders of factors II, V and X. These cause defective secondary haemostasis leading to reduced fibrin formation.[26] Deficiencies in the normal inhibitors of fibrinolysis, such as alpha 2-antiplasmin or plasminogen activator inhibitor (PAI), may also cause excess bleeding.

A number of acquired disorders of haemostasis can also manifest as excessive menstrual bleeding. The most common of these are idiopathic thrombocytopaenic purpura, vitamin K deficiency states, drug-related thrombocytopaenia, liver disease, and platelet function defects.

Dysfunctional uterine bleeding

DUB is a common condition, in fact the commonest condition, causing excessive menstrual bleeding. It is used to describe cases where underlying pelvic pathology, systemic disease and complications of pregnancy have been excluded as the cause. It is therefore said to be a diagnosis of exclusion. Menstrual cycles associated with DUB can be classified as either ovulatory or anovulatory.[4] Anovulatory DUB is defined when menstrual cycles are irregular and is a frequent occurrence

Table 1.3 — Local endometrial factors involved in menorrhagia

Abnormality	Local endometrial factors altered
Defective vasculature	Reduced endothelin
	Increased nitric oxide and PAF
	Altered prostaglandin production, $\uparrow PGE_2$, $\uparrow PGI_2$
Defective haemostasis	Increased fibrinolysis
	Altered platelet function
Defective endometrial repair	Increased VEGF expression
	Increased matrix degradation
Other factors	Increased lysosome numbers and activity
	Increased cytokine, TNF and macrophage production

just post-menarche and the years preceding the menopause, as well as in women with polycystic ovarian syndrome. Ovulatory DUB is defined when the menstrual cycles are regular and occurs in approximately 80% of cases. Although it is not clearly understood, the disturbances of molecular mechanisms in the endometrium appear to be responsible.

Factors implicated as being responsible for DUB can be seen as disturbances in specific mechanisms, mentioned earlier in the chapter, that are involved in the control of menstrual blood loss. These are disturbances in local endometrial haemostasis, disturbances in vascular events and disturbances in endometrial repair and regeneration (see Table 1.3).

Haemostasis

Haemostasis is the mechanism whereby the coagulation system with formation of platelet/fibrin plug and fibrinolysis (the process whereby fibrin clot is broken down to fibrin degradation products) occur to control bleeding. However, it has been known for some time that haemostasis in the menstrual endometrium differs from that in other parts of the body. Studies on the endometrium have demonstrated the absence of these platelet–fibrin haemostatic plugs after the first day of menstruation and the complete intra–vascular localisation of these plugs suggesting rapid degradation by active fibrinolysis. Further increased fibrinolytic activity could also result in excessive menstrual bleeding (see Fig. 1.2). Evidence from objective MBL studies and endometrial studies does suggest that enhanced fibrinolytic activity has a major role in women with DUB. Women with bleeding disorders suffer from excessive menstrual blood loss. Increased fibrinolytic activity has been shown in the endometrium of women with increased MBL. Both the menstrual fluid and the endometrium in women with objective menorrhagia have higher levels of tissue plasminogen activator (tPA). Finally, tranexamic acid, an inhibitor of fibrinolysis, has been demonstrated to reduce menstrual blood loss by about 50%.[27]

Vascular disturbances

Evidence from Markee's study demonstrated that regulation of blood loss during menstruation is mediated primarily by the specialised endometrial spiral arterioles. Those factors that regulate the vascular tone are therefore implicated in the control of menstrual bleeding, and aberrations in their production and function may be a cause for menorrhagia. Those widely studied are the prostaglandins, endothelins, nitric oxide and platelet-activating factor (PAF).

Prostaglandins

Prostaglandins are vaso-active peptides involved in the vascular control of the spiral arterioles. They have both vasoconstricting and vasodilating properties and are thought to play an important role in the control of endometrial bleeding. These prostaglandins are produced via the arachidonic pathway involving the enzyme prostaglandin synthetase to produce thromboxane A_2 (TXA_2) in platelets and prostacyclin (PGI_2) in endothelial and smooth muscle cells. The endometrium produces mainly prostaglandins PGF_2 and PGE_2, with smaller amounts of PGI_2 and TXA_2. TXA_2 and PGF_2 are vasoconstrictors whilst PGI_2 and PGE_2 have the opposite effect of vasodilation. TXA_2 is also a promoter of platelet adhesion while PGI_2 acts as an inhibitor of platelet adhesion. The interaction between the prostaglandins synthesised helps in the control of blood loss during menstruation and shifts in the production of these peptides to ones of vasodilatory has been suggested as important in the pathogenesis of menorrhagia.[13] Evidence from the endometrium of women with menorrhagia has shown significantly higher levels of prostaglandins PGE_2 and PGF_2 and their metabolites. Others have questioned the significance of these observations and suggested that the prostaglandin ratio of prostacyclin to thromboxane and PGE_2 to PGF_2 may be more important. Other evidence comes from objective blood loss studies which report a reduction in MBL by 30% when prostaglandin synthesis inhibitors were taken during menstruation.

Endothelins, PAF and nitric oxide

Endothelins are potent vasoconstrictors produced by the endometrium. They have been implicated in menorrhagia although there is no direct data for their role in control of menstruation. It has been suggested that PAF, being a vasoconstrictor and platelet aggregator, may also play a role in the control of the endometrial vascular bed. PAF stimulates release of PGE_2 from the endometrium during the secretory phase but suppresses the release of PGF_2 from the endometrium in the proliferative phase giving a possible role in changing the ratio of PGE_2/PGF_2 prostaglandin production.

Recent studies have focused on the free radical nitric oxide as being important in the local control of endometrial function, including implantation and menstruation. Its actions include inhibition of platelet adhesion, vasodilation, as well as being an important mediator of paracrine interactions.[28] The discovery of nitric oxide generating enzymes NOS within the endometrium have lead to suggestions that NO might be involved in the initiation and control of menstrual bleeding and determine the degree of menstrual bleeding.[29]

Endometrial repair

The endometrium undergoes regeneration during menstruation. This is largely controlled by local factors such as angiogenic growth factors, matrix metalloproteinases (MMPs) and macrophages. Disturbances in this process may contribute to changes in the volume of menstrual blood loss and menorrhagia.

Angiogenic growth factors

Angiogenesis, the mechanism of new growth and development of blood vessels, is important for the regeneration of the endometrial vasculature and menstrual loss. The growth factors involved are vaso-active endothelial growth factor (VEGF), fibroblast growth factor (FGF), epidermal growth factor (EGF), transforming growth factor (TGF) and tumour necrosis factor (TNF). All promote endothelial cell proliferation, migration and facilitate changes needed in the extracellular matrix for new vessel formation. VEGF is a major angiogenic factor in the development of blood vessels. Its multiple actions include proliferation and migration of endothelial cells, vasodilation of the vasculature and stimulation of nitric oxide release from endothelial cells. VEGF also induces the release of prostacyclin, another vasodilatory agent, by activating phospholipase A2 in the arachidonic pathway. As well as its effects on the endothelial cell, VEGF is thought to influence the local coagulation in the endometrium by increasing the expression of plasminogen activators leading to the release of plasmin.

Given all the above possible actions potentially controlling menstruation, disturbances of VEGF expression could, therefore, lead on to alterations in menstrual blood volume and menorrhagia.

Matrix metalloproteinases

The extracellular matrix is important in promoting the structural integrity of the endometrium. It includes components such as fibronectins, collagens, laminin, hyaluronic acid and proteoglycans. MMPs are a family of enzymes that, together, degrade the components of the extracellular matrix causing endometrial regression and breakdown. They are activated by the withdrawal of progesterone and migratory leucocytes and appear to be under the stimulus of TNF and interleukin 9. Their expression has been implicated in the role of menstruation. It has been suggested that prolonged or excessive tissue degradation due to MMP activity may result in increased MBL.[30]

Lysosomes

These are intracellular membrane bound vacuoles that contain destructive enzymes and are involved in endometrial remodelling and regeneration. Their activity increases in the late secretory phase and during early menstruation. Their activity is also increased in women with ovulatory DUB and with excess bleeding in IUCD use.[24]

Other factors

Macrophages and polymorphonuclear leucocytes may be implicated in the control of menstrual blood loss and excess blood loss. Increased leucocyte infiltration has been observed in the endometrium of women with menorrhagia secondary to IUCD use. Both PAF and PGE_2, potent vasodilators are released by macrophages. These may stimulate the release of free oxygen radicals which could lead to local destruction of tissue.[24,30]

Summary

Menorrhagia is a common problem. Causes can be associated with pelvic pathology and coagulopathies but, in the majority of cases, DUB is the underlying diagnosis. We are still a long way from understanding the mechanisms involved although, from recent studies, it does appear that disturbances of local endometrial events may govern excess bleeding in DUB. Hopefully though, through continuing research, we may be able to unravel some of the mystery and offer the most effective treatment and improve the overall quality of life for women.

References

1. Short RV. The evolution of human reproduction. *Proc R Soc Lond* 1976; 195: 3–24.

2. Shaw RW, Brickley MR, Evans L, Edwards MJ. Perceptions of women on the impact of menorrhagia on their health using multi-attribute utility assessment. *Br J Obstet Gynaecol* 1998; 105: 1155–1159.

3. Hallberg L, Hagdahl AM, Nilsson L, Rybo G. Menstrual blood loss: a population study. *Acta Obstet Gynecol Scand* 1966; 45: 320–335.

4. Prentice A. Medical management of menorrhagia. BMJ 1999; 319: 1343–1345.

5. Bradlow J, Coulter A, Brooks P. *Patterns of Referral* 1992. Oxford Health Services Research Unit.

6. Coulter A, Klassen A, McPherson K. How many hysterectomies should purchasers buy? *Eur J Public Health* 1995.

7. Barer AP, Fowler WM. The blood loss during normal menstruation. *Am J Obstet Gynecol* 1936; 31: 979–986.

8. Cole SK, Billewicz WZ et al. Sources of variation of menstrual blood loss. *J Obstet Gynaecol Br Comm* 1971; 78: 933–939.

9. Gath D, Osborn M, Bungay G et al. Psychiatric disorder and gynaecological symptoms in middle aged women: a community survey. *Br Med J* 1987; 294: 213–218.

10. Rees MCP. The role of menstrual blood loss measurements in the management of complaints of excessive menstrual bleeding. *Br Med J* 1991; 98: 327–328.

11. Fraser IS, Arachchi GJ. Aetiology and investigation of menorrhagia. In: S Sheth, C Sutton (Eds) *Menorraghia*, Chapter 1, pp 1–9, 1984. ISIS Medical Media.

12. Chimbria TH, Anderson A, Turnbull C. Relation between measured blood loss and patients subjective assessment of loss, duration of bleeding, number of sanitary towels, uterine weight and endometrial surface area. *Br J Obstet Gynaecol* 1980; 87: 603–609.

13. Smith SK. Angiogenesis, vascular endothelial growth factor and the endometrium. *Hum Reprod Update* 1998; 4(5): 509–519.

14. Lumsden MA, Wallace EM. Clinical presentation of uterine fibroids. *Bailliere Clin Obstet Gynaecol* 1998; 12(2): 177–195.

15. Vollenhoven BJ, Lawrence AS, Healy DL. Uterine fibroids: a clinical review. *Br J Obstet Gynaecol* 1990; 97: 285–298.

16. Fraser IS, McCarron G, Markham R. Objective measurement of menstrual blood loss in women with a complaint of menorrhagia associated with pelvic disease or coagulation disorder. *Obstet Gynecol* 1986; 68: 630–633.

17. Nishida M. Relationship between the onset of dysmenorrhoea and histological findings in adenomyosis. *Am J Obstet Gynecol* 1991; 165.

18. Aziz R. Adenomyosis: current perspectives. *Obstet Gynecol Clin North Am* 1989; 16: 221–235.

19. Ferenczy A. Pathophysiology of adenomyosis. *Hum Reprod Update* 1998; 4(4): 312–322.

20. Quinn MA, Kneale B, Fortune DW. Endometrial carcinoma in pre-menopausal women: a clinico-pathological study. *Gynecol Oncol* 1985; 20: 298–306.

21. Rybo G. Variations of menstrual blood loss. *Res Clin Forum* 1982; 4: 81–89.

22. Farquahar CM, Lethaby A, Sowter M, Verry J, Baranyai J. An evaluation of risk factors for endometrial hyperplasia in premenopausal women with abnormal menstrual bleeding. *Am J Obstet Gynecol* 1999; 181(3): 525–529.

23. Wang IY, Russell P, Fraser IS. Endometrial morphometry in users of intrauterine contraceptive devices and women with ovulatory dysfunctional bleeding: a comparison with normal endometrium. *Contraception* 1995; 51(4): 243–248.

24. Wang IY, Fraser IS, Barsamian SP, Manconi F, Stree DJ, Cornillie FJ, Russell P. Endometrial lysosomal enzyme activity in ovulatory dysfunctional bleeding, IUCD users and post partum women. *Mol Hum Reprod* 2000; 6(3): 258–263.

25. Ragni MV, Bontempo FA, Hassett AC. Von Willebrand disease and bleeding in women. *Haemophilia* 1999; 5(5): 313–317.

26. Ewenstein BM. The pathophysiology of bleeding disorders presenting as abnormal uterine bleeding. *Am J Obstet Gynecol* 1996; 175(3): 770–777.

27. Lethaby A, Augood C, Duckitt K. Nonsteriodal anti-inflammatory drugs for heavy menstrual bleeding. *Cochrane Database* 1998.

28. Cameron IT, Campbell S. Nitric oxide in the endometrium. *Human Reprod Update* 1998; 4(5): 565–569.

29. Zervon S, Klentzeris LD, Old RW. Nitric oxide synthase expression and steroid regulation in the uterus of women with menorrhagia. *Mol Hum Reprod* 1999; 5(11): 1048–1054.

30. Fraser IS, Hickey M. Dysfunctional uterine bleeding. In: I Fraser, R Jansen, R Lobo, M Whitehead (Eds) *Estrogens and Progestogens*, pp 419–435, 1998. London: Churchill and Livingston.

2

Diagnosing menorrhagia

Jenny Higham

Menorrhagia is a familiar complaint to the gynaecologist. It is the most common reason for referral alone or in combination with other menstrual symptoms in premenopausal women. Around 20% of women at one time in their lives are likely to complain of excessively heavy periods. Having a label of 'menorrhagia sufferer' is likely to precipitate as a minimum, long-term medical therapy and modest to radical surgical intervention. One would expect, therefore, that robust means of diagnosis would have been developed and routinely applied in clinical practice. In reality this is far from the case.

What methods are employed to establish this frequent clinical complaint?

History

Normally the gynaecologist will have been given an indication and at times a very accurate description of the extent of the problem by the General Practitioner referral letter. A number of questions are routinely put to the woman, as described below. It is useful to explore the evidence as to whether these are actually fruitful enquiries in relation to establishing the nature of condition.

Are your periods heavy? How many sanitary towels and/or tampons do you use per period? Do you need double protection?

Certainly, subjective impression alone is not reliable — result illustrates how a woman's impression that she is suffering with heavy loss is not borne out by objective measurement. These results show the measured menstrual blood loss of 207 women who had a complaint of excessively heavy periods. Half the women had loss of less than 80 ml (the objective definition of menorrhagia), those women with most florid histories from the lower losers.[1]

Which are the heaviest days?

The pattern of menstrual loss is similar in both women with normal loss, and with normal loss and genuine menstruation.[2] It is somewhat suspicious if a woman has no lightening of loss as the period progresses and complains of great drama on every day of bleeding. A rare exception to this is an arteriovenous malformation which can produce torrential arterial type haemorrhage. This condition may be congenital or acquired following surgery such as evacuation, molar pregnancy and even post-caesarean section. If this diagnosis is suspected, then even 'simple' such as diagnostic curettage should be avoided as they can provoke life-threatening haemorrhage.

How long do you bleed for?

The duration of bleeding may be a useful enquiry to estimate the limitation/annoyance factor in the woman's life. Certainly protracted loss of more than seven days places restrictions in some activities such as sex and exercise for some women. My own data from women presenting to me with a normal clinical examination certainly suggested that with duration of bleeding, especially when more than 6–7 days, is likely to be associated with the genuine diagnosis of menorrhagia.[1]

Is the cycle regular?

The regularity of the cycle is a useful enquiry in establishing whether they are likely to be ovulatory or not. In reality, more than 80% of women with regular menorrhagia will be ovulating. Clinically an irregular cycle in the women in her late 40s may suggest the potential proximity of the menopause, a factor which may be used in counselling, although predicting the timing of the onset of the menopause is notoriously difficult. Certainly there is more evidence that progestogens are of value in the erratic heavy anovulatory bleeders which may reduce flow in addition to precipitating a more regular bleeding pattern.[3]

Do you pass clots of blood? How large are these clots?

The passage of clots is not easily measured and this blood is often lost down the toilet pan at the time of changing sanitary items. Most women if complaining of heavy loss will answer 'yes' to this question. What is more likely to be of interest is the additional information as to the estimate of size. Some women describe a drop the size of the fist of their hand or a baby's head. Whilst to others it is a tiny slither of coagulation a couple of millimetres in size. Certainly, the genuine woman giving the former description could be losing more than 80 ml in a single clot alone.

Do you experience flooding (uncontrollable loss which may soil underwear/bed linen)?

Flooding and episode of soiling normally is lost again from formal measurements but is an indicator of how her periods are impeding her life, not to underestimate the embarrassment of soiled clothes/bed linen and the obvious expense in replacement of ruined items.

Do you experience pain with your periods? How much do your periods affect your daily life, i.e. are you housebound or need to take days off work?

There is no good published evidence to prove that genuine menorrhagia is either more or less painful. 'Menstrual debility', however, will be much influenced by the presence of pain. Severe dysmenorrhoea may well warrant more extensive investigations such as laparoscopy.

Have you ever been pregnant?

The effect of intrauterine pregnancy on blood loss has been studied. Reports are not always 100% in concordance but the overall view would seem to be that increased numbers of pregnancies increase the measured blood loss on the few occasions this has been studied. Older women of course have a greater opportunity to have been pregnant and, therefore, could this not just be an age effect alone? It would appear not. There is an effect of pregnancy on a population basis over and above that of age. Both age and pregnancy act in population statistics terms, to increase the volume of menstrual blood loss.[1]

What do you use for contraception?

Contraceptive method is an obligatory question in the sexually active women. First, to establish the likelihood of a pregnancy or its complications affecting the individual. Secondly, it is well known that an inert or copper containing intrauterine device increases blood loss by around 30% and may be an iatrogenic cause of menorrhagia. The combined oral contraceptive pill is a potentially good treatment of excess loss and/or irregular and painful loss but obviously inappropriate to offer to the woman already taking it.

Do you have bleeding in between your periods or after sex?

Intermenstrual or post-coital bleeding may have important clinical significance. Menorrhagia can be found in association with other pathology and it is the duty of the gynaecologist to exclude serious pathology such as endometrial hyperplasia or endometrial or cervical cancer.

Do you have any particular tendency to bleeding or bruising elsewhere?

A generalised bleeding tendency, especially in women with menarchal onset and continuing menorrhagia is relevant or when other symptoms are suggestive. It is rarely going to be the cause in the 40-year old woman that presents with a 6-month history of heavy periods with no suspicious previous history such as post-partum haemorrhage or other bleeding episodes.

Examination

In the region of 50% of women who complain of menorrhagia have a general and gynaecological examination which is unremarkable.

What specific thoughts should run through one's head whilst assessing the menorrhagia sufferer?

General diseases are rare as a specific cause of menorrhagia but a few are of relevance. Are there stigmata of thyroid dysfunction or other major disease such as renal or liver dysfunction, a bleeding diathesis or SLE? If systemic disease is suspected, it should be investigated and given appropriate treatment. If not, our conventional remedies may well not work and the patient will also thank you for the potential benefits to her general health.

The gynaecological condition that is frequently associated in textbooks with menorrhagia is endometriosis, well known to be more prevalent in the pain sufferer and in fact there is no good objective evidence that it is a good cause of menorrhagia in itself. Acute pelvic inflammatory disease is a condition that may precipitate menorrhagia but the chronic disorder, involving scarring and adhesions, is more likely to induce pain. It is the duty of the competent gynaecologist to exclude a gross bleeding malignancy on the cervix but it is unlikely to be found in the presence of cyclical bleeding. What may be more likely is a polyp may be seen protruding through os. Although no good studies exist matching blood loss with such structural abnormalities, clinically, one is aware of a reported marked improvement in bleeding with the removal of large lesions which occupy a significant percentage of the cavity. If on examination a pelvic mass is found, the differential diagnosis obviously includes fibroids. Although research remains to be done in the area, those that are submucous in nature and indenting the cavity are frequently, clinically, associated with a high menstrual blood loss.

Prolapse of course may warrant treatment in its own right. The further examination of the uterine cavity and endometrial sampling will be dealt with in the next chapter. Finally, it is not unheard of to find a forgotten intrauterine contraceptive device. On the rare occasion it is a satisfying and a quick cure to remove the device (ensuring, of course, you are not going to precipitate legal action in the event of an unwanted pregnancy!).

Investigations

Here I shall only concentrate on the initial tests as much will be covered in the next chapter.

A full blood count

Overall, there is a negative correlation between haemoglobin level and volume of menstrual blood loss with increased likelihood of anaemia at above 60–80 ml of blood per period. A haemoglobin alone is not a diagnostic, however, many women compensate if on an adequate diet and vitamin and mineral supplementation is a common phenomenon. Also women can be anaemic from causes other than their menses, with haemoglobinopathies such as thalassaemia trait overlooked. There is no place for denying women treatment or being 100% sure she has menorrhagia on the basis of a single haemoglobin estimation alone. The remaining parameters of white cell indices and platelets may, on occasion, give rise to a surprise diagnosis of leukaemia or thrombocytopaenia which, if severe enough, will lead to menorrhagia.

Ferritin

Long-standing menorrhagia is likely to lead to a chronic iron deficiency. A serum ferritin will, therefore, be low. It should encourage adequate supplementation.

Semi-quantitative methods

Patient completed records

Familiar to gynaecologists are the menstrual calendars where patients record the dates and make an assessment of the heaviness of flow on each day, usually, by filling in a grid with the higher the column the greater the perceived loss. In 1990 the pictorial blood loss assessment chart (PBAC) method of assessment was published[4] and further explored and found to be useful by Janssen and colleagues.[5] The chart depicts lightly, moderately and heavily stained sanitary towels and tampons. The score being greater for the more densely stained items. Episodes of flooding and the passage of clots are recorded. Such a technique does give a total numerical score which enable comparisons 'before and after' treatment. This feature and the

attractiveness of not having to actually measure blood loss has led to a widespread use of the chart in clinical research.

The PBAC technique will always be attractive as it avoids the need for collections of sanitary wear, however, the agreement is far more variable at the higher scores and the larger blood volumes. In addition, there have been large changes in the types of sanitary protection available on the market with items with 'wings', dry top cover sheets and a central core containing an absorbent gel all of which reduce the accuracy of the PBAC method. Prof. PMS O'Brien and colleagues have advanced the principle of patient recorded data and converted it to an electronic format called the menstrual symptometrics.[6] This technique has modified and improved on the PBAC method to take account of potential detracting factors and also accurately records other menstrual symptomatology including the pre-menstrual syndrome and dysmenorrhoea. Data is inserted daily into a hand held palm top computer by the patient and at the end of the month there is the ability to down load the prospectively acquired data and give an immediate picture of menstruation.

Measuring menstrual blood loss

A variety of measurement techniques have been developed to quantify menstrual blood loss. They fall into four main categories:

1. weight estimates of sanitary wear,
2. radioisotope methods,
3. iron determination,
4. haemoglobin determination.

This list is not exhaustive as there are other individual reports of novel approaches that have never become universally employed.

Weight estimates

Weighing is a simple method of determining the total menstrual fluid loss. It relies on the accurate measurement of sanitary items before and after use. It has the potential drawback of not being specific for blood and can be misleading in the event of significant urinary incontinence. The contribution of blood to menstrual discharge has been shown to vary considerably ranging between 1.6% and 82%, with a mean of 36%.[7]

The following techniques are more specifically directed towards the blood component of menstrual loss.

Radioisotope methods

Labelling of peripheral red blood cells with both iron and chromium have been described. The pre- and post-menses fall in total body radioisotope has been used to calculate the menstrual loss. Alternatively, the level of radioisotope in the collected menstrual protection has also been tried. Both techniques when initially developed lacked accuracy, which with practice have the potential to be overcome. The fact that they are no longer routinely used is likely to be a reflection of the reticence for women to volunteer for such studies.

Iron determination

Both a chemical assay and spectrophotometric techniques have been employed to extract the iron form soiled sanitary material. The iron content being directly proportional to the blood content of the collection. Despite the apparent success of the method, as described in studies published in the 1960s and 1970s the technique appears to have been abandoned.

Haemoglobin determination

Determining the content of haemoglobin in soiled sanitary collections has become the established 'gold standard' technique for objective menstrual loss measurements.[8] In an alkaline solution the haemoglobin molecule is converted into a coloured haematin molecule. The density of colour in the brown solution that is produced when sanitary collections are mixed in a sodium hydroxide solution can be accurately measured with a spectrophotometer. A sample of venous blood is incubated in parallel to the menstrual collection and, knowing the optical density of this solution and having accurately measured the volume of alkaline sodium hydroxide solution added to the menstrual collection, then by a simple calculation, the volume of menstrual blood can be calculated.

Although minor modification of this technique (the employment of alternative solutions such as dilute acid and detergents have been described), fundamentally, the technique of measuring the colour of solution that is produced and comparing it with the venous blood concentration remains. Thus the majority of publications concerning population based menstrual measurement and assessments of the efficacy of medical or surgical treatments have relied upon this alkaline haematin technique.

Measurement techniques such as the alkaline haematin technique are technically challenging but are not popular, both amongst the technicians who may need to carry them out or the patients who find it inconvenient to collect during menstruation, especially when out and about. This combination of factors has lead to the vast majority of women have treatments, both medical and surgical, on the basis of subjective information alone.

Conclusion

In the majority of clinicians' hands the diagnosis of menorrhagia remains a subjective one. It is important to remember that this will lead to many women getting unnecessary treatment and information is frequently inadequate for meaningful research studies.

If you really need to know the menstrual blood loss volume, the best method still remains the alkaline haematin or similar technique, until perhaps the use of palm top computers for this purpose becomes a more routine phenomenon.

References

1. Higham JM, Shaw RW. Clinical associations with menstrual blood loss. *Eur J Obstet Gynecol Reprod Biol* 1999; 82: 73–76.
2. Haynes PJ, Anderson ABM, Turnbull AC. Patterns of menstrual blood loss in menorrhagia. *Res Clin Forums* 1979; 1(2): 73–78.
3. Fraser IS. Treatment of ovulatory and anovulatory dysfunctional uterine bleeding with oral progestogens. *Aust N Z Obstet Gynaecol* 1990; 30: 353–356.
4. Higham JM, O'Brien PMS, Shaw RW. Assessment of menstrual blood loss using a pictorial chart. *Br J Obstet Gynaecol* 1990; 97: 734–739.
5. Janssen CA, Scholten PC, Heintz AP. A simple visual assessment technique to discriminate between menorrhagia and normal menstrual blood loss. *Obstet Gynecol* 1995; 85: 977–982.
6. Wyatt K, Dimmock P, Crowe J, Jones P, Hays-Gill B, Francoise B, O'Brien PMS. Presented to the Blair Bell Society December 1999. The Menstrual Symptometrics.
7. Fraser IS, McCarron G, Markham R, Resta T. Blood and total fluid content of menstrual discharge. *Obstet Gynaecol* 1985; 65: 194–198.
8. Hallberg L, Nilsson L. Determination of menstrual blood loss. *Scand J Clin Lab Invest* 1964; 16: 244–248.

3

The role of ultrasound in investigating menorrhagia

K. Jermy, T.H. Bourne and K.D. Jones

Introduction

In the majority of women with menorrhagia there is no identifiable underlying organic cause and it can be classified as dysfunctional uterine bleeding (DUB).[1] However, DUB is a diagnosis made after pelvic or systemic pathology has been excluded. Rare systemic causes of excess menstrual bleeding, such as abnormal thyroid function and haematological diseases, can be excluded with appropriate blood tests. The most common organic intra-uterine causes of menorrhagia can be excluded with hysteroscopic or ultrasound examination and tissue sampling. The development of transvaginal ultrasonography (TVS) has enabled the gynaecologist to obtain high-resolution images of the uterus and ovaries. This has facilitated the accurate diagnosis of intra-cavity focal pathology, such as submucous fibroids and endometrial polyps. Endometrial cancers, endometrial hyperplasia, adenomyosis and, rarely, oestrogen producing ovarian tumours can also be detected. This is achieved with high frequency transducers (6–7.5 MHz) located inside probes which can be placed in close proximity to the pelvic organs. Abdominal probes are used to visualise pelvic masses that extend beyond the focal length of the vaginal probe (approximately 10 cm). The use of saline hydrosonography (s-HS) further enhances the views of the endometrial cavity and endometrium by acting as a negative contrast agent. Colour flow Doppler can provide additional information about blood flow and vascularity. Because of these advances in technology, it has become feasible to use TVS as a primary diagnostic tool in the investigation of menorrhagia.

Furthermore, we believe that if TVS and s-HS are made available at every consultation and used in combination with blind endometrial biopsy, most patients with abnormal uterine bleeding can be appropriately managed during a single clinic visit.

Instruments and ancillary devices

Ultrasound machine

For most clinics a small, portable machine is all that is required. This must have a vaginal probe and a 3.5 MHz abdominal probe. Facilities for image capturing should be available, either as hard copy or to a computer. For general uses a Doppler facility is not necessary. An adequate machine will thus be available from the low end of the market in terms of price and it is likely that their cost will continue to fall.

Computer database systems

A number of commercial database systems exist for the storage of data, including digital images. This allows a written report to be generated, immediately, for the referring physician and patient and also allows access to previous images for easy comparison either following surgery or the conservative management of, e.g., ovarian cysts.

Improving picture definition and resolution

The control panel

The more sound that a transducer receives the brighter the image. The gain or volume of ultrasound is usually controlled by a series of slides which control slices of the image approximately 2 cm thick. It is the gain control settings that determine the quality of the image displayed. The image can also be magnified, thus decreasing the margin of error when measurements are made.

Sonohysterography

s-HS is a simple technique involving the instillation of sterile saline into the uterine cavity. All the required equipment can be found in a routine gynaecology clinic except for the catheter used to access the uterine cavity. We use a 5 French paediatric nasogastric feeding tube. This is first primed with sterile saline. The 20 ml syringe is then removed and the catheter is grasped at the tip with sponge holding forceps and passed through the cervical os using a vulsellum for counter traction if required. The syringe is then reattached and the saline gently instilled. Alternatives to the feeding tube include a modified pipelle du Cornier (its rigidity helps insertion) and thin balloon catheters either urinary or custom made (e.g. Goldstein sonohysterography catheter, Cook Ob/Gyn IN, USA). The presence of a balloon helps to reduce backflow of saline and maintain uterine distension. These devices tend to be more expensive, are not readily available and distension of the balloon at the internal cervical os can cause increased discomfort.

Safety features

Infection

There is a small risk of transmission of infection as the trans-vaginal probe comes into contact with mucous membranes. This is reduced by the use of an appropriate cover for the transducer, usually a glove or condom. It is estimated that up to 7%[2] of covers will sustain perforations and contamination of the probe may also occur on removing the cover after use. Because of this, appropriate cleaning of the transducer must occur between patients. Sterilisation of the probe is not practical and disinfection using a germicidal cloth (e.g. 70% alcohol) or spray, after first wiping off the gel, is effective. The probe is then left to air dry for at least 5 min. Basic hygiene measures, such as washing hands after each case and ensuring that contaminated gloves do not come into contact with the ultrasound machine, must be used to minimise cross infection. The risk of pelvic infection following s-HS is very small, if it occurs at all. Despite this, in our clinic we recommend the use of prophylactic antibiotics in all potentially fertile women to minimise this risk. Sonohysterography should not be performed in the presence of overt pelvic infection.

Shock

Cervical or anaphylactic shock may occur during the ultrasound examination and resuscitation equipment should be available in all gynaecological clinics. The equipment should be in good order and the clinic staff should be able to use it. Typically, cervical shock occurs when the cervix is instrumented and the patient becomes hypotensive and bradycardic. An anaphylactic reaction can occasionally occur to the latex in the probe cover.

Analgesia requirements

TVS is a well tolerated procedure. Even when sonohysterography is performed, the routine use of analgesia is not advocated. In one series 98% of patients undergoing TVS and 87% of patients undergoing s-HS reported either no or minimal discomfort.[3] However, equipment should be available to provide a paracervical block when indicated with some cases of cervical stenosis or at the patient's request.

Performing the scan and definitions

After inserting the probe into the vagina, the uterus and subsequently the adnexae are surveyed in the sagittal and coronal planes.

The uterine cavity

Endometrium

Maximum endometrial thickness is the distance (in mm) from one myometrial/endometrial interface to the other across the cavity of the uterus. A thickness >12 mm for pre-menopausal patients and >5 mm for post-menopausal patients is typically used to indicate the possible presence of intra-cavity pathology. This measurement excludes intra-cavity fluid but includes any tissue. It is usually obtained just below the fundus. If cut-off values derived from the measurement of endometrial thickness are ever to be widely accepted as a method for excluding endometrial pathology, then the issue of reproducibility is of vital importance. It is particularly relevant with reference to operators with different levels of experience with ultrasound. The fact that neither experienced nor inexperienced examiners will always identify the endometrium makes it important to consider such findings potentially pathological. In such instances hydrosonography is indicated.[4] If the endometrium can still not be visualised, then hysteroscopy with directed biopsy should be performed.

Polyps

A polyp is defined as a smooth-margined, echogenic mass of variable size and shape often with a homogeneous texture, but sometimes cystic in nature. The structure must emerge from the endometrium but not disrupt the myometrial–endometrial interface.

Submucous fibroids

These are defined as round structures of mixed echogenicity emanating from the endometrium. They cause disruption of the inner circular muscle layer, protruding into the uterine cavity to a varying degree and have a cover of intact endometrium.[3,5–7]

Adenomyosis

The presence of one or more of the following is required to diagnose adenomyosis:

1. thickening and asymmetry of the anterior and posterior myometrial walls;

2. increased echotexture of the myometrium;

3. hetrogeneous indistinctly marginated areas in the myometrium.[8]

Results of studies

What are the standard techniques for assessing the endometrium against which TVS and s-HS can be compared? For many years the most widely used technique for obtaining a sample of endometrium for histological evaluation was dilatation and curettage (D&C). However, this procedure has numerous limitations. The operation of D&C has a false negative rate of between 2% and 6% for diagnosing endometrial cancer and hyperplasia.[9,10] Such figures also hold true for other methods of obtaining an endometrial sample such as the Vabra (Berkeley Medevices, Berkeley, CA, USA) and Pipelle (Milex Products, Chicago, IL, USA).[11] These problems arise due to sampling errors. Stock and Kanbour[10] demonstrated this point by performing

D&C immediately prior to hysterectomy in 50 women. They showed that in 30 out of the 50 patients (60%), less than half of the cavity was sampled. More recently, the evaluation of endometrial pathology with direct vision has become possible with hysteroscopy. This can be used in both an outpatient and inpatient setting. The procedure allows for directed biopsies to be taken, thereby minimising the theoretical risk of sampling errors. However, this concept pre-supposes that the operator will recognise areas of endometrial abnormality under direct vision. This is not always the case. Furthermore, many outpatient hysteroscopes have no operating channel with which to take biopsies and sampling is still in effect 'blind'. Nevertheless, the literature suggests that hysteroscopy provides an increase in diagnostic information. Gimpleson and Rappold[12] studied 276 patients who underwent both hysteroscopy and D&C. Hysteroscopy yielded more information in 44 patients whilst D&C gave more accurate information in only nine patients. The use of hysteroscopy seems to offer particular advantages for the diagnosis of endometrial polyps and submucous myomas. Several patients in this study had been previously treated with multiple curettage procedures before their endometrial pathology was found with the hysteroscope. Therefore, it is against hysteroscopy that TVS must be compared if its true role in the assessment of the endometrium is to be determined (Table 3.1).

Table 3.1 — Comparison of TVS in the evaluation of the uterine cavity in women (pre- and post-menopausal) with abnormal uterine bleeding

Authors	n	TVS		SHS		Hysteroscopy	
		Sens	Spec	Sens	Spec	Sens	Spec
Endometrial polyps							
Schwarzler et al	98	56	97	84	97	92	100
Bernard et al	59	–	8	91	–	–	–
Widrich et al	64	–	–	100	81	94	90
Submucosal myomas							
Schwarzler et al	98	82	98	94	98	88	100
Bernard et al	159	–	–	90	95	–	–
Widrich et al	64	–	–	92	98	100	96
Fedele et al	65	100	94	–	–	100	96
Endometrial hyperplasia/carcinoma							
Schwarzler et al	98	67	89	87	91	90	91
Bernard et al	159	–	–	89/40	96/100	–	–
Widrich et al	64	–	–	86	97	43	100

Sens — sensitivity; Spec — specificity.

Endometrial assessment

TVS is a highly sensitive method for detecting endometrial abnormalities[13–15]. In the assessment of post-menopausal bleeding, the finding of a regular endometrial echo with a thickness of less than 5 mm has been shown to have a high negative predictive value for the presence of pathology.[16] However, the pre-menopausal endometrium is a dynamic structure and wide variations in the endometrial thickness have been associated with pathology.[17] The most consistent measurements are taken in the proliferative phase when the endometrium is at its thinnest and most echolucent.[18] With all measurements of the endometrial echo, it is important to visualise it as a three-dimensional structure, so as to avoid missing focal irregularities. Three-dimensional ultrasound has an established role in the assessment of congenital uterine abnormalities[19] and it may be that it has a role in improving the visualisation of acquired conditions of the uterine cavity as well.

The endometrial outline should be regular and uninterrupted, whatever the thickness. A thick, secretory endometrium on unenhanced TVS will often disguise endometrial pathology. In contrast, a periovulatory 'triple line' endometrium will offer the best unenhanced views of the uterine cavity. TVS affords good myometrial/endometrial interface definition. This is important in the assessment of suspected endometrial carcinoma. Most benign and cancerous lesions of the endometrium will manifest themselves morphologically as polyps. These tend to be hyperechoic or cystic structures distorting the endometrial echo. Colour Doppler may demonstrate a single feeding blood vessel to the structure.

Uterine myomas

Advances in the management of uterine myomas have resulted in a need to provide accurate pre-treatment information concerning their size, quantity and location. This is especially true with the increasing use of minimally invasive techniques of fibroid resection. The ultrasound appearances of myomas are varied. Before the menopause, they tend to be a well defined heterogeneous or hypoechoic uterine mass in nature. TVS can be an inaccurate method of mapping large uterine fibroids and magnetic resonance imaging (MRI) may provide added information. MRI is indicated when fibroid embolisation is planned as it allows the accurate assessment of fibroid shrinkage and the distinction of intra-mural fibroids from adenomyosis.[20] TVS is used in conjunction with abdominal scanning to ensure pedunculated subserosal fibroids are not missed. Submucosal fibroids project into the uterine cavity and distort the endometrium. Their accurate classification allows selection for transcervical resection in appropriate cases. Fedele et al[15] demonstrated the sensitivity of TVS for the diagnosis of submucosal fibroids to be 100%, with a sensitivity of 94%. Hysteroscopy (outpatient), performed on the same population, had a sensitivity and specificity of 100% and 96% respectively in their diagnosis. The only criticism of TVS in this study was its apparent inability to differentiate endometrial polyps from submucosal fibroids. All of the scans were performed in the secretory phase of the cycle. Endometrial polyps tend to be hyperechoic structures, easily masked by a thick secretory endometrium. By performing the scans during the proliferative phase, the distinction between intra-cavity fibroids and polyps is easier to make. The PPV was as high as 92%.[3]

Adenomyosis

This is a condition characterised by the presence of endometrial glands and stroma in the myometrium which may have a diffuse or focal distribution. It can be difficult to distinguish adenomyosis from intramural myomas. It is an important distinction to make because the definitive management of adenomyosis is hysterectomy, whereas myomas can be treated with the conservation of the uterus. The reported sensitivity and specificity of TVS in diagnosing diffuse adenomyosis is 80% and 74% respectively and 8% and 98% for focal lesions.[21] However, MRI scanning has been shown to be significantly better than TVS in the diagnosis of adenomyosis ($p < 0.02$).[8] For this reason MRI remains the diagnostic modality of choice if fibroid embolisation is planned but it does add considerably to the overall cost of the treatment.

Saline sonohysterography

This technique involves the introduction of a monographic negative contrast agent into the uterine cavity, to enhance routine TVS in the identification of uterine cavity pathology. The examination should ideally be performed in the proliferative phase of the menstrual cycle, once menstruation has ceased. This not only enhances views of the uterine cavity, but also reduces the risk of disturbing an early intra-uterine pregnancy.

Indications for s-HS

- Thickened endometrium.
- Poor views of the endometrium due to an axial position of uterus and large myomas distorting the uterine cavity.
- Preoperative localisation, assessment of size and relation to the uterine cavity of submucous fibroids/endometrial polyps.

Complications

- Failure to complete the procedure — this usually occurs due to cervical stenosis, or in the presence of multiple large fibroids. The problems encountered with a patulous cervix may be overcome by using either a balloon catheter or infusing the saline solution faster. Overall failure rates ranging from 1.8%[22] to 4.6%[23] are quoted.
- Infection — there are no reports of infection following s-HS.
- There is no evidence to support the theoretical concern that instillation of fluid into the uterine cavity, either at hysteroscopy or saline sonohysterography, may promote dissemination of endometrial carcinoma.[24]

Advantages

- s-HS is cheaper than hysteroscopy both in terms of the initial capital cost and running costs.
- It is less painful.
- Visualisation with s-HS is not limited to the uterine cavity but also allows a panoramic view of the myometrium, fallopian tubes, ovaries and Pouch of Douglas.

The 'One Stop' Ultrasound Based Clinic

In-patient hysteroscopy and curettage, under general anaesthesia, is no longer considered an acceptable first line management strategy for the management of abnormal uterine bleeding.[25,26] This had led to the creation of out-patient hysteroscopy clinics.[27–29]

However, recent data has suggested that ultrasound may be as effective as hysteroscopy for the detection of focal endometrial pathology. This is particularly true if out-patient hysteroscopy is carried out with blind endometrial sampling rather than directed biopsy.

Therefore, it is important to establish which approach should be used as a first line test to evaluate abnormal uterine bleeding.

We have established a one stop clinic for the management of women with abnormal uterine bleeding based on TVS and s-HS. Our management strategy for women with menorrhagia is summarised in Figure 3.1. We have reported our experience with the first 93 patients attending the clinic (submitted for publication). In the clinic, patients are seen with the intention of performing a scan (TVS), s-HS, endometrial biopsy and blood tests. The findings are then recorded on a computer database (Viewpoint) and a management plan formulated.

TVS has been compared to hysteroscopy for the detection of intra-uterine lesions.[30] In pre-menopausal women, the sensitivity and specificity of TVS compared poorly with the results of out-patient hysteroscopy, 60% and 88% respectively.[31] These findings have been supported by other studies.[32,33] However, there is a wide variation in the sensitivity and specificity which can be as high as 94% and 89%.[30] When TVS and hysteroscopy are used in combination the accuracy of diagnosis of uterine disease increases[35] and, therefore, the role of TVS is largely seen as an initial diagnostic method[37] prior to hysteroscopy.

However, the combination of TVS with s-HS has made ultrasound without hysteroscopy a potential first line investigation.[3,5–7,37–40] A recent study[3] has shown that compared to TVS alone, TVS plus s-HS increases the sensitivity from 67% to 87%, the specificity from 89% to 91%, the positive predictive value from 88% to 92% and the negative predictive value from 71% to 86%. These findings are supported by other studies, where the sensitivity and the specificity of s-HS compared to hysteroscopy, have been reported as 90% and 83%[40] and 99% and 88%[41]. A randomised study comparing TVS plus s-HS with office hysteroscopy for endometrial assessment has been carried out.[41] This showed that the sensitivity and specificity of ultrasonography was 85% and 100% respectively. The corresponding values for office hysteroscopy were 77% and 92%.

TVS was acceptable to most patients attending the clinic (95.7% of patients). This is supported by data from a randomised trial[41] which clearly demonstrated that more patients preferred TVS to hysteroscopy ($P < 0.001$). This is an extremely important observation when considering which investigation should be used as a first line test. The patients attending our clinic who did not undergo TVS were either virgo intacta or

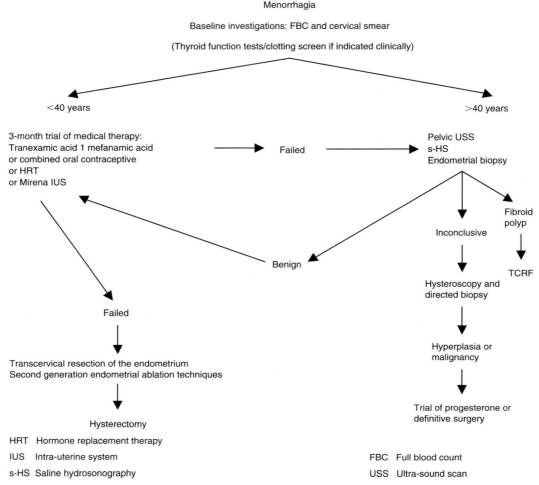

Menorrhagia

Baseline investigations: FBC and cervical smear

(Thyroid function tests/clotting screen if indicated clinically)

<40 years

>40 years

3-month trial of medical therapy:
Tranexamic acid 1 mefanamic acid
or combined oral contraceptive
or HRT
or Mirena IUS

Failed

Pelvic USS
s-HS
Endometrial biopsy

Fibroid
polyp

Inconclusive

Benign

TCRF

Failed

Hysteroscopy and
directed biopsy

Transcervical resection of the endometrium
Second generation endometrial ablation techniques

Hyperplasia or
malignancy

Hysterectomy

Trial of progesterone or
definitive surgery

HRT   Hormone replacement therapy

IUS   Intra-uterine system

s-HS   Saline hydrosonography

FBC   Full blood count

USS   Ultra-sound scan

Figure 3.1 — Flow diagram of the management of women with menorrhagia.

chose to undergo no further intervention after referral to the clinic.

We did have to perform an in-patient hysteroscopy in 16.3% of patients because of an inability to take endometrial biopsies. This is a higher rate of in-patient admissions than rates reported by other clinics of 3%[27] and 8.3%.[29] We were able to detect intra-mural and subserosal fibroids (21.3% of patients) and submucous fibroids (6.7% of patients) distinguish between them. This is important in planning a surgical procedure because submucous fibroids which project <50% into the uterine cavity cannot be resected hysteroscopically. The patients with adenocarcinoma of the endometrium (3.4% of patients) were all post menopausal and had an endometrial thickness of >5 mm and positive biopsies. This is a similar prevalence of pathology to previously published work from the unit,[3] and compares to detection rates reported in hysteroscopy clinics.

Having ultrasound available at every consultation also facilitates the incidental diagnosis of adnexal pathology. Adnexal pathology was detected in 12 (13.5%) of patients in this study. We were able to manage 89.2% of the patients on the basis of a single visit. The benefits are clear. It avoids repeated out-patient visits and decreases in-patient episodes. This in turn decreases the waiting list for hospital out-patient appointments and for surgery. Patients are diagnosed and treated at the same time and therefore they begin treatment sooner. Medical therapy was the first line treatment in 50.5% of patients and another 17.2% only required reassurance. This is in keeping with the Royal College of Obstetricians and Gynaecologists recommendations for the management of pre-menopausal women.[25,26] However, most of the patients seen in the clinic had not received any previous medical treatment in the community.

Although the clinic has not been formally assessed in terms of cost, it is likely that these are less than with any other management strategy because most gynaecology departments already have ultrasound equipment. The main limiting factor in the UK is that radiographers and not gynaecologists perform ultrasound scans.

Conclusions

Trans-vaginal ultrasonography is highly sensitive in the diagnosis of intra-cavity pathology, but lacks specificity in many cases.[16,17] s-HS has been shown to be a highly sensitive and specific technique in the identification of both the normal uterine cavity and the characterisation and localisation of intra-cavity pathology. This optimises management strategies, whether expectant, medical, minimally invasive or more radical surgical techniques. The advantages and disadvantages are summarised in Table 3.2. The use of a non-invasive diagnostic technique prevents unnecessary surgical intervention which can be applied as the primary diagnostic tool in the 'One Stop' clinic setting.

Table 3.2 — A summary of the advantages and disadvantages of using trans-vaginal ultrasound as the first line test to evaluate abnormal uterine bleeding

Advantages	Disadvantages
Well tolerated, safe, reproducible and cheap	User dependent
No preparation required before the procedure (full bladder, etc.)	Can be lacking, in specificity for focal lesions
Ovarian and uterine structures as well as endometerial morphology can be assessed	Blind endometrial biopsy required
Can be integrated into a 'one stop' gynaecology setting, allowing an immediate initial diagnosis	
Specificity can be increased by the instillation of saline into the uterine cavity	

References

1. Higham JM. Medical treatment of menorrhagia. *Progress in Obstetrics and Gynaecology* Vol. 9, Chapter 21; 335–345.

2. Jimenez R, Duff P. Sheathing of the endovaginal probe: Is it adequate? *Infect Dis Obstet Gynecol* 1997; 1: 37–39.

3. Schwarzler P, Concin H, Bosch H, Berlinger A, Wohlgenannt K, Collins WP, Boume TH. An evaluation of sonohysterography and diagnostic hysteroscopy for the assessment of intra-uterine pathology. *Ultra-sound Obstet Gynecol* 1998; 11: 337–342.

4. Granberg S, Boume TH. Trans-vaginal ultrasonography of endometrial disorders in postmenopausal women. *Ultrasound Quarterly* 1995; 13: 16–24.

5. Parsons AK, Lense J. Sonohysterography for endometrial abnormalities: Preliminary results. *J Clin Ultra-sound* 1993; 21: 87–95.

6. Wildrich T, Bradley LD, Mitchinson AR, Collins R. Comparison of saline infusion sonography with office hysteroscopy for the evaluation of the endometrium. *Am J Obstet Gynecol* 1996; 174: 1327–1334.

7. Bronz L, Suter T, Rusca T. The value of trans-vaginal sonography with and without saline instillation in the diagnosis of uterine pathology in pre- and post-menopausal women with abnormal bleeding or suspect monographic findings. *Ultra-sound Obstet Gynecol* 1997; 9: 53–58.

8. Ascer SM, Arnold LL, Patt RH, Schruefer JJ, Bagley AS, Semelka RC, Zeman RK, Simon JA. Adenomyosis: prospective comparison of MR imaging and trans-vaginal sonography. *Radiology* 1994; 190: 803–806.

9. Holst J, Koskela O, von Schoultz B. Endometrial findings following curettage in 2018 women according to age and indications. *Ann Chir Gynaecol* 1983; 72: 274–277.

10. Stock R, Kanbour A. Prehysterectomy curettage. *Obstet Gynecol* 1975; 45: 537–541.

11. Koonings P, Moyer D, Grimes D. A randomised clinical trial comparing Pipelle and Tis-U-Trap for endometrial biopsy. *Obstet Gynecol* 1990; 75: 293–295.

12. Gimpleson R, Rappold H. A comparative study between panoramic hysteroscopy with directed biopsies and dilatation and curettage. *Am J Obstet Gynecol* 1988; 158: 489–492.

13. Smith P, Bakos O, Heirner G, Ulrnsten U. Trans-vaginal ultrasound for identifying endometrial abnormality. *Acta Obstet Gynecol Scand* 1991; 70: 591–594.

14. Mendelson E, Bohm-Vaelez M, Joseph N, Neiman H. Endometrial abnormalities: evaluation with trans-vaginal ultrasonography. *AJR* 1988; 150: 139–142.

15. Fedele L, Bianchi S, Dorta M, Brioschi D, Zanotti F, Vercellini P. Trans-vaginal ultrasonography versus hysteroscopy in the diagnosis of uterine submucosal myomas. *Obstet Gynecol* 1991; 77: 745–748.

16. Granberg S, Wikland M, Karlsson B, Norstrom A, Friberg LG. Endometrial thickness as measured by endovaginal ultrasonography for identifying endometrial abnormality. *Am J Obstet Gynecol* 1991; 164: 47–52.

17. Dijkhuizen F, Brohnann H, Potters A, Bongers M, Heintz A. The accuracy of trans-vaginal ultrasonography in the diagnosis of endometrial abnormalities. *Obstet Gynecol* 1996; 87: 345–349.

18. Goldstein SR. Use of ultrasonography for triage of peri-menopausal patients with unexplained uterine bleeding. *Am J Obstet Gynecol* 1994; 170: 565–570.

19. Jurkovic D, Geipel A, Gruboeck K, Jauniaux E, Nutecei M, Campbell S. Three dimensional ultrasound for the assessment of uterine anatomy and detection of congenital anomalies: a comparison with hydrosonography and two-dimensional sonography. *Ultra-sound Obstet Gynecol* 1995; 5: 233–237.

20. Goodwin Sc, Walker WJ. Uterine artery embolisation for the treatment of uterine fibroids. *Curr Opin Obstet Gynaecol* 1998; 10(4): 315–320.

21. Fedele L, Bianchi S, Dorta M, Arcaini L, Zanotti F, Carinelli S. Trans-vaginal ultrasonography in the diagnosis of diffuse adenomyosis. *Fert Steril* 1992; 58: 94–97.

22. Bernard JP, Lecuru F, Darles C, Robin F, deBievre P, Taurelle R. Saline contrast sonohysterography as first-line investigation for women with uterine bleeding. *Ultra-sound Obstet Gynecol* 1997; 10: 121–125.

23. Widrich T, Bradley LD, Mitchinson AR, Collins RL. Comparison of saline infusion sonography with office hysteroscopy for the evaluation of the endometrium. *Am J Obstet Gynecol* 1996; 174: 1327–1334.

24. De Vore G, Schwartz P, Morris J. Hysterography: a five year follow-up in-patients with endometrial carcinoma. *Obstet Gynecol* 1982; 60: 369–372.

25. Royal College of Obstetricians and Gynaecologists (1994). In-patient treatment — D&C in women aged 40 or less. RCOG Guidelines No. 3.

26. Royal College of Obstetricians and Gynaecologists (1999). The Management of Menorrhagia in Secondary Care. RCOG Guidelines No. 5.

27. Basckett TF, O'Connor H, Magos AL. A comprehensive one-stop menstrual problem clinic for the diagnosis and management of abnormal uterine bleeding. *Br J Obstet Gynecol* 1996; 103: 76–77.

28. Coats PM, Haines P, Kent SH. Flexible hysteroscopy: an outpatient evaluation in abnormal uterine bleeding. *Gynaecol Endoscopy* 1997; 6: 229–235.

29. Roman JD, Trivedi AN. Implementation of an outpatient hysteroscopy clinic at Waikato Women's Hospital report of the first 60 cases. *New Zeal Med J* 1999; 1091: 253–255.

30. Emanuel MH, Verdel MJ, Wamsteker K, Lammes FB. A prospective comparison of trans-vaginal ultrasound and diagnostic hysteroscopy in the evaluation of patients with abnormal uterine bleeding: clinical implications. *Am J Obstet Gynecol* 1995; 172: 547–552.

31. Pal 1, Lapensee L, Toth TL, Isaacson KB. Comparison of office hysteroscopy, trans-vaginal ultrasonography and endometrial biopsy in evaluation of abnormal uterine bleeding. *J Soc Laparoendoscopic Surg* 1997; 1: 125–130.

32. Alcazar JL, Laparte C. Comparative study of trans-vaginal ultrasonography and hysteroscopy in postmenopausal bleeding. *Gynecol Obstet Inves* 1996; 41: 47–49.

33. Giusa-Chiferi MG, Goncalves WJ, Baracat EC, de Albuquerque Neto LC, Bortoletto CC, de Lirna GR. Trans-vaginal ultrasound, uterine biopsy and hysteroscopy for post menopausal bleeding. *Int J Gynaecol Obstet* 1996; 55: 39–44.

34. Indman PD. Abnormal uterine bleeding. Accuracy of vaginal probe ultrasound in predicting abnormal hysteroscopic findings. *J Reprod Med* 1995; 40: 545–548.

35. Feng L, Xia E, Duan H. Diagnosis of uterine disease by combined hysteroscopic and ultrasonography. *Chinese J Obstet Gynaecol* 1996; 31: 334–337.

36. Mortakis AE, Mavrelos K. Trans-vaginal ultrasonography and hysteroscopy in the diagnosis of endometrial abnormalities. *J Am Assoc Gynaecol Laparoscopists* 1997; 4: 449–452.

37. Lev-Toaff AS, Toaff ME, Lin JB, Merton DA, Goldberg BB. The value of sonohysterography in the diagnosis and management of uterine bleeding. *Radiology* 1996; 201: 179–184.

38. Goldstein SR, Schwartz LB. Evaluation of abnormal vaginal bleeding in perimenopausal women with endovaginal ultrasound and saline infusion sonohysterography. *Ann New York Acad Sci* 1997; 828: 208–212.

39. Saidi ME, Sadler RK, Theis VD, Akright BD, Farhart SA, Villanueva GR. Comparison of sonography, sonohysterography and hysteroscopy for evaluation of abnormal uterine bleeding. *J Ultra-sound Med* 1997; 16: 587–591.

40. Bernard JP, Lecuru F, Darles C, Robin F, de Bievre P, Taurelle R. Saline contrast sonohysterography as first-line investigation for women with uterine bleeding. *Ultrasound in Obstet Gynaecol* 1997; 10: 121–125.

41. Timmerman D, Deprest J, Boume T, Van den Berghe I, Collins WP, Vergote I. A randomised trial on the use of ultrasound or office hysteroscopy for endometrial assessment in postmenopausal patients with breast cancer who were treated with tarnoxifen. *Am J Obstet Gynecol* 1998; I: 62–70.

4

Role of hysteroscopy in the management of menorrhagia

Majella G. Okeahialam and Peter J. O'Donovan

Introduction

Menorrhagia may be defined as excessive menstrual loss. Objectively, this means measured menstrual loss in excess of 80 ml per menstrual cycle.[1] In clinical practice, it is not possible to routinely perform an objective assessment of menstrual loss, and menorrhagia is therefore taken to be a complaint of excessive menstrual loss. A significant population of women complaining of menorrhagia will have a measured blood loss less than 80 ml per cycle. Menorrhagia is a major reason for gynaecological referral. Various methods have been developed for the objective assessment of menstrual loss. These have not been very helpful in the clinical management of menorrhagia.

Menorrhagia may start anytime from menarche through the reproductive years to menopause and in postmenopausal women on hormone replacement therapy. It can start suddenly or run a chronic course. Recent evidence suggests that most excessive uterine bleeding is due to local endometrial and myometrial dysfunction.[2] In the peri-menopausal period and beyond, meticulous evaluation of the uterine cavity and uterine body is essential and histological evaluation of the endometrial sample is mandatory.[3]

During the normal menstrual cycle, proliferation of endometrium is induced by the effect of oestrogens while progestogens induce secretory differentiation.[4] For menstruation to occur, there is extensive arteriolar vasoconstriction and bleeding occurs as vessels dilate.

The causes of menorrhagia can vary from a dysfunctional aetiology to the existence of pelvic pathology and rarely to systemic disorders. Apart from the social and psychological effects of menorrhagia, the severity can be assessed by estimation of the haemoglobin level and other blood indices and the effect on the iron status. Menorrhagia is the commonest cause of iron deficiency anaemia in the reproductive age women.[5]

Available methods for the evaluation of menorrhagia include traditional dilatation and curettage under anaesthesia, outpatient blind endometrial biopsy, hysteroscopy, transvaginal ultrasonography with or without colour flow Doppler, 3-dimensional ultrasonography and sonohysterography. Computerised tomography (CT) and magnetic resonance imaging (MRI) have also been used occasionally to evaluate menorrhagia. These have been used alone or in combination to assess the uterine cavity. Some of these methods of endometrial assessment are yet to undergo rigorous clinical evaluation before they can be recommended for routine use. At present, hysteroscopy and ultrasonography, used alone or in combination, are standard methods of endometrial assessment.

Aetiology of menorrhagia

The causes of menorrhagia can be categorised into three main groups, namely:

- dysfunctional uterine bleeding (DUB),
- bleeding due to pelvic pathology,
- medical disorders including coagulation defects.

DUB is a diagnosis of exclusion. Pelvic causes of menorrhagia include:

- uterine fibroids;
- adenomyosis;
- endometrial polyps;
- endometriosis;
- endometritis;
- presence of intra-uterine contraceptive device (IUCD);
- endometrial hyperplasia;
- rarely, endometrial cancer.

Large submucous fibroids and pedunculated fibroid polyps are associated with the heaviest degree of loss.[6] The endometrial pathologies that can be diagnosed by hysteroscopy include:

- submucous fibroids,
- polyps,
- hyperplasia,
- malignancy.

Hysteroscopy will also help in confirming the dysfunctional aetiology of menorrhagia.

Systemic diseases occasionally cause menorrhagia. Systemic causes of menorrhagia can vary from

- von Willebrand's disease and other blood factor deficiency states;
- hypothyroidism;
- autoimmune disorders like idiopathic thrombocytopaenia and systemic lupus erythomatosis;
- chronic liver disease;
- use of anticoagulants like wafarin;
- rarely, leukaemia.

Unsuspected pregnancy bleeding can present like an acute episode of menorrhagia or complicate an ongoing chronic menorrhagia. Menorrhagia can occur in postmenopausal women taking hormone replacement therapy.

How to investigate menorrhagia

A detailed general examination, including abdominal and pelvic examination to exclude local lower genital tract and pelvic abnormalities, is necessary prior to any investigation.[7]

A full blood count and estimation of the serum ferritin level in anaemic patients will help to determine the severity of the menorrhagia. When the history is suggestive of systemic illness, investigation can be directed to the suspected disease, e.g. thyroid function test if there is suspicion of hypothyroidism.

Only young women with menorrhagia that is refractory to treatment require invasive investigations like hysteroscopy, whereas hysteroscopy is mandatory in women during the peri-menopausal years.[3]

In some patients, despite very detailed and exhaustive investigation, no apparent cause for the menorrhagia can be identified and the aetiology is therefore labelled as DUB.

Hysteroscopy plays a pivotal vital role in the evaluation of the uterine cavity in any woman suffering with menorrhagia. Although transvaginal scan is a very good method of screening for intra-uterine pathology, abnormal uterine pathology can only be confirmed by direct visualisation of the uterine cavity by hysteroscopy.[3] This will define the pathology, its location and extent, and help in the choice of treatment.

Hysteroscopes and ancillary equipment

With the decline in the use of dilation and curettage, hysteroscopy has emerged as the gold standard for evaluation of the uterine cavity. Hysteroscopy offers an optimal assessment of the whole endometrial surface.[8–10] The technical advancement in fibre-optics and camera systems and the availability of various forms of hysteroscopes in the form of rigid, semi-rigid and flexible types and small calibre hysteroscopes has made hysteroscopy a very attractive method for the comprehensive assessment of the uterine cavity. Hysteroscope can be used both for the diagnosis and treatment of intra-uterine pathology

Hysteroscopy can be performed using a flexible, rigid or semi-rigid telescope. Rigid hysteroscopes can have a single-flow channel in the outer sheath for the inflow of the distension medium and sometimes with an additional outflow channel (continuous flow) for operative procedures. Flexible and semi-rigid hysteroscopes are usually single-flow systems.

Hysteroscopy can be performed for diagnostic or operative purpose. It can be performed as an outpatient procedure with or without analgesia or under general anaesthesia. Fluid or carbon dioxide (CO_2) gas can be used for distension of the uterine cavity.

The distal end of the hysteroscope can have either a 0° or 30° lens. The diameter of the hysteroscope can vary from 2.5 to 8 mm when fully assembled. Diagnostic hysteroscopes of 4 mm or less may be more acceptable for outpatient purposes as there may be no need for cervical dilatation.

CO_2 is the most commonly used gas for the distension of the uterine cavity during hysteroscopy. This can be delivered in a continuous and controlled manner using a CO_2 insufflator.

Low viscosity fluids are presently popular distension media for hysteroscopy. For diagnostic purposes, normal saline is adequate while glycine is ideal for therapeutic purposes. Other fluids that can be used for hysteroscopy are 4% or 5% sorbitol and 5% dextrose. The distension fluid may be delivered by gravity, pressure cuffs or electronically controlled pumps.

Lighting for the hysteroscope can be generated via a xenon or halogen light source. A video camera for the display of the image on a display screen is essential for modern hysteroscopy. Video printer or recorders are also vital accessories.

Contraindications to hysteroscopy include:

- acute pelvic inflammatory disease,
- acute endometritis,
- suspicion of pregnancy.

Profuse uterine bleeding is a relative contraindication to hysteroscopy, although a continuous flow hysteroscopy will improve visibility. Hysteroscopy in the second half of the cycle in patients not using adequate contraception is discouraged as an early pregnancy can be disturbed.[3]

Overview on hysteroscopy

Hysteroscopic assessment of the uterine cavity can detect small submucous fibroids, polyps and focal sites of malignancy that might be missed by ultrasonography or blind biopsy.[9] Being able to perform hysteroscopy in an outpatient setting has increased the attraction to the procedure. Outpatient hysteroscopy is acceptable to the majority of patients,[11] it is safe, simple[12] and considerably reduces the need for hospital admission. It is cost effective and can be performed with minimal facilities.[13] Hysteroscopy offers the advantage of directed biopsies to specific site in the uterine cavity, but experience is required for proper assessment of the endometrial cavity. Endometrial biopsy is not required routinely in young adolescent women with menorrhagia. It is advisable in those where there is no obvious endometrial cause for the menorrhagia to exclude an incidental hyperplasia. Endometrial sampling is mandatory in women of 35 years or older because of the possibility of pre-malignant and malignant changes in the endometrium. If the uterine cavity looks normal at hysteroscopy, endometrial biopsy can be obtained with any disposable plastic endometrial sampling device.

Saline hysteroscopy is said to produce less discomfort than gas hysteroscope.[11,14] Apart from offering optimal endometrial assessment, hysteroscopy is capable of distinguishing between hyperplasia, polyps and submucous fibroids.[15]

Hysteroscopy with directed biopsy is a satisfactory method of evaluating the endometrial cavity. When no endometrial pathology is seen at hysteroscopy, experienced hysteroscopists may not take an endometrial biopsy but, as a general rule, an endometrial biopsy is usually advisable. Appropriate patient selection, adequate training of staff, satisfactory instrumentation maintenance and trained ancillary staff will help to maximise the benefits of the procedure and reduce complications.

Menorrhagia occurs in about 12% of women with periods.[17] In the majority of patients, the menstrual loss returns to normal after removal of the polyps. The aetiology and mechanism whereby polyps cause menorrhagia is not known.[16] The polyps can be sessile or pedunculated and may be single or multiple. Hysteroscopy can visualise small polyps that may be missed by techniques (Fig. 4.1).

Endometrial cancer is a rare cause of menorrhagia, but about 40% of women found to have endometrial cancer prior to menopause will present with menorrhagia.[17] At hysteroscopy, endometrial carcinoma can appear as a polypoid lesion with atypical vessels or as a diffused lesion of the endometrium (Fig. 4.2). Hysteroscopy offers the advantage of directed biopsy of suspicious isolated lesions of the endometrium.

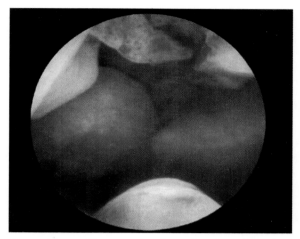

Figure 4.1 — Hysteroscopic view of endometrial polyps. Reproduced from Basic Gynaecological Endoscopy by Patricia Wilson with her kind permission.

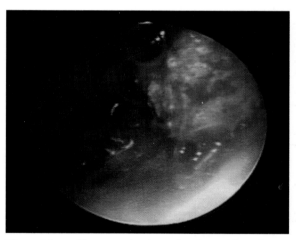

Figure 4.2 — Hysteroscopic view of endometrial carcinoma. Courtesy of Mr VN Chilaka MRCOG, Leicester General Hospital, Leicester, UK.

Hysteroscopy is very helpful in the differentiation of submucous fibroids from polyps. Submucous fibroid appears as a dense, white mass protruding into the endometrial cavity with a network of vessels running over the surface. Submucous fibroids can be pedunculated, single or multiple can cause gross distortion of the endometrial cavity.

Hysteroscopy offers the chance of resecting submucous fibroids hysteroscopically or vaporising it with laser or bipolar diathermy.

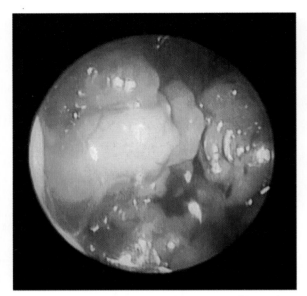

Figure 4.3 — Hysteroscopic view of severe atypical hyperplasia. Courtesy of Mr VN Chilaka MRCOG. Leicester General Hospital, Leicester, UK.

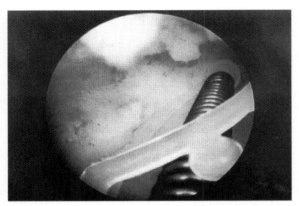

Figure 4.4 — Missing multiload IUCD found at hysteroscopy. Reproduced from Diagnostic Hysteroscopy: a practical guide by de Gruyter. With kind permission of the publisher.

Endometrial hyperplasia is characterised by abnormal endometrial proliferation. This may or may not have atypical cellular changes. The presence of atypical, cellular architecture increases the risk of malignancy. At hysteroscopy, hyperplastic endometrium looks thick and may be cystic (Fig. 4.3). The hyperplasia may be focal or diffused. Hysteroscopy can suspect a hyperplastic endometrium, but only histology of the endometrial sample can confirm or grade the hyperplasia. Hysteroscopy offers the opportunity of visualising this abnormal endometrium and taking a biopsy.

An IUCD can be forgotten inside the uterine cavity and the patient can present with menorrhagia (Fig. 4.4). Hysteroscopy offers the opportunity to make the diagnosis and also remove the IUCD at the same time.

Therapeutic hysteroscopy

The treatment of menorrhagia hysteroscopically ranges from resection of polyps and submucous myoma to resection or ablative procedures of the endometrium. These will be discussed in other chapters. Hysteroscopy offers the opportunity of visualising missing IUCD inside the uterine cavity. As this may be the cause of the menorrhagia, it also offers the opportunity of removing

it at the same time, if required. Prior to ablative procedures of the endometrium, hysteroscopy is necessary to evaluate the feasibility of the procedure and to obtain an endometrial biopsy to confirm benign histology of the endometrium prior to the ablative procedure.

Safety and complications of hysteroscopy

When performed by experienced personnel, complications are not common in diagnostic hysteroscopy.[15] Cervical laceration can occur from instruments used for grasping the cervix and during dilatation of the cervix. Uterine perforation or creation of false passages can occur either with the hysteroscope or dilator if cervical dilatation is necessary. Visceral damage can follow uterine perforation. Uterine perforation in an awake patient at outpatient hysteroscopy and performed by experienced personnel should be a rarity. Infection following diagnostic hysteroscopy is very uncommon. CO_2 embolism is a very rare complication which can cause circulatory collapse. Vasovagal attacks can follow outpatient hysteroscopy. Inadvertent intra-vascular injection of local anaesthetic can cause collapse. Fluid overload is a dangerous complication that can follow therapeutic hysteroscopy. Painful uterine contractions can also follow hysteroscopy. Haemorrhage and infection can also complicate hysteroscopy. Screening the at-risk population prior to hysteroscopy can help to reduce the risk of pelvic infection following the procedure.

Conclusion

Menorrhagia is one of the most common gynaecological complaints prior to menopause. Precise diagnosis of this very common problem is difficult. Satisfactory management can only be achieved through perception of the patient's tolerance to bleeding and use of techniques such as transvaginal ultrasonography and outpatient hysteroscopy and endometrial biopsy to try and achieve a diagnosis. The type of investigation required should be tailored to the specific needs of the individuals.

Young women with little possibility of major pathology are best evaluated with less invasive techniques such as ultrasonography. They can be offered hysteroscopy if ultrasonography suspects endometrial pathology or if they do not respond to conventional medical treatment. Peri-menopausal women with menorrhagia are best evaluated by hysteroscopy preferably in an outpatient setting and in addition to endometrial biopsy. The use of ultrasound in conjunction with hysteroscopy is very helpful in the evaluation of women with menorrhagia.

Hysteroscopy has a major role to play in the diagnosis and treatment of menorrhagia. Majority of benign intra-uterine pathology which can cause menorrhagia can be treated hysteroscopically, thus avoiding major surgery.

References

1. Hallberg L, Hogdahl AM, Nilsson L, Rybo G. Menstrual blood loss — a population study. *Acta Obstet Gynecol Scand* 1996; 45: 320–351.

2. Sheppard BL, Bonnar J. Pathophysiology of menorrhagia. In: S Sheth, C Sutton (Eds) *Menorrhagia*, Chapter 2, pp 11–22, 1999. ISIS Medical Media.

3. Wamsteker K. Endoscopy: hysteroscopy. In: Ivo Brosens, Kees Wamsteker (Eds) *Diagnostic Imaging and Endoscopy in Gynaecology: A Practical Guide*, pp 17–38, 1997. WB Saunders Company Ltd.

4. Read C. Managing the menopause 111. In: David Barlow, Peter Collins (Eds) A *Practical Guide to Long Term HRT*, pp 73–83, 1997. Novo Nordisk Pharmaceuticals Ltd.

5. Cohen BJB, Gobor J. Anaemia and menstrual blood loss. *Obstet Gynecol Surv* 1980; 35: 597–602.

6. Fraser IS, Arachchi. Aetiology and investigation of menorrhagia. In: S Sheth, C Sutton (Eds) *Menorrhagia*, Chapter 1, pp 1–10, 1999. ISIS Medical Media.

7. Thorneycroft IH. Practical aspects of HRT. *Prog Cardiovas Dis* 1995; xxxviii(3): 243–252.

8. Spencer CP, Cooper AJ, Whitehead MI. Management of abnormal bleeding in women receiving hormone replacement therapy. *Br Med J* 1997; 315: 37–42.

9. Downes E, Al-Azzawi F. The predictive value of outpatient hysteroscopy in a menopause clinic. *Br J Obstet Gynaecol* 1993; 100: 1148–1149.

10. Gimpleson RJ, Rappold HO. A comparative study between panoramic hysteroscopy with directed biopsies and dilatation and curettage: a review of 276 cases. *Am J Obstet Gynaecol* 1988; 158(81): 489–492.

11. Nagele F, O'Connor H, Davies A, Badawy A, Mohamed H, Magos A. 2500 outpatient diagnostic hysteroscopies. *Obstet Gynaecol* 1996; 88(1): 87–92.

12. Coats PM, Haines P, Kent ASH. Flexible hysteroscopy: an outpatient evaluation in abnormal uterine bleeding. *Gynaecol Endosc* 1997; 6: 229–235.

13. De Jong P, Doel F, Falconer A. Outpatient diagnostic hysteroscopy. *Br J Obstet Gynaecol* 1990; 97: 229–303.

14. Nagele F, Bournas N, O'Connor H, Broadbent M, Richardson R, Magos A. A comparison of carbon dioxide and normal saline for uterine distension during outpatient hysteroscopy. *Fertil Steril* 1996; 65: 305–309.

15. Raju KS, Taylor RW. Routine hysteroscopy for patients with high risk of uterine malignancy. *Br J Obstet Gynaecol* 1986; 93: 1259.

16. Van Bogaert LJ. Clinicopathologic findings in endometrial polyps. *Obstet Gynecol* 1988; 71: 771–773.

17. Quinn M, Naele B, Fortune DW. Endometrial carcinoma in pre-menopausal women: a clinicopathological study. *Gynecol Oncol* 1985; 20: 298–306.

5

Current treatment options: An evidence-based approach

Anne E. Lethaby, Neil P. Johnson and Cynthia M. Farquhar

Introduction

Although medical therapy is usually the first option for treating heavy menstrual bleeding (HMB), it is not always effective and some of the most effective treatments may cause unacceptable side effects. When medical treatment fails or women no longer wish to be on long-term therapy, hysterectomy has been the procedure of choice and is one of the few surgical procedures associated with an almost 100% success rate. Although high levels of satisfaction are reported following hysterectomy[1] it is, nevertheless, a major surgical procedure with significant physical and emotional complications and high costs. Complications associated with hysterectomy range from 21% to 43%[2,3] and full recovery may take up to 12 weeks.[3] By 28 days, only 67% of women who undergo vaginal hysterectomy have returned to their normal levels of activity.[4]

In the mid-1980s less invasive surgical techniques, or minimal access surgery, were introduced with the purpose of removing the entire thickness of the endometrium (endometrial ablation) while leaving the uterus intact and producing amenorrhoea or hypomenorrhoea. According to the physics of the technology used endometrial ablation systems may be divided into five categories:

1. laser,
2. monopolar and bipolar electrical,
3. heated fluid,
4. cryotherapy,
5. microwave and radiofrequency energy.

The endometrial tissue may be removed under direct hysteroscopic view. These direct hysteroscopic techniques, known collectively as 'first generation' endometrial ablation techniques, include transcervical endometrial resection (TCRE), rollerball endometrial ablation and endometrial laser ablation (ELA) and are described in detail elsewhere. More recently, in order to minimise the need for technical skill and the complications of hysteroscopic surgery, a number of less invasive or 'second generation' endometrial ablative techniques have been introduced where the procedure is performed blind without direct hysteroscopic visualisation.

Destruction of the endometrium was developed as an alternative to hysterectomy where the indication was HMB. It has been suggested that endometrial destruction techniques avoid the need for hysterectomy in about 80% of the women treated.[5] When this procedure was introduced, it was hoped that hysterectomy rates would decline and cost savings would be made.[5,6]

Unfortunately, this prediction has not come true. For example, a recent retrospective study in the UK, between 1989 and 1996,[7] reported that hysterectomy rates had remained relatively steady since the introduction of endometrial ablation and rates of endometrial ablation had declined slightly since 1992 and 1993. The authors concluded that endometrial destruction appears to have added an alternative operative technique for menorrhagia and an increase in the total number of procedures for this condition. In addition, many women undergoing endometrial ablation require additional surgery after their initial treatment which reduces the cost differential between ablation and hysterectomy.[8]

This chapter examines the evidence for the current endometrial destruction methods for menorrhagia and makes comparisons of the currently available techniques and these techniques compared with hysterectomy and medical therapy options. Research-based evidence varies widely in terms of quality, reliability, and validity and ranking of the evidence should aid in interpretation and comparison of studies. Accordingly, the studies that are assessed here will be graded according to the SIGN grading system which is used in the development of evidence-based clinical guidelines (Table 5.1).[9] The SIGN grade awarded to

Table 5.1 — Levels of evidence[10]

1[++]	High quality meta-analyses, systematic reviews of RCTs, or RCTs with a very low risk of bias
1[+]	Well-conducted meta-analyses, systematic reviews, or RCTs with a low risk of bias
1[−]	Meta-analyses, systematic reviews, or RCTs with a high risk of bias
2[++]	High quality systematic reviews of case–control or cohort studies
High quality case–control or cohort studies with a very low risk of confounding or bias and a high probability that the relationship is causal
2[+]	Well-conducted case–control or cohort studies with a low risk of confounding or bias and a moderate probability that the relationship is causal
2[−]	Case–control or cohort studies with a high risk of confounding or bias and a significant risk that the relationship is not causal
3	Non-analytic studies, e.g. case reports, case series
4	Expert opinion

each study will be specified in square brackets in the text. Properly designed randomised controlled trials (RCTs) or systematic reviews are the highest level of evidence and results from these studies will be considered superior to those of others. Results from relevant outcomes of the randomised trials that were identified from searches are summarised in Table 5.2.

Hysteroscopic endometrial ablation versus hysterectomy

Hysteroscopic ablative techniques (mostly TCRE) have been compared with hysterectomy (mostly abdominal) in a Cochrane systematic review (Ref. 10 [1^{++}]). The review pooled results from five RCTs involving a total of 752 participants and follow-up ranged from 4 months to 4 years. HMB was eliminated by hysterectomy but, at 1-year follow-up, bleeding was not reduced from pre-surgical levels in 13% of women undergoing endometrial ablation. After longer follow-up, however, the differences between hysterectomy and endometrial ablation appeared to narrow, possibly because of re-treatment in the endometrial ablation group or women reaching the menopause.

There were high satisfaction rates for both types of surgery. Satisfaction rates, however, were significantly higher among women undergoing hysterectomy up to 2 years after surgery but this did not persist at longer follow-up. Most quality of life measures were not significantly different between groups but more women who had a hysterectomy had an improvement in their general health 1 year after surgery. Improved social functioning, improved general health perception and reduced pain were also significantly different 2 years after surgery for these women compared with those who had endometrial ablation. Duration of surgery and recovery time, as measured by hospital stay and time to return to work, were all significantly reduced in women undergoing endometrial ablation but, because of excessive statistical heterogeneity, the summary measures are unreliable. Nevertheless, each of the individual trials separately reported significant differences between groups for these outcomes. It is unclear whether the difference of 23 min in duration of surgery is clinically important, but a difference of 5 days in hospital stay and 4.5 weeks in return to work are likely to represent a financial and social benefit to women.

Most complications, in particular sepsis, blood transfusion, urinary retention, anaemia, pyrexia, vault, and wound haematoma and cautery of hypergranulation were more common in women having a hysterectomy but fluid overload was more likely in women having endometrial ablation. There was a clear difference between the groups in the likelihood of requiring repeat surgery. In one study, by 4 years 38% of those who had endometrial ablation had required repeat surgery compared to 1% of those randomised to hysterectomy although 76% of all endometrial ablation patients still avoided a hysterectomy (Ref. 8 [1^{++}]). Initially, treatment costs were significantly lower for these women but the difference in costs over time between both surgical groups narrowed to 5–11% because of the cost of re-treatment.

The review concluded that there was good evidence that hysteroscopic endometrial destruction techniques provided an alternative to hysterectomy which should be offered to women with menorrhagia. High satisfaction rates, shorter operation time and hospital stay, earlier recovery and reduced post-operative complications were all benefits of endometrial ablation but re-treatment was necessary as much as 38% of the time.

Hysteroscopic endometrial ablation techniques

Transcervical resection of the endometrium

Endometrial resection with a cutting loop (TCRE) is considered by many to be the standard reference technique for hysteroscopic treatment of abnormal uterine bleeding. This technique has certainly been the most intensively studied in terms of therapeutic benefit but it requires a high level of surgical skill. The major operative risks with this technique are fluid overload, uterine perforation and haemorrhage.

Concern over these complications prompted the Department of Health in the UK to undertake a prospective audit (known as Mistletoe) of the currently used endometrial ablation techniques in England and Wales (Ref. 11 [3]) and a similar smaller study in Scotland with the aim of determining the incidence and nature of complications. The total complication rate for all techniques (mostly hysteroscopic) in the Mistletoe audit was only 4.4% and was linked to the experience of the operator. However, endometrial destruction by rollerball or laser were significantly safer than TCRE

Table 5.2 — RCTs of comparisons of endometrial destruction methods or with hysterectomy or medical therapy

Authors (Reference)	Year of publication	Intervention(s)	n	Amenorrhoea rate	Proportion satisfied	Re-treatment rate
Pinion et al (14)	1994	1. Laser ablation or TCRE	105	45%	80%	37%
Aberdeen Endometrial Ablation Trials Group (8)	1999	2. Hysterectomy (mostly abdominal)	99	98% (4 years)	91% (at 4 years)	1% (at 4 years)
O'Connor et al (52)	1997	1. TCRE	116	21%	85%	22%
		2. Hysterectomy (50% abdominal and 50% vaginal)	46	100% (at 3 years)	96% (at 3 years)	5% (at 2 years)
Gannon et al (53)	1991	1. TCRE	25	64%	Not determined	16%
		2. Hysterectomy (abdominal)	26	100% (at 1 year)		0% (at 1 year)
Dwyer et al (54)	1993	1. TCRE	99	30%	79%	32%
		2. Hysterectomy (abdominal)	97	100% (at 2 years)	93% (at 2 years)	0% (at 2 years)
Crosignani et al (29)	1997a	1. TCRE	45	23%	87%	12%
		2. Hysterectomy (vaginal)	47	100% (at 2 years)	95% (at 2 years)	0% (at 2 years)
Crosignani et al (26)	1997b	1. TCRE	35	26%	94%	9%
		2. LNG–IUS	35	18% (at 1 year)	85% (at 1 year)	12% (at 1 year)
Bhattacharya et al (13)	1997	1. Laser ablation	188	23%	90%	16%
		2. TCRE	184	22% (at 1 year)	91% (at 1 year)	20% (at 1 year)

(continued)

Table 5.2 — (*continued*)

Authors (Reference)	Year of publication	Intervention(s)	n	Amenorrhoea rate	Proportion satisfied	Re-treatment rate
Vercellini et al (19)	1999	1. Endometrial vaporisation	47	36%	96%	Not determined
		2. TCRE	44	48%	93%	
Kittelsen and Istre (27)	1998	1. TCRE	30	70%	Not determined	14%
		2. LNG-IUS	30	36%		20%
				(at 1 year)		(at 2 years)
Cooper et al (23, 24, 41)	1997 1999a,b	1. Medical therapy for menorrhagia	94	30%	57%	Not determined
		2. TCRE	93	38%	79%	
				(at 2 years)	(at 2 years)	
Meyer et al (31)	1998	1. ThermaChoice™ balloon ablation	128	15.2%	96%	1.6% (hyst)
		2. Rollerball ablation	117	27.2%	99%	2.5% (hyst)
				(at 1 year)	(at 1 year)	(at 1 year)
Romer et al (34)	1998	1. Cavaterm™ balloon ablation	10	90%	100%	Unknown
		2. Rollerball ablation	10	90%	100%	
				(at 1 year)		
Corson et al (37)	1999	1. Vesta™ ablation	150	31.8%	Not determined	Not determined
		2. TCRE + rollerball	126	39.6%		
				(at 1 year)		
Cooper et al (24, 41)	1999a,b	1. Microwave ablation	129	40%	77%	0%
		2. TCRE	134	40%	75%	0%
				(at 1 year)	(at 1 year)	(at 1 year)

(2.1% and 2.7% vs 6.4%). This difference in complication rates was not found, however, in either the Scottish audit of 978 cases (Ref. 12 [3]) or a randomised trial of 372 women comparing ELA with TCRE (Ref. 13 [1[+]]).

Endometrial laser ablation

Only two RCTs have compared ELA and TCRE (Refs 13, 14 [1[+ +]]). One trial, after 1-year follow-up, reported no clear differences in operative complications (23% vs 19.5%), satisfaction rates (90.3% vs 89%) or need for further treatment (20% vs 16%) although re-treatment in women undergoing laser ablation was more likely to be repeat ablation compared to hysterectomy in women undergoing TCRE.[13] There were also no significant differences in recovery time or symptom relief. However, the procedure of TCRE was faster (difference of 9 min) and cheaper (difference of £167 per procedure) in the short term than ELA.

An earlier RCT also compared laser ablation with TCRE in subgroups. Satisfaction and complication rates, improvement in menstrual symptoms, operating time, recovery time, need for further surgery and change in quality of life were not significantly different between groups but the trial was insufficiently powered to produce meaningful results for these comparisons.[15]

Uncontrolled case series of TCRE and laser ablation have reported long-term results (Refs 15 [3]; 16 [3]). In the former study, the hysterectomy rate in 525 women undergoing TCRE with a mean follow-up of 31 months was only 9% and 80% avoided further surgery.[15] In the Phillips series, 746 women were monitored for up to 6 years and the rate of repeat surgery was 15% with a predicted hysterectomy rate of 21% at 6.5 years.[16] Results from these studies must be viewed with caution because of the lack of randomisation, incomplete follow-up and potential for bias. There is some evidence of bias as the need for further surgery was lower than that reported by the randomised trials of the procedure.

Rollerball ablation

Women undergoing rollerball ablation in a randomised trial comparing GnRHa with danazol as pre-treatment regimens (Ref. 17 [1[+]]) were followed up 5–6 years after their surgery to assess the long-term outcome of reduction in menstrual blood loss (Ref. 18 [1[+]]). High levels of amenorrhoea (50% and 42% respectively) and a significant reduction of menstrual bleeding from baseline persisted in a proportion of the original study group (some women had become post-menopausal and had hysterectomies). The authors concluded that, with careful preselection of menorrhagic women, rollerball ablation has excellent long-term outcomes.

Vaporising electrode

Endometrial ablation using a cylindrical vaporising electrode has been compared with TCRE (Ref. 19 [1[+ +]]). One operator performed all procedures without intra-operative complications but, although no fluid overload was detected, distension fluid deficit was significantly higher in the women undergoing TCRE. Operating time was only slightly faster in the vaporisation group (difference 1.5 min). There was an appreciable between-group difference in the percentage of women with no or minimal operating difficulties (91% in the vaporisation group and 70% in the TCRE group, $p < 0.014$, OR = 4.5). Experimental studies have concluded that the vaporising electrode is a safe, rapid and easy method of ablation that allows treatment of submucous fibroids (Refs 20 [3]; 21 [3]).

Summary

The hysteroscopic endometrial ablation methods have been compared in randomised comparisons and generally have similar efficacy and safety profiles. Garry concluded that 'endometrial ablation is now one of the most carefully evaluated of surgical procedures'[5] but these first-generation techniques may cause operative complications, they require a degree of surgical skill and are limited to women who have completed their families.

Hysteroscopic endometrial ablative techniques versus medical treatment

TCRE has also been compared with medical therapies for menorrhagia. In practice, many clinicians feel that a trial of medical treatment is appropriate in women with menorrhagia before attempting surgery of any kind.[22] After pre-operative endometrial thinning, TCRE was compared with medical treatment in terms of clinical status and quality of life after 4 months and 2 years (Refs 23 [1+]; 24 [1+]). Women were randomly allocated to either TCRE or medical treatment but choice of medical treatment was determined by the gynaecologist and so the outcomes could only be validly compared between TCRE and medical treatment as a whole. Some types of medical therapy may have been more effective or acceptable than others but the trial design was not appropriate for drawing these types of conclusions. At 4 months, women allocated to TCRE were more likely to be totally or generally satisfied (76% vs 27%), to find the treatment acceptable (93% vs 36%) and willing to have the treatment again (93% vs 31%). Significant differences between the two groups persisted at 2 years although the differences had narrowed. Women undergoing TCRE were more likely to be totally or generally satisfied (79% vs 57%), to find the treatment acceptable (93% vs 77%) and willing to recommend the treatment (78% vs 24%). There was extensive re-treatment in both randomised arms. Of women in the medical treatment group, 59% had undergone TCRE, hysterectomy or both and 17% in the TCRE group had undergone further surgery. It is probably not valid to draw the conclusion that TCRE was more successful than medical treatment as a whole because the medical treatment assigned was not randomised and so direct comparisons with a particular type of drug were not possible. However, there is also a suggestion from this trial that women failing medical treatment and undergoing a successful TCRE are less satisfied (as measured by change in quality of life scores) than those randomly allocated to initial TCRE. If true, this would have implications for the current practice of an initial trial of medical therapy for women with menorrhagia before considering surgery.

The levonorgestrel-releasing intrauterine system (LNG-IUS) has recently been shown to be an effective medical therapy for menorrhagia (Ref. 25 [1+]). This medical treatment has been compared to TCRE in two RCTs (Refs 26 [1++]; 27 [1+] 28 and has also been considered as an alternative to hysterectomy (Ref. 28 [1+]).

The LNG-IUS was compared to TCRE in 70 women in specialised medical centres in Italy in terms of reduction of monthly bleeding, satisfaction rates and health-related quality of life.[29] Both treatments were highly effective in reducing menstrual blood loss at 1 year of follow-up (in the lower range of normal) although scores were significantly lower for women in the TCRE group. There were no significant differences in degree of satisfaction and health-related quality of life perception but the power of the study was not sufficient to detect differences for these outcomes. Side effects were more likely in women in the LNG-IUS group.

Another RCT compared TCRE with the LNG-IUS in 60 women with a follow-up extending to 2 years.[27] The following outcomes were assessed: Pictorial Blood Loss Assessment Chart (PBAC) score at 12 months, treatment success measured as PBAC score <75 at 2 years (failure was a premature surgical intervention for TCRE or second expulsion for LNG-IUS or, in both groups, withdrawal because of an adverse event related to treatment). By 12 months, the PBAC score was significantly reduced from baseline in both groups but significantly less bleeding was achieved in the TCRE group (median PBAC score of 17 in the LNG-IUS group and 0.5 in the TCRE group, $p = 0.02$). Moreover, treatment success was more likely in the TCRE group (93% vs 67%, $p = 0.012$). The PBAC score, however, may not be an accurate outcome measure for evaluating menstrual blood loss. Although this score has been used in a number of trials, a recent prospective study was unable to validate this measure (Ref. 30 [3]).

In the Kittelsen trial, adverse events occurred in both groups. Six women in the LNG-IUS group discontinued treatment because of irregular bleeding or continuous spotting, abdominal pain or expulsion of the device. In the TCRE group, four women underwent repeated resection during the follow-up period of 24 months and another two women had menopausal symptoms during follow-up so success of the procedure could not adequately be assessed.

In summary, there is some evidence that TCRE is more effective than LNG-IUS in reducing HMB. This conclusion needs to be confirmed by additional studies but a RCT in the UK comparing the LNG-IUS with TCRE (SMART Study) has recently been abandoned because of recruitment difficulties. No evidence was identified where endometrial ablation was compared to any other medical therapy.

Second-generation endometrial ablative techniques

To reduce the technical skill required to perform endometrial ablation with direct visualisation by hysteroscope and to minimise the invasiveness of the procedures, several second-generation techniques are currently under investigation. There are a variety of methods, most of which do not require visualisation of the cavity. Their rationale is a reduction in the risk of complications by avoiding the need for uterine distension with fluid, a decrease in the rate of uterine perforation because the instrumentation remains stationary and a lower requirement for surgical prowess. Most of these are still experimental although RCTs have evaluated the thermal balloon and microwave methods.

Balloon devices

The thermal transfer balloon methods rely on a combination of heating and pressure within the uterine cavity to achieve destruction of the endometrium and the superficial myometrium. The two products that are being actively used are Cavaterm™ (Wallsten Medical, Morges, Switzerland) and ThermaChoice™ (Gynecare Products Division, Ethicon, Inc., Menlo Park, CA).

ThermaChoice™ was compared with rollerball in a randomised study of 255 women with regular uterine cavities of <30 ml (Ref. 31 [1^{++}]). Treatment time was longer with rollerball but 27% of the women became amenorrhoeic compared with 15% of the women undergoing ThermaChoice™ ablation. Menstrual blood flow was significantly reduced from baseline in both methods. Over 80% of women in both groups had their menstrual blood loss reduced to normal bleeding or less, defined as PBAC < 100 (80.2% balloon and 83.4% rollerball ablation). Intra-operative complications occurred in 3.2% of hysteroscopic rollerball patients but there were no complications in the ThermaChoice™ group. Post-operatively, there was a minor complication rate of 2.4% for rollerball and 2.9% for balloon therapy. Twelve centres were used in this study so the quality of hysteroscopic surgery may not have been constant and no pre-operative thinning was used. Satisfaction rates in both groups were high (85.6% of women were highly satisfied with the balloon procedure compared to 86.7% of women having rollerball).

This study was followed up 12 months later by an uncontrolled study of 296 women (Ref. 32 [3]). Mean cavity length in the study was 8.5 cm and women with fibroids or other irregular uterine cavities were excluded. The amenorrhoea rate (15%) was similar to that reported in the above RCT and a further 17% had spotting. The success of the procedure, defined as a reduction in blood flow from menorrhagia to eumenorrhoea or less, ranged from 88% to 91% over the year's follow-up, although 10% requested subsequent

surgery. The balloon method was simple to use. Thirty-nine per cent of the women were treated under local anaesthesia and the time to complete the procedure was <30 min in 71% of the women. There was an overall minor complication rate of 3% (cystitis, low grade endometritis and haematometra).

A non-randomised prospective study in France compared the ThermaChoice system with hysteroscopic TCRE (Ref. 33 [2^{+}]). Mean operative time for women having balloon ablation was half that required for TCRE (20 min vs 45 min, $p < 0.05$) but the postoperative bleeding pattern was similar in the two groups, apart from higher rates of eumenorrhoea in the balloon ablation group (38% vs 14%, $p = 0.0006$). Failure rates related to bleeding were similar (15.1% vs 17.6%). There were no intra-operative complications in either group and minimal post-operative complications. Failure of treatment was associated with age <43 years in the TCRE group and retroverted uterus in the balloon ablation group. Overall, success rates of both procedures were consistently similar up to 3 years after treatment.

The ThermaChoice™ system is also being compared with LNG-IUS in an ongoing RCT in New Zealand. Results will not be known until about mid-2001.

The Cavaterm™ balloon device has not been so thoroughly investigated. A small German RCT with 20 women compared the Cavaterm™ method with rollerball after endometrial thinning with GnRHa (Ref. 34 [1^{-}]). Identical results were reported for both groups (amenorrhoea and hypomenorrhoea, 90%) and all women were satisfied with the treatment after a follow-up of 9–15 months. A small prospective uncontrolled pilot study of 50 women with a limited follow-up period assessed efficacy and safety of the Cavaterm™ method and reported a low complication rate (two women required antibiotics for suspected endometritis) and a high rate of amenorrhoea (68%) (Ref. 35 [3]). The authors of this study are currently conducting an RCT of Cavaterm™ versus hysteroscopic laser ablation.

Balloon ablation is not suitable for all women with HMB. All of the above studies required that women have no obvious uterine cavity structural abnormalities and women were thoroughly sampled to exclude unresolved hyperplasia or cancer. This requirement could prevent use of the system in up to 30% of women who can be treated by hysteroscopic methods (Ref. 12 [3]). In the Amso study, improved results were associated with smaller uterine cavities and higher balloon pressures. Balloon-based technologies also have the theoretical disadvantage that not all parts of the uterine cavity will be equally treated. Also, increasing the treat-ment time from 8 to 12–16 min has been demonstrated not to increase the efficacy (Ref. 36 [2$^+$]).

Electrical devices

The VestaDUB is a monopolar electrical device with 12 electrodes attached to a balloon. The balloon acts as a mechanism to get the electrodes into contact with the endometrium. A multi-centre, RCT of the Vesta™ system versus TCRE and rollerball is currently under-way in the US and some interim results have been reported (Ref. 37 [1$^+$]). Thirty-eight per cent of poten-tial participants were excluded from the trial because of uterine pathology in the form of myoma or polyps. All randomised women ($n = 276$) had 2 weeks of pre-operative treatment with oral contraceptive pills. After 12 months, the average PBAC score reduction was 94% in the Vesta™ group and 91% in the resection and rollerball group. Similar amenorrhoea scores were reported for both groups, 32% and 40% respectively. Success, as defined by a PBAC score <76 was achieved in 88% and 83% respectively. Comparisons were also made between the Vesta group and data from registra-tion studies on ThermaChoice™ presented to the FDA in the US. Although these results represent a lower grade of evidence since there was no randomisation for the ThermaChoice™ group, the Vesta™ system had a greater mean per cent decrease in PBAC score (93% vs 85.5%, $p = 0.001$) and a significantly greater percent-age of women in this group had amenorrhoea (33.3% vs 13.2%, $p < 0.001$).

A second-generation bipolar electrical device, Novacept™, is still experimental but a large, randomised multi-centre study comparing Novacept™ to roller-ball is currently underway in the US.

Microwave endometrial ablation

Microwave endometrial ablation (MEA™) uses an 8 mm diameter probe emitting microwaves with a fre-quency of 9.2 GHz that restricts penetration to a max-imum of 6 mm. In a pilot study, Sharp demonstrated that the average treatment time was 2 min 12 s and 83% of women were satisfied 6 months after treatment (Ref. 38 [3]). Results from an experimental non-randomised trial of 43 women undergoing micro-wave ablation between 1994 and 1995 with 3 years of follow-up showed that the technique was simple to learn and perform and women reported high rates of satisfaction (Ref. 39 [3]). Three women had re-treatment

with the same procedure and four women had hys-terectomies. A satisfaction rate of 87.5% at 1 year and a failure rate of 12.5% (2/16) were reported in another small prospective study (Ref. 40 [3]).

A RCT comparing MEA™ to TCRE was recently undertaken in Aberdeen in 263 women (Ref. 41 [1^{++}]). Entry criteria were less exclusive than for balloon therapy; uterine size was restricted to the size of a 10-week pregnancy but no exclusion was made for fibroids or irregular uterine cavities. Pre-operative endometrial thinning was undertaken. MEA™ was faster than TCRE with an operation time of 11 min (15 min with TCRE, $p = 0.001$) and with fewer complications. The amenorrhoea rate was identical in both groups at 40% with hypomenorrhoea in a further 50% in each group. The primary outcome of the study was patient satisfaction and rates were high for both procedures (at 12 months, 77% of women in the microwave group and 75% of women in the TCRE group were totally or generally satisfied with their treatment). Acceptability of treatment rates was over 90% for both techniques and quality of life was also improved. Intra-operative difficulties were minimal although equipment failure was significantly more likely in the microwave group. Haemorrhage occurred in five women undergoing TCRE but none in the microwave group.

As with many other second-generation techniques, an advantage of the microwave technique is that up to 85% of procedures can be performed under local anaesthetic (D. Parkin, personal communication). Another RCT is currently in progress at the same cen-tre comparing microwave endometrial ablation under local anaesthetic with the same technique under gen-eral anaesthetic in order to assess the true acceptability of local anaesthetic treatment.

Radiofrequency electromagnetic energy

Ablation with radiofrequency electromagnetic energy using an intrauterine probe was first described in 1990 (Ref. 42 [3]). Treatment appears to be fast, simple and effective but there are concerns about safety. Com-plications such as superficial skin burns and vesico-vaginal fistulae have been reported (Ref. 43 [3]) and cost is high.

Cryoablation

Cryoablation has been reported as a potential treatment for menorrhagia but there is insufficient data to evaluate this method. In one study, 63% of women were completely satisfied with their treatment at 3–18 months follow-up but none were amenorrhoeic and 33% subsequently underwent hysterectomy (Ref. 44 [3]).

Hydro ThermAblator™

Only one of the newer ablative techniques requires the use of a hysteroscope. The Hydro ThermAblator™ circulates low pressure hot saline directly into the uterine cavity under hysteroscopic control (Ref. 45 [3]) but evaluation of this technique has been minimal. Nevertheless, the authors suggest that it may be safer than laser or electrosurgical methods. A potential advantage is the ability to treat women where the size of the uterus is irregular. In an earlier method, the EnAbl™ system, there was a significant risk of escape of heated fluid through the fallopian tubes into the peritoneal cavity causing peritoneal or bowel injuries (Ref. 46 [3]).

Photodynamic therapy

Studies of photodynamic therapy aiming at selective destruction of the endometrium by interactions between light and a photosensitiser have not produced encouraging results (Ref. 47 [3]) and the technique is still experimental.

Laser endometrial ablation

The Nd:YAG laser has also been used non-hysteroscopically to produce interstitial hyperthermia at a temperature of 102°C for 5 min. The ELITT™ method, pioneered by Donnez, does not require direct contact with the endometrium in order to induce coagulation (Ref. 48 [3]). In an unpublished study, 99 women were treated by the ELITT™ system and a high rate of combined amenorrhoea/spotting (91%) was reported at 12 months follow-up. No measures of satisfaction were given and two women were required to undergo subsequent hysterectomy. Few details have been given about this study and clearly RCTs are required before conclusions can be reached about efficacy and safety of this method.

Pre-operative endometrial thinning

Complete endometrial removal is an important determinant of the success of the various endometrial ablation techniques. During the menstrual cycle, the endometrial thickness of the uterus varies from as little as 1 mm in the immediate post-menstrual phase to 10 mm or more in the late secretory phase.[49] Since the available endometrial ablative techniques are most effective if the thickness is <4 mm, surgery is best performed either in the immediate post-menstrual phase or after administration of hormonal agents that are known to induce endometrial thinning or atrophy. There are significant practical difficulties in arranging surgery at the optimum time of the menstrual cycle and, moreover, the thickness of the endometrium varies in individual women. Consequently, the role of hormonal thinning agents prior to endometrial surgery has been investigated.

A Cochrane systematic review reported that endometrial thinning by GnRHa and, to a lesser extent, danazol, prior to hysteroscopic surgery improves both the operating conditions for the surgeon and short-term post-operative outcome (Ref. 50 [1++]). Surgery was significantly shorter (a difference of 5 min) and more easily performed and there was a higher rate of amenorrhoea post-surgery in women pre-treated with GnRHa compared with no treatment (relative risk (RR) 1.7, 95% confidence interval (CI) 1.5–2.1). However, there were no differences in complication rates or women's feelings of satisfaction with the procedure and uncertainty over the long-term effects of this pre-operative treatment. Disadvantages of pretreatment, however, are high cost and side effects; cost effectiveness analysis is needed to include these factors.

Little data was available to assess the role of pre-operative endometrial thinning prior to second-generation ablation. A small RCT with 30 peri-menopausal menorrhagic women assessed the effectiveness and safety of balloon ablation without pre-treatment compared with delayed ablation after pre-treatment with GnRHa (Ref. 51 [1+]). Pre-treatment had no significant effect on the success of ablation or on the rate of complications. Further research is required to clarify the role of pre-treatment prior to ablation.

Discussion

Conclusions about the efficacy, safety and acceptability of the endometrial ablation methods are tenuous until more randomised high quality research is performed. A number of methodological deficiencies need to be addressed:

1. Many of the second-generation endometrial ablation methods do not appear to be so promising.

Uncontrolled series of these methods report good results in terms of reduction in menstrual bleeding but no efforts are made to control for bias, follow-up is usually limited and no valid conclusions can be reached based on these studies alone. RCTs are needed for rigorous evaluation.

2. Decisions must be made about meaningful and valid outcome measures. Donnez claims that it is sensible to consider amenorrhoea as a reliable and uniform early indicator of the success of a procedure because its definition is clear and objective — no bleeding. Others suggest that amenorrhoea need not be an end point. Liu suggests that peri-menopausal women like to experience less menstrual flow but still appreciate a regular bleed to re-affirm that they are not at the end of their menstrual life. In a survey of women who had undergone endometrial ablation, amenorrhoea did not seem to be a critical therapeutic endpoint. Moreover, many of the RCTs evaluating treatments measure menstrual blood loss prior to and after treatment to assess efficacy but objective reduction in menstrual blood loss does not necessarily correlate with the woman's perception of the clinical effectiveness of the treatment administered. Thus, satisfaction with and acceptability of the treatment are more important measures indicating success.

3. Another problem is the use of simple proportions to estimate the rates of outcome measures such as subsequent hysterectomy, satisfaction and amenorrhoea. Since these outcomes are time dependent, the use of simple proportions is likely to underestimate the true event rates. Survival analyses for hysterectomy rates but not satisfaction or amenorrhoea rates would overcome this limitation.

4. Generalisability of the current research is compromised by the use of a selective study population. Many of the women who enter trials are recruited from gynaecological outpatient clinics after failure with medical treatment for their HMB administered by their general practitioners at an earlier time. Chien suggests that bias is produced when the study population has already been exposed to an intervention which may have altered the natural history of the disease. It is also important to undertake 'pragmatic' controlled trials where entry is based on a subjective complaint of unacceptable menstrual loss to increase general applicability of the results.

In spite of these methodological concerns, there is good evidence that hysteroscopic endometrial ablation offers an alternative to hysterectomy for menorrhagia. As newer less invasive methods of hysterectomy (e.g.

vaginal hysterectomy) become more widely used this conclusion may need to be re-evaluated. There has not, however, been a consequent reduction in the numbers of hysterectomies performed. Coulter has suggested that this may be because there is a lower threshold for minimal access surgery and these procedures are also being employed as an alternative to medical therapy although this suggestion has not been confirmed.

Second-generation ablative methods clearly need more extensive and rigorous evaluation with well-powered RCTs before confident conclusions may be reached about their effectiveness, safety and acceptability when compared with the more traditional methods of hysteroscopic ablation. The balloon methods look promising but they cannot be used in all women with menorrhagia. The microwave method is less restrictive but its use still needs careful and long-term evaluation.

Whilst it is clear that only a small proportion of gynaecologists will be adequately trained to perform first-generation endometrial ablation procedures, the lower level of surgical skill required to perform the second-generation procedures should, in time, permit these to be offered to most women with HMB. The first-generation techniques, however, are likely to retain their place for women who have, for example, submucous fibroids or endometrial polyps. For this reason, pre-operative hysteroscopy or ultrasound assessment of the endometrial cavity would seem advisable even though the evaluation of the necessity of the assessment is yet to be reported.

The choice of treatment will ultimately be driven by consumer demand. Women's perception of their menstrual loss is highly subjective and many women with menstrual blood loss within the normal range feel that their quality of life is reduced to such an extent that they will undergo inconvenient medical therapy or highly invasive surgery. In fact, only one in seven women will refuse surgery even if they are shown to have a menstrual blood loss within the normal menstrual range. The IPMEN study, a multi-centre RCT to assess the costs and benefits of using structured information and analysis of the preferences of women with menorrhagia, is currently in progress. It should make clear how the provision of information impacts on decision-making. Initial results suggest that shared decision-making affects the strength of women's preferences for the treatment they would or would not choose but may not alter the decision made.

Ultimately, the role and responsibility of clinicians is to provide an informed effective framework of options based on carefully graded evidence for women with menorrhagia. Treatment choice must be based on evidence. This evidence is still being gathered but it is entirely possible, that some time in the future, endometrial ablative surgery may become a first option in menorrhagic women who no longer wish to be fertile.

References

1. Weber AM, Walters MD, Schover LR, Church JM, Piedmonte MR. Functional outcomes and satisfaction after abdominal hysterectomy. *Am J Obstet Gynecol* 1999; 181: 530–535.

2. Dicker RC, Greenspan JR, Strauss LT et al. Complications of abdominal and vaginal hysterectomy among women of reproductive age in the United States. *Am J Obstet Gynecol* 1982; 144: 841–848.

3. Clarke A, Black N, Rowe P, Mott S, Howle K. Indications for and outcome of total abdominal hysterectomy for benign disease: a prospective cohort study. *Br J Obstet Gynaecol* 1995; 102: 611–620.

4. Van den Eeden SK, Glasser M, Mathias SD, Colwell HH, Pasta DJ, Kunz K. Quality of life, health care utilisation and costs among women undergoing hysterectomy in a managed care setting. *Am J Obstet Gynecol* 1998; 178: 91–100.

5. Garry R. Endometrial ablation and resection: validation of a new surgical concept. *Br J Obstet Gynaecol* 1997; 104: 1329–1331.

6. Magos A. Management of menorrhagia: hysteroscopic techniques offer a revolution in treatment. *Br Med J* 1990; 300: 1537–1538.

7. Bridgman SA, Dunn KM. Has endometrial ablation replaced hysterectomy for the treatment of dysfunctional uterine bleeding? National figures. *Br J Obstet Gynecol* 2000; 107: 531–534.

8. Aberdeen Endometrial Ablation Trials Group. A randomised trial of endometrial ablation versus hysterectomy for the treatment of dysfunctional uterine bleeding: outcome at four years. *Br J Obstet Gynecol* 1999; 106: 360–366.

9. Scottish Intercollegiate Guidelines Network. *Grading System for Recommendations in Evidence-Based Clinical Guidelines*, March 2000.

10. Lethaby AE, Shepperd S, Cooke I, Farquhar C. *Endometrial Resection and Ablation Versus Hysterectomy for Heavy Menstrual Bleeding (Cochrane Review)*. The Cochrane Library, Issue 2, 2000. Oxford: Update Software.

11. Overton C, Hargreaves J, Maresh M. A national survey of the complications of endometrial destruction for menstrual disorders: the Mistletoe study. *Br J Obstet Gynaecol* 1997; 104: 1351–1359.

12. Scottish Hysteroscopy Audit Group. A Scottish audit of hysteroscopic surgery for menorrhagia: complications and follow up. *Br J Obstet Gynaecol* 1995; 102: 249–254.

13. Bhattacharya S, Cameron IM, Parkin DE. A pragmatic randomised comparison of transcervical resection of the endometrium with endometrial laser ablation for the treatment of menorrhagia. *Br J Obstet Gynaecol* 1997; 104: 601–607.

14. Pinion SB, Parkin DE, Abramovich DR, Naji A, Alexander DA, Russell IT, Kitchener HC. Randomised trial of hysterectomy, endometrial laser ablation and transcervical endometrial resection for dysfunctional uterine bleeding. *Br Med J* 1994; 309: 979–983.

15. O'Connor H, Magos A. Endometrial resection for the treatment of menorrhagia. *New Eng J Med* 1996; 335(3): 151–156.

16. Phillips G, Chien PF, Garry R. Risk of hysterectomy after 1000 consecutive endometrial laser ablations. *Br J Obstet Gynaecol* 1998; 105: 897–903.

17. Fraser IS, Healy DI, Torode H, Song JY, Mamers P, Wilde F. Dept Goserelin and danazol pre-treatment before rollerball endometrial ablation for menorrhagia. *Obstet Gynecol* 1996; 87: 544–550.

18. Teirney R, Arachchi G, Fraser IS. Menstrual blood loss measured 5–6 years after endometrial ablation. *Obstet Gynecol* 2000; 95: 251–254.

19. Vercellini P, Oldani S, Yaylayan L et al. Randomised comparison of vaporizing electrode and cutting loop for endometrial ablation. *Obstet Gynecol* 1999; 94: 521–527.

20. Vercellini P, Oldani S, de Giorgi O et al. Endometrial ablation with a vaporizing electrode. II. Clinical outcome of a pilot study. *Acta Obstet Gynecol Scand* 1998; 77: 688–693.

21. Brooks PG. Resectoscopic myoma vaporizer. *J Reprod Med* 1995; 40: 791–795.

22. Macdonald R. Modern treatment of menorrhagia. *Br J Obstet Gynaecol* 1990; 97: 3–7.

23. Cooper KG, Parkin DE, Garratt AM et al. A randomised comparison of medical and hysteroscopic management in women consulting a gynaecologist for treatment of heavy menstrual loss. *Br J Obstet Gynaecol* 1997; 104: 1360–1366.

24. Cooper KG, Parkin DE, Garratt AM et al. Two-year follow up of women randomised to medical management or transcervical resection of the endometrium for heavy menstrual loss: clinical and quality of life outcomes. *Br J Obstet Gynaecol* 1999a; 106: 258–265.

25. Irvine GA, Campbell-Brown MB, Lumsden MA, Heikkila A, Walker JJ, Cameron IT. Randomised comparative trial of the levonorgestrel intrauterine system and norethisterone for treatment of idiopathic menorrhagia. *Br J Obstet Gynaecol* 1998; 105: 592–598.

26. Crosignani PG, Vercellini P, Apolone G, de Giorgi O, Cortesi I, Meschia M. Endometrial resection versus vaginal hysterectomy for menorrhagia: long-term clinical and quality-of-life outcomes. *Am J Obstet Gynecol* 1997b; 177: 95–101.

27. Kittelsen N, Istre O. A randomized study comparing levonorgestrel intrauterine system (LNG IUS) and transcervical resection of the endometrium (TCRE) in the treatment of menorrhagia: preliminary results. *Gynaceol Endosc* 1998; 7: 61–65.

28. Lahteenmaki P, Haukkamaa M, Puolakka J, Riikonen U, Sainio S, Suvisaari J, Nilsson CG. Open randomised study of use of levonorgestrel releasing intrauterine system as alternative to hysterectomy. *Moth Baby J* 1998; 316: 1122–1126.

29. Crosignani PG, Vercellini P, Mosconi P et al. Levonorgestrel-releasing intrauterine device versus hysteroscopic endometrial resection in the treatment of dysfunctional uterine bleeding. *Obstet Gynecol* 1997a; 90: 257–263.

30. Reid PC, Coker A, Coltart R. Assessment of menstrual blood loss using a pictorial chart: a validation study. *Br J Obstet Gynaecol* 2000; 107: 320–322.

31. Meyer WR, Walsh BW, Grainger DA et al. Thermal balloon and rollerball ablation to treat menorrhagia: a multi-centre comparison. *Obstet Gynecol* 1998; 92: 98–103.

32. Amso NR, Strabinsky SA, McFaul P, Blanc B, Pendley L, Neuwirth R. Uterine thermal balloon therapy for the treatment of menorrhagia: the first 300 patients from a multi-centre study. *Br J Obstet Gynaecol* 1998; 105: 517–523.

33. Gervaise A, Fernandez H, Capella-Allouc S et al. Thermal balloon ablation versus endometrial resection for the treatment of abnormal uterine bleeding. *Hum Reprod* 1999; 14 (11): 2743–2747.

34. Romer T. Die therapie rezidivierender menorrhagien — Cavaterm-ballon-koagulation versus Roller-ball-endometriumkoagulation — eine prospecktive randomisierte Vergleichsstudie [The treatment of recurrent menorrhagias — Caveterm™-balloon-coagulation versus Roller-ball-endometrial ablation — a prospective randomised comparative study]. *Zentralbl Gynakol* 1998; 120: 511–514.

35. Hawe JA, Phillips AG, Chien PF, Erian J, Garry R. Cavaterm thermal balloon ablation for the treatment of menorrhagia. *Br J Obstet Gynaecol* 1999; 106: 1143–1148.

36. Bongers MY, Mol BWJ, Brolmann HAM. Comparison of 8 versus 16 minutes heating in the treatment of menorrhagia with hot fluid balloon ablation. *J Gynaecol Surg* 1999; 15: 143–148.

37. Corson SL, Brill AI, Brooks PG et al. Interim results of the American Vesta trial of endometrial ablation. *J Am Assoc Gynecol Laparosc* 1999; 6(1): 45–49.

38. Sharp N, Cronin N, Feldberg I, Evans M, Hodgson D, Ellis S. Microwaves for menorrhagia: a new and fast technique for endometrial ablation. *Lancet* 1995; 346: 1003–1004.

39. Hodgson DA, Feldberg IB, Sharp N et al. Microwave endometrial ablation: development, clinical trials and outcomes at three years. *Br J Obstet Gynaecol* 1999; 106: 684–694.

40. Milligan MP, Etokowo GA. Microwave endometrial ablation for menorrhagia. *J Obstet Gynaecol* 1999; 19(5): 496–499.

41. Cooper KG, Bain C, Parkin DE. Comparison of microwave endometrial ablation and transcervical resection of the endometrium for treatment of heavy menstrual loss: a randomised trial. *Lancet* 1999b; 354: 1859–1863.

42. Phipps JH, Lewis BV, Roberts T et al. Treatment of functional menorrhagia by radiofrequency induced thermal endometrial ablation. *Lancet* 1990; 335: 374–375.

43. Thijssen RFA. Radiofrequency induced endometrial ablation: an update. *Br J Obstet Gynaecol* 1997; 104: 608–613.

44. Pittrof R, Majid S, Murray A. Transcervical endometrial cryoablation (ECA) for menorrhagia. *Int J Gynaecol Obstet* 1994; 47: 135–140.

45. das Dores GB, Richart RM, Nicolau SM, Focchi GR, Cardeiro VC. *J Am Assoc Gynecol Laparosc* 1999; 6(3): 275–278.

46. Richart RM, Dores GB, Nicolau SM et al. Histologic studies of the effects of circulating hot saline on the uterus before hysterectomy. *J Am Assoc Gynecol Laparosc* 1999; 6(3): 269–273.

47. Gannon MJ, Johnson N, Roberts JH et al. Photosensitization of the endometrium with topical 5-aminolevulenic acid. *Am J Obstet Gynecol* 1995; 173: 1826–1828.

48. Donnez J, Polet R, Mathieu P-E, Konwitz E, Nisolle M, Casanas-Roux F. Endometrial laster interstitial hyperthermy: a potential modality for endometrial ablation. *Obstet Gynecol* 1996; 87(3): 459–464.

49. Weingold AB. Gross and microscopic anatomy. In: NG Kose, AB Weingold, PM Gershenson (Eds) *Principles and Practice of Clinical Gynaecology*, pp 3–32, 1990. New York: Churchill Livingstone.

50. Sowter MC, Singla AA, Lethaby A. *Pre-operative Endometrial Thinning Agents before Hysteroscopic Surgery for Heavy Menstrual Bleeding (Cochrane Review)*. The Cochrane Library, Issue 2, 2000. Oxford: Update Software.

51. Lissak A, Fruchter O, Mashiach S, Brandes-Klein O, Sharon A, Kogan O, Abramovici H. Immediate versus delayed treatment of preimenopausal bleeding due to benign causes by balloon thermal ablation. *J Am Assoc Gynecol Laparosc* 1999; 6(2): 145–150.

52. O'Connor H, Broadbent JAM, Magos AL, McPherson K. Medical Research Council randomised trial of endometrial resection versus hysterectomy in management of menorrhagia. *Lancet* 1997; 349: 897–901.

53. Gannon MJ, Holt EM, Fairbank J, Fitzgerald M, Milne MA, Crystal AM, Greenhalf JO. A randomised trial comparing endometrial resection and abdominal hysterectomy for the treatment of menorrhagia. *Br Med J* 1991; 303: 1362–1364.

54. Dwyer N, Hutton J, Stirrat GM. Randomised controlled trial comparing endometrial resection with abdominal hysterectomy for the surgical treatment of menorrhagia. *Br J Obstet Gynaecol* 1993; 100: 237–243.

6

Classifying endometrial ablation techniques

Claude A. Fortin

Introduction

Endometrial ablation is now a mature recognised and accepted alternative to hysterectomy for the treatment of abnormal uterine bleeding. Introduction of operative hysteroscopy has offered the long awaited solution to the destruction of the endometrium. Hysteroscopic electrosurgical and laser ablation techniques are achieving high satisfaction rates. Being skill dependant with a steep learning curve, these procedures have not challenged enough hysterectomy. Therefore starting in the mid-90s, different ablative devices from various energy sources were designed. After revision of the ideal for endometrial ablation we shall try to classify them.

Endometrial ablation ideal

1. Effective
   - Completely destroy the basal layer
   - Predictable results
2. Short procedure
3. Easy to perform
   - Negligible learning curve
4. Safe
   - Rare complications
5. Reduced post-operative recovery
6. Suitable for office setting or out patient
7. Well tolerated
8. High satisfaction rate
9. Cost effective
   - Treat majority of patients

Terminology for endometrial ablation

- 1st Generation: iterative hysteroscopic
- 2nd Generation: blind global
- 3rd Generation: pseudovisual

1st Generation: iterative hysteroscopic surgery (Laser, TCRE and Rollerball)

Advantages	Disadvantages
Less invasive procedure	Steep learning curve
Reduced anaesthesia time	Limited to GA

Less complications	Patient safety concerns
Quicker recovery	Fluid overload
Treats irregular cavities	Perforation
Cost effective	Gas embolism
High satisfaction	Haemorrhage

2nd Generation: blind global treatment systems

- Balloon technology
- Radio frequency
- Cryotherapy
- Interstitial laser

Advantages	Disadvantages
Addresses patient safety	Treats mostly normal cavities
No distension fluids	Cavity size limitations
Reduced risk of perforation	Deployment problems
Negligible learning curve	Post-operative cramping
Easy and usually fast	Lack of long-term studies
Effective	
High satisfaction	

3rd Generation: visual and pseudovisual

- Circulating hot saline
- Microwave ablation

Advantages	Disadvantages
Treats irregular cavities and fibroids	Histology absent
Reduced learning curve	Cramping issues
Rare cavity size limitations	
Effective and safe	
Iterative	

Conclusion

From various energy modes to different devices, new endometrial ablation techniques are evolving towards continuous improvement in order to reduce hysterectomy rates for benign uterine disorders.

This simple classification should provide adequate information for the gynaecologist to make an informed choice in his (her) treatment options.

7

Hysteroscopic endometrial laser ablation technique

David Hunter

Introduction

Surgical ablation of the endometrium was not a new concept when Goldrath described laser photovaporisation of the endometrium in 1981.[1] In 1882 Tilt had attempted endometrial ablation using a solution of silver nitrate to destroy 'that diseased cavity' with disastrous results.[2] Following this aborted attempt at treatment of menstrual dysfunction, others used steam under pressure, various combinations of chemicals and cryotherapy in order to induce amenorrhoea but none of the methods became accepted because of the serious side effects of the treatments.[3,4]

The introduction of the hysteroscope, first by Pantaleoni in the 1860s and then popularisation of the use of the hysteroscope as a diagnostic tool in the 1960s and 70s[5,6] revolutionised the investigation of abnormal uterine bleeding and allowed for directed therapeutic, as well as diagnostic, procedures to be performed as opposed to the blind treatments which, up until that time, had been all that was available. The first description of intra-uterine surgical intervention under vision was that of Neuwirth and Amin when they resected submucous fibroids using a modified urologists' resectoscope and diathermy loop in 1973.[7]

Lasers had been used for a number of other medical indications outside gynaecological practice (mainly in the field of ophthalmology). However, it was 1981 before Goldrath published on the potential for destruction of the endometrium using this energy source[1] and the concept of endometrial laser ablation was born.

Laser is an acronym for **l**ight **a**mplification by the **s**timulated **e**mission of **r**adiation, which describes how the energy is derived. An electron is encouraged to leave its orbit around an atom by the application of an electrical voltage differential. When the electron returns to its orbit the atom releases a photon packet of energy. These photon packets are collimated (all of the light waves are in phase and synchronous) and the laser light is produced in a parallel non-divergent beam. This may be in the visible or non-visible spectrum depending on the wavelength of the light produced. The wavelength is dependent upon the material from which the laser light is produced. For instance, the neodymium: yttrium–aluminium–garnett (Nd:YAG) laser wavelength is 1060 nm and for carbon dioxide is 10,600 nm. The wavelength determines the characteristics of the laser, e.g. the mode of transmission (flexible fibre for Nd:YAG and KTP, rigid arms with mirrors and coupling devices for CO_2) and the tissue effects. It is these characteristics that make laser so useful.

Each wavelength of light produced has specific properties and therefore different effects. When using the light produced by the Nd:YAG laser, 25–30% of the inherent energy scatter is forward, 30–40% is reflected and only 30–45% of the energy is absorbed by the tissue being treated.[8] Considering all wavelengths of light energy, this is a relatively high proportion of forward scatter allowing for a controlled depth of thermal injury (glandular structures within the myometrium, up to 4 mm, are reliably destroyed by the delivery of Nd:YAG laser energy). It is this controlled depth of thermal injury which contributes to the low perforation rate and the excellent safety record of endometrial laser ablation. The carbon dioxide laser, on the other hand, has more lateral spread of energy with a lower proportion of forward scatter and the light is absorbed by water so cannot penetrate the irrigating solution within the uterus (the deep endometrial glandular structures survive). KTP:YAG produces much less depth of thermal injury and is also unsuitable.

Instruments, ancillary devices, safety features and dimensions

The use of a laser in theatre legally requires certain safety features to be used to reduce the risks of injury to theatre personnel and the patient as a result of inadvertent exposure to laser radiation. A laser safety committee is required and only those surgeons and staff authorised to use the laser can do so. Theatre rooms where the laser is in use should be locked or the entrances to the theatre should be clearly marked with 'CAUTION' signs stating that a laser is being used and the windows are blacked out. In particular, there is a risk of damage to the cornea and retina of the surgeon, other operating theatre personnel or patient should the laser be discharged whilst the tip of the laser is outside the uterine cavity or if the transmitting fibre is damaged. In order to avoid damage to the eyes of theatre personnel, the use of protective spectacles or goggles, which are specific to the wavelength of light produced by each of the types of laser used, is mandatory. In addition, the electrical supply to the laser generator requires a specific electrical socket and lead capable of delivering a current of 40 A and voltage of 415 V.

To maintain the clear field of vision under which all of the hysteroscopic techniques for endometrial ablation must be performed, a three channel operating hysteroscope is necessary. Inflow and outflow channels permit

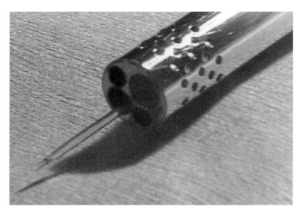

Figure 7.1

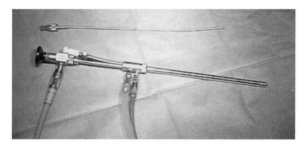

Figure 7.2

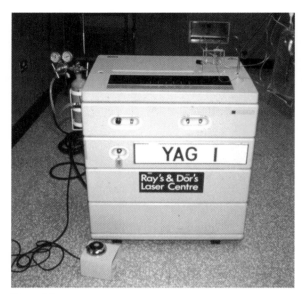

Figure 7.3

Monitoring System, AQUINTEL Inc., Mountainview, CA, USA). The maximum intra-uterine pressure is initially set at 75 mmHg with a flow rate of 250 ml/min. These settings are altered according to the patient's mean arterial pressure, amount of bleeding and the quality of the image obtained. Fluid loss due to spillage is limited by the use of a plastic drape to ensure that as much 'leaked' fluid as possible is returned to the fluid monitoring device. Fluid deficit is calculated automatically (by weight), displayed continuously and recorded at least every 5 min throughout the operative procedure.

One of the advantages of laser ablation is that normal saline can be used as the distension medium. This is an isotonic electrolytic solution which is much safer in overload than hypotonic non-ionic solutions such as glycine, sorbitol and mannitol. Overload with these solutions is effectively a water overload resulting in hyponatraemia and reduced osmolality.

The laser employed in this unit is an Nd:YAG laser (Surgical Laser Technology, Malvern, PA, USA) used in the contact mode with a maximum power output of 80 W. The energy is delivered through a 600 μm bare quartz fibre, Fibre transmission of more than 95% is essential for economic use of the generator and adequate therapeutic effect. The laser generator is bulky and heavy and because of its size is removed from the theatre when not in use (Fig. 7.3).

The entire endometrium is treated under direct vision and general anaesthesia (regional anaesthesia may be

the maintenance of continuous flow of fluid with the evacuation of blood, tissue fragments and gas produced by the vaporisation of tissue. A separate channel is necessary for the delivery of the laser fibre. The typical external diameter of the scope is approximately 8 mm with an operating channel of 5 French gauge although good quality smaller diameter scopes (approximately 5.5 mm) are now becoming available. In Middlesbrough the procedure is performed using a Weck–Baggish operating hysteroscope sheath with a 0° straightforward scope (Weck; ER Squibb and Sons, New York City, New York, USA) under video control (Figs 7.1 and 7.2). A good quality camera and video system such as the Olympus OTV-SX digital signal processing camera system with three chip camera and cold light source (Olympus CLV-S20) are recommended. An inadequate view is dangerous. The cold light source, video and camera equipment are all placed on a single video stack situated to the patient's right side and the surgeon's monitor at the head of the operating table.

Fluid infusion and monitoring with pressure controlled, continuous flow of normal saline is maintained with a WOM hysteroflator (HYS-SURGIMAT) and an Aquasens fluid monitoring system (AquaSens Fluid

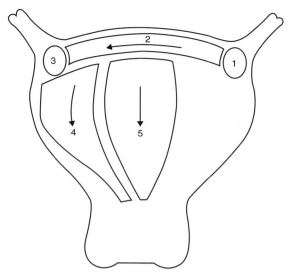

Figure 7.4

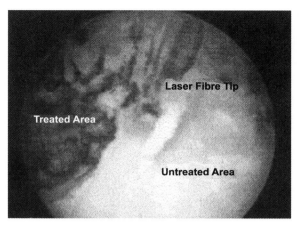

Figure 7.5

used but this would be rather infrequent). The procedure commences with the treatment of the cornua, then the fundus, anterior, lateral and posterior walls in a systematic fashion, ablating towards the internal cervical os but not to within the endocervical canal (ablation of the cervical epithelium results in a high number of cases of haematometra) (Fig. 7.4). Complete obliteration of the cavity will result in a surgically induced Ashermann's syndrome.

Safety features

Although inherently a safe device, if used incorrectly the Nd:YAG laser is capable of producing a burn in any tissue, the depth of which depends on the duration of thermal insult and power output of the generator. The inherent safety features of the laser system are its high proportion of forward scatter of energy and the mechanism by which the laser is discharged or fired (the foot pedal is guarded and once placed at the surgeon's foot can only be depressed by the surgeon when the laser is in operational mode). The safe use of the laser is dependent upon adequate training of all theatre staff responsible for the care of the patient. To reduce the incidence of serious complications there are a number of important basic safety principles that must be followed. The operating surgeon and scrub nurse should:

1. Ensure that the cervix has been dilated without the creation of a false passage either in the endometrium or the myometrium and that uterine perforation

has not occurred. If the uterine cavity cannot be explored without the creation of a false passage, or if the uterus has been perforated, the procedure should be abandoned and the patient asked to return at a subsequent date for a second attempt at cervical dilatation and endometrial ablation or listed for hysterectomy.

2. Never discharge the laser unless the tip of the laser fibre is within the hysteroscopic field of vision.

3. Always keep the tip of the fibre in motion when the laser is being discharged. In particular, the laser should only be discharged when the tip of the fibre is being dragged *towards* the operating surgeon, *never* if the laser fibre is being introduced into the uterine cavity (Fig. 7.5).

4. Treat each area within the uterus once only.

5. Ensure that the laser is on standby mode or that the power has been switched off prior to withdrawing the fibre tip from the uterine cavity and, conversely, only switch the generator to operational mode when the tip of the fibre is within the uterine cavity.

6. Monitor the fluid deficit at least every 5 min throughout the procedure (no matter how rapid or prolonged). If the fluid deficit exceeds 1500 ml, 20 mg frusemide should be administered intravenously and a self retaining urinary catheter inserted to accurately assess urinary output. If the fluid deficit exceeds 2500 ml the procedure should be abandoned, the patient should remain in hospital overnight and be reviewed in the outpatient department to assess the effect of the treatment administered.

As with electrosurgical devices, any laser is a potentially dangerous instrument and should only be used when the surgeon and ancillary staff have been adequately trained in its use.

Practical aspects of treatment

Endometrial preparation

The laser may be used in the contact or non-contact mode. When used in the contact mode the laser is dragged over the endometrium producing a 'furrow' of approximately 1 mm depth with 5 mm of thermal necrosis beyond. Using the non-contact (blanching technique) the fibre does not touch the endometrium and the laser is activated from 2 to 3 mm off the endometrial surface to produce visible blanching. The dragging technique is the more commonly used because it is easier to view the already treated areas during the procedure (i.e. the furrows) but both can safely and reliably induce thermal necrosis to a depth of 4–5 mm. The depth of thermal injury induced by the passage of the laser fibre tip is dependent on the power output of the generator, the transmission of energy to the tip of the fibre, the speed of passage of the tip and the pressure with which the laser is applied to a soft tissue. When the endometrium has been poorly prepared, the required depth of thermal necrosis necessary for therapeutic effect is greater as glandular elements of the basal layer of the endometrium can be up to 16 mm from the endometrial surface. To ensure therapeutic effect in such circumstances each area requires repeated treatments or the power density delivered to each area must increase (by slowing the passage of the tip of the fibre or by increasing the power output of the laser). Any one or combination of these factors will increase the risk of a full thickness burn through the myometrium. For this reason, thin or prepared atrophic endometrium is preferred.

Operating lists timed according to the patient's bleeding episodes presents an extreme administrative challenge which precludes performing ablation timed with the patient's menstrual cycle. Similarly, because mechanical preparation by curettage induces bleeding (which obscures the surgeon's view), radical curettage is not used as a preparatory technique.

Chemical induction of hypo-oestrogenism is the preferred method of endometrial preparation. This is typically achieved using gonadotrophin releasing hormone analogues or danazol. Danazol reliably inhibits follicular maturation and hence induces hypo-oestrogenism

but side effects at therapeutic doses may be severe. A single gonadotrophin releasing hormone analogue implant lasting for 4 weeks will adequately prepare the endometrium and only one-third of women will suffer menopausal side effects. This is undoubtedly more expensive than oral danazol (approximately £60 vs £30) but compliance is ensured and the endometrium is consistently thinned.

Few studies have compared the effect of the various agents used for endometrial preparation specifically prior to ELA, mainly because ELA is performed much less frequently than either TCRE or rollerball ablation. The randomised controlled trial of gonadotrophin releasing hormone analogue (goserelin) against danazol undertaken by Garry addresses this issue.[9] In this study, endometrial thickness measured by ultrasound, subjective assessment of the adequacy of endometrial preparation by the operating surgeon and histological evidence of endometrial glandular and stromal inactivity were assessed. Other factors, including uterine volume, duration of surgery and volume of distension medium absorbed, were also recorded. There was no significant difference in the endometrial thickness as assessed by ultrasound (1.0 mm vs 1.0 mm) but the proportion of inactive glands in the group pre-treated with goserelin was higher. Although the proportion of women judged subjectively to have well prepared endometrium was only slightly higher with goserelin, the treatment time for this group was significantly shorter. In addition, when two injections of goserelin were administered, the patient satisfaction rate was significantly higher but this finding has not been reproduced in any other study.

The use of danazol or gonadotrophin releasing hormone analogues remains a matter of personal and economic choice.

Donnez uses a second GnRH analogue injection 2 weeks prior to surgery so that the patient remains hypo-oestrogenic during the healing phase postoperatively. He claims an improved amenorrhoea rate.[10]

Inclusion and exclusion criteria

Endometrial laser ablation can be performed when medical therapy has failed or as an alternative to medical treatment, insertion of an intrauterine progesterone releasing device or hysterectomy. There are few absolute contra-indications to ELA. A uterine size of more than 12 weeks and the presence of large fibroids do not preclude treatment if the surgeon is experienced and the patient is aware that the procedure may be performed in two or even three stages.

Similarly, the presence of septa, fibroids or polyps does not contraindicate endometrial laser ablation, indeed, treatment is relatively more likely to be successful if uterine abnormalities are present.[11]

Inclusion criteria

- Excessive menstrual loss (dysfunctional uterine bleeding, fibroids, benign polypi)
- Family completed
- Bleeding primary complaint (not pain or premenstrual syndrome).

Exclusion criteria

- Uterine size more than 12 weeks (relative contraindications)
- Large (>5 cm) submucous fibroids
- Concomitant gynaecological pathology
- Dysmenorrhoea primary complaint
- Patient request for amenorrhoea (absolute contraindications)
- Endometrial hyperplasia or carcinoma (all stages of endometrial atypia)
- Active pelvic inflammatory disease or other pelvic infection.

Duration of treatment

In the series of Phillips and Garry,[11] the average treatment time for all patients (including those with fibroids) was 22 min. For patients without fibroids the treatment time is shorter. The time to prepare the patient in theatre is minimal but no adjustments to the patient's position are necessary once the patient has been placed in the lithotomy position with the legs slightly abducted and flexed at the hip. The theatre scrub nurse and operating surgeon assemble the instruments as the patient is positioned. 'Turnover' time is approximately 35 min per patient. Patients require a single injection of gonadotrophin releasing hormone analogue one calendar month pre-operatively and this can be administered at the general practitioner's surgery.

Analgesic requirements

Patients not contraindicated to non-steroidal anti-inflammatory agents are consented to receive rectal diclofenac (100 mg) which is inserted at the conclusion of the procedure. In addition, 20 ml 0.5% bupivacaine is injected radially into the cervix to reduce post-operative cramping pain. Garry has shown that this significantly reduces the need for post-operative opioids.[12] Only patients with serious medical conditions, or those with no carer at home remain in hospital overnight. The vast majority of procedures are performed as day cases (>90%). The procedure is not performed in the outpatient setting because of the duration of treatment and the need for uterine distension which is a potent cause of intra-operative pain.

Results of *ex vivo/in vitro* studies

In addition to describing the technique of endometrial laser ablation in 1981, Goldrath described the effect of the procedure on the endometrium and underlying myometrium. This suggested a 4–5 mm depth of thermal necrosis using the Nd:YAG laser and the dragging method. The myometrium is thinnest at the cornua (approximately 10–12 mm) and this ensures a 5 mm 'buffer' of healthy non-treated myometrium to protect extra-uterine visceral structures.

Davis reported similar tissue effects with a power output of 80 W using the Nd:YAG laser and shallower depth of tissue destruction with lesser power outputs.[13]

Duffy's study of the effects of electrical thermal injury on the depth of tissue necrosis remains the only other documented example of tissue injury at endometrial ablation for all of the first generation devices (ELA, TCRE and rollerball).[14]

Results of treatment

It is now 20 years since Goldrath's description of the technique which allows for comment on long-term follow-up of patients (the longest follow-up of any of the ablation technologies). In addition to Goldrath's published data, a number of other case series have been reported with variable numbers of patients/procedures and follow-up periods (12 months to 12 years) with amazingly consistent results (amenorrhoea approximately 35–40% and patient satisfaction 85%).

Goldrath reported results of 427 ablations in 407 women in 1995.[8] Excellent results were obtained in 379 (89%) patients and only 35 (8.2%) had poor outcomes. Goldrath has also found that the addition of a single injection of medroxyprogesterone acetate intraoperatively almost doubles the rate of amenorrhoea (69% vs 37%, $p < 0.00001$) and that the number of failures when such adjuvant therapy is administered was also significantly lower ($p < 0.04$).

Garry, Erian and Grochmal's series of 859 women followed up for at least 6 months reported excellent results and follow-up for up to 3 years.[15] The rate of minor complications was low (transient fluid overload 0.4%, infection 0.4% and perforation 0.3%) and there were no major complications requiring laparotomy. The mean treatment time was 24 min, 60% of patients were amenorrhoeic and 32% had continuing but acceptable bleeding. Of the 39 who had ongoing menorrhagia, 26 responded to a second laser ablation, only 13 (3%) underwent hysterectomy.

In Jourdain's series of 137 patients, 17 (13.3%) subsequently underwent hysterectomy and 85% were satisfied with the treatment outcome but the mean follow-up was only 32 months. Of the satisfied women, 35 (29.2%) had had menopause since the procedure.[16] Jourdain attributed most of the failures in this series to the presence of adenomyosis or fibromas but in other series the presence of fibromas increased the likelihood of successful outcome.

The largest reported number of procedures from a single centre is that of Phillips and Garry from South Cleveland.[11] This group reported on 1000 consecutive ablations on 873 patients. A single ablation was performed on 746 women, 124 (14.2%) underwent two procedures and three (0.4%) underwent two repeat ablations. Using a survival curve analysis to compensate for variable follow-up times, it was determined that the hysterectomy rate (for all indications for hysterectomy) at 6.5 years was 21% (95% CI 16–27%). After adjusting for confounding due to age and dysmenorrhoea the only factors affecting risk of subsequently undergoing hysterectomy were having a repeat ablation which increased the relative risk (RR 2.93; 95% CI 1.59–5.40; $p = 0.0015$) and the presence of intra-uterine fibroids or polypi which reduced the risk (RR 0.26; 95% CI 0.08–0.86; $p = 0.0082$).

Pinion's randomised trial of hysterectomy, TCRE and ELA describes a series of 204 patients who would otherwise have been treated with hysterectomy for menorrhagia.[17] Randomisation was in the ratio hysterectomy:hysteroscopic surgery, 1:1, with half of the patients in the hysteroscopic surgery arm undergoing TCRE and the others being treated with ELA. There were no reported statistically significant differences between the TCRE and ELA groups. There was less operative and early morbidity in the hysteroscopic surgery group and a more rapid recovery than in the hysterectomy group (2–4 weeks vs 2–3 months,

$p < 0.001$). Seventeen (17%) patients in the hysteroscopic treatment arm subsequently underwent hysterectomy and eleven a repeat hysteroscopic procedure. Seventy eight percent (78%) (75/96) and 89% (79/89) of patients in the hysteroscopic surgery and hysterectomy groups were satisfied ($p < 0.001$) at 12 months and 95% and 90% respectively felt that there had been an acceptable improvement in their symptoms.

Bhattacharya's trial of ELA versus TCRE is the only trial of significant size directly comparing first generation minimal access techniques in a randomised controlled fashion.[18] Women with menorrhagia and without fibroids were randomised to receive treatment with TCRE ($n = 184$) or ELA ($n = 188$). TCRE was significantly quicker, but there were no differences in intra-operative morbidity or clinical outcomes, improved bleeding patterns being observed in 95% and 94% of patients in the TCRE and ELA groups respectively. Although there was no reported statistically significant difference in the rates of further surgical intervention (20% vs 16%) only nine women (5%) required hysterectomy in the ELA group as opposed to 25 (14%) in the TCRE group. Satisfaction rates at 1 year were similar (90% ELA, 91% TCRE).

Complications and rates of adverse incidences

Procedure related complications are rare if the safety principles outlined above are followed. The risk of uterine perforation at cervical dilatation or insertion of blunt instruments is approximately 1% at dilatation for curettage. The reported incidence at ELA is somewhat lower at 0–0.4%.[18,19] Uterine perforation intra-operatively, either with the hysteroscope or with the tip of the laser fibre, will occur very infrequently in the normal uterus but when myomectomy (particularly with submucous fibroids with a large intra-mural component) is performed the risk increases depending on the site and size of the myoma.

A comprehensive analysis of complications associated with each of the ablation techniques was performed by the Clinical Audit Unit of the Royal College of Obstetricians and Gynaecologists as the MISTLETOE study.[19] Of a total of more than 10,000 ablations and resections, 1793 laser ablations were performed. The overall rates of immediate complications (haemorrhage, perforation, cardio-respiratory and visceral burn) with laser and rollerball ablation were significantly lower than with resection alone. In resection with ball and radiofrequency ablation, the incidence of intra-operative fluid absorption was significantly higher. There was a highly significantly lower rate of emergency surgical intervention during laser than all of the other techniques assessed (0.34% vs 1.11% (rollerball), 1.36% (loop and ball), 2.39% (loop alone) and 2.86% (radiofrequency ablation)).

Fluid absorption is known to occur in almost all patients undergoing hysteroscopic endometrial ablation procedures. The intra-operative absorption of fluid was studied in detail by Garry et al.[20] This group have demonstrated that the rate of fluid absorption is dependent upon the rate of fluid flow through the uterus, the intra-uterine pressure and the depth of thermal injury. All of these factors must be carefully controlled throughout the procedure. The fluid used should be an electrolyte containing solution — NaCl 0.9% is ideal. This reduces the risk of electrolyte disturbance, particularly dilutional hyponatraemia, which is common when non-electrolytic solutions are used (TUR syndrome) and may cause serious neurological sequelae and even death. What is defined as excessive fluid absorption varies from unit to unit. In our unit, when the fluid deficit is more than 1500 ml, a stat dose of frusemide is administered intravenously and a urinary catheter inserted and the urinary output is then deducted from the fluid deficit. If the fluid deficit then exceeds 2500 ml, the procedure may be abandoned (depending on the urinary output and the patient's condition) and the therapeutic response awaited with an incomplete ablation. If the patient is dissatisfied with the result a further ablation or hysterectomy is scheduled.

Extra-uterine visceral thermal injury has not occurred in South Cleveland Hospital unit where almost 2000 procedures have been performed. Such injuries are extremely serious and may require laparotomy with segmental bowel resection or even the creation of a stoma. Of greater concern is when such injuries are not diagnosed intra-operatively and the patient may then present in a moribund state a number of days later with faecal peritonitis.

Vascular injury is uncommon.[19] Uterine vessel injury is more common than major pelvic vessel injury. Bleeding from within the uterus intra- or post-operatively can usually be controlled with electrocautery or tamponade from the inflated balloon of a urinary catheter. However, if this fails to arrest haemorrhage, hysterectomy may rarely become necessary.

Post-operative endometritis is uncommon (<1%). Patients are advised to expect a sero–sanguinous discharge for up to six weeks post-operatively. Intra-operative antibiotics are used routinely in this unit and the incidence of endometritis is 0.2%. There are few episodes of serious infection and low incidence rate of re-admission to hospital.

An exceedingly rare, but potentially fatal, complication of laser ablation is gas embolism: this has been reported with the use of a carbon dioxide cooled coaxial fibre and an exposed tip.[21] As with all hysteroscopic procedures, this complication can occur as a result of intra-vasation of gas produced by vaporisation of endometrium, gas within the fluid infusion set and direct intra-vasation of room air through venous sinuses in the cervix if these are traumatised by cervical dilatation and particularly if the patient is placed in the head down position.

Late complications include:

1. failure with recurrence of menorrhagia;
2. pelvic pain as a result of the tubal syndrome;
3. dysmenorrhoea (often secondary to the presence of adenomyosis or endometriosis);
4. the formation of granulomata within the uterine cavity.[22]

Assessment of the cavity in the woman who has been amenorrhoeic but then bleeds, is not without its difficulties as pockets of endometrium may be obscured to the hysteroscopist by scarring within the cavity.

Costs

The initial cost of setting up a laser to use for endometrial laser ablation is high. Modifications to a theatre or the construction of a purpose built theatre run into many thousands of pounds. Laser systems vary in price from £50,000 to more than £80,000 and such a high initial outlay explains why the technique has been relatively poorly adopted (in comparison with TCRE and rollerball). However, once installed, the equipment can be used repeatedly and the cost of disposables and replacement of laser fibres is low. The more frequently the equipment is used, the less expensive the treatment becomes. At South Cleveland Hospital the estimated theatre cost per case is £200, including laser depreciation and fibre usage. In addition, the majority of the procedures are performed as day cases so hospital 'hotel' costs remain low.

Bhattacharya estimated that ELA would cost £145 per patient more than TCRE.[18] However, the costing will be very much reduced in centres with frequently used laser as the major cost is in its introduction. This excess costing also ignores the higher complication rate for TCRE and need for further treatment as outlined in the MISTLETOE study.

Conclusions

Endometrial laser ablation is an efficacious method of endometrial destruction for the treatment of menstrual dysfunction, intra-cavitary fibroids and polyps. Morbidity and mortality associated with the procedure are low but the learning curve is longer than with many of the newer second generation devices. The technique has a long track record and more than 75% of women will avoid the need for a subsequent hysterectomy.

Advantages and disadvantages

Advantages	Disadvantages
Safety, lowest laparotomy, perforation and hysterectomy rates of all first generation procedures	Initial cost of set-up Learning curve Longer operation time
Low risk of fluid overload	
Effective with long-term follow-up	
Very few exclusions, pathology can be treated specifically	

References

1. Goldrath MH, Fuller TA, Segal S. Laser photovaporization of the endometrium for the treatment of menorrhagia. *Am J Obstet Gynaecol* 1981; 140: 14–19.

2. Tilt EJ. Radio frequency endometrial ablation. In: CJG Sutton (Ed.) *New Surgical Techniques in Gynaecology*, pp. 18–19, 1991. Carnforth: The Parthenon Publishing Group.

3. Hardt W, Genz T. Atmocausis vaporisation. Most severe internal burns following intrauterine use of steam. *Geburtshilfe Frauenheilkd* 1989; 49: 293–295.

4. Droegmueller W, Greer B, Makowski E. Cryosurgery in patients with dysfunctional uterine bleeding. *Obstet Gynaecol* 1971; 38: 256–258.

5. Lindemann HJ. Historical aspects of hysteroscopy. *Fertil Steril* 1973; 24: 230–243.

6. Hamou J. Microhysteroscopy. A new procedure and its original applications in gynaecology. *J Reprod Med* 1981; 26: 375–382.

7. Neuwirth RS, Amin HK. Excision of submucous fibroids with hysteroscopic control. *Am J Obstet Gynaecol* 1973; 126: 95–99.

8. Goldrath MH. Hysteroscopic endometrial ablation. *Obstet Gynaecol Clin North Am* 1995; 22: 559–572.

9. Khair A, Shelley-Jones D, Garry R. A prospective randomised trial comparing a GnRH Analog, Zoladex, and Danazol as agents for priming the endometrium prior to endometrial laser ablation. *J Am Assoc Gynaecol Laparosc* 1994; 1: S17.

10. Donnez J, Vilos G, Gannon MJ, Maheux R, Emanuel MH, Istre O. Goserelin acetate (Zoladex) plus endometrial ablation for dysfunctional uterine bleeding: a 3 year follow up evaluation. *Fertil Steril* 2001; 75: 620–622.

11. Phillips G, Chien PF, Garry R. Risk of hysterectomy after 1000 consecutive endometrial laser ablations. *Br J Obstet Gynaecol* 1998; 105: 897–903.

12. Garry R, Shelley-Jones D, Mooney P, Phillips G. Six hundred endometrial laser ablations. *Obstet Gynaecol* 1995; 85: 24–29.

13. Davis JR, Maynard KK, Brainard CP, Purdon TF, Sibley MA, King DD. Effects of thermal endometrial ablation: clinicopathologic correlations. *Am J Clin Pathol* 1998; 109: 96–100.

14. Duffy S, Reid PC, Smith JH, Sharp F. *In vitro* studies of uterine electrosurgery. *Obstet Gynaecol* 1991; 183: 22–27.

15. Garry R, Erian J, Grochmal SA. A multi-centre collaborative study into the treatment of menorrhagia by Nd:YAG laser ablation of the endometrium. *Br J Obstet Gynaecol* 1991; 98: 357–362.

16. Jourdain O, Joyeux P, Lajus C, Sfaxi I, Harle T, Roux D, Dallay D. Endometrial Nd:YAG laser ablation by hysterofibroscopy: long term results of 137 cases. *Eur J Obstet Gynecol Reprod Biol* 1996; 69: 103–107.

17. Pinion SB, Parkin DE, Abramovich DR, Naji A, Alexander DA, Russell IT, Kitchener HC. Randomised trial of hysterectomy, endometrial laser ablation, and transcervical endometrial resection for dysfunctional uterine bleeding. *Br Med J* 1994; 309: 979–983.

18. Bhattacharya S, Cameron IM, Parkin DE, Abramovich DR, Mollison J, Pinion SB, Alexander DA, Grant A, Kitchener HC. A pragmatic randomised comparison of transcervical resection of the endometrium with endometrial laser ablation for the treatment of menorrhagia. *Br J Obstet Gynaecol* 1997; 104: 601–607.

19. Overton C, Hargreaves J, Maresh M. A national survey of the complications of endometrial destruction for menstrual disorders: the MISTLETOE study. *Br J Obstet Gynaecol* 1997; 104: 1352–1359.

20. Hasham F, Garry R, Kokri MS, Mooney P. Fluid absorption during laser ablation of the endometrium in the treatment of menorrhagia. *Br J Anaesth* 1992; 68: 151–154.

21. Kelly M, Matthews HM, Weir P. Carbon dioxide embolism during laser endometrial ablation. *Anaesthesia* 1997; 52: 65–67.

22. Silvernagel SW, Harshbarger KE, Shevlin DW. Post-operative granulomas of the endometrium: histological features after endometrial ablation. *Ann Diagnostic Pathol* 1997; 1: 82–90.

8

Hysteroscopic electrosurgical resection and rollerball

Peter Scott and Adam Magos

Introduction

Hysteroscopic endometrial ablation with electro-surgery was introduced as a less invasive alternative to hysterectomy in the management of abnormal uterine bleeding of benign origin. Although Nd:YAG laser ablation was described 2 years before electrosurgical treatment,[1,2] the literature concerning endometrial ablation by electrosurgery is more detailed and thorough, perhaps because the obvious cost advantage has meant that it is more widely practised. There is now a large volume of data regarding technique, complications, short and long-term outcome, as well as randomised comparisons with medical treatments, other methods of ablation and hysterectomy. Endometrial resection and rollerball ablation, the two basic techniques, must be one of the most intensively studied surgical treatments in modern medical practice.

Equipment

The initial hysteroscopic electrosurgical technique, for the purposes of treating abnormal uterine bleeding by destroying the endometrium, was first formally described by DeCherney in 1983.[2] The initial technique involved coagulation of the endometrium, using the loop electrode of a single channel resectoscope with Hyskon distension, in women with intractable uterine haemorrhage who were not suitable for hysterectomy. Exactly when actual resection of the endometrium was first tried is not clear from the literature, but DeCherney and Neuwirth in the USA and Hamou in France must be considered the early pioneers. Hamou, having an engineering background, modified the American technique by using a continuous flow resectoscope and sterile 1.5% glycine solution as the distending medium, a similar combination to the one described earlier by Hallez, also working in Paris, for hysteroscopic myomectomy.[3,4] Using a continuous flow resectoscope with a low viscosity fluid has become the standard equipment for most gynaecologists performing resectoscopic surgery.

The cutting loop is an inefficient electrode for coagulating (cf. cutting) the endometrium and it was only a matter of time before the rollerball was suggested as a more logical alternative. The first series was published in the English literature by Vancaillie but a Japanese publications claims priority in terms of timing.[5,6] Rollerball ablation has proved itself to be an easier and safer technique than resection but is not ideal for women with submucous fibroids, a common finding in women with menorrhagia. Whether one uses a cutting loop or rollerball has become largely a matter of personal preference and many now use both the rollerball for the uterine fundus and the cutting loop to treat the body of the uterus.[7]

The equipment commonly used is a 26 French gauge continuous flow passive handle resectoscope with a 4 mm forward oblique endoscope and a 24 French gauge cutting loop. The use of a passive handle mechanism ensures that the cutting loop is inside the sheath at rest and, consequently, accidental trauma is unlikely. Distension of the uterine cavity for adequate visualisation of the fundus is achieved by using an irrigation pump to maintain an intrauterine pressure of 80–120 mmHg. Insufficient intrauterine pressure provides inadequate uterine distension and over distension can lead to problems of excessive fluid absorption. To maintain a continuous flow of uterine irrigant, a suction device is attached to the outflow of the resectoscope to generate a negative pressure of around 50 mmHg. The suction pressure may be increased if the view is too cloudy and decreased if uterine distension is inadequate prior to increasing the distension pressure. The distension media commonly used is sterile 1.5% glycine although other non-conductive media can be used for example mannitol, sorbitol/mannitol.

Endometrial preparation

For ablation to be successful, the basal layer of the endometrium needs to be destroyed. Normal endometrium varies in thickness during the menstrual cycle from 3 to 12 mm.

There are two views with respect to the pre- and, to some extent, post-operative use of endometrial suppressants such as danazol or GnRH analogues. With endometrial resection, pre-treatment is not vital and Hamou, for instance, argues strongly against it. In contrast, we have found that endometrial suppression makes the surgery easier and faster thereby reducing fluid absorption, with the result that we prefer a 6–8 week course prior to surgery.[8] Pre-treatment also reduces the volume of tissue to be removed, improves the view which increases safety and is associated with less bleeding. Others advocate suction curettage immediately before ablation.[9] Certainly, an endometrial thickness >4 mm is likely to mean that rollerball ablation will not achieve full thickness endometrial destruction.[10] There is also some evidence that endometrial suppression, post-surgery, may improve the rate of amenorrhoea.[11,12]

Patient selection

Prior counselling ensures that the patient has completed her family, has menorrhagia sufficient to warrant surgery and understands the remote possibility of the procedure converting to a hysterectomy. Periods should be regular as irregular menstruation will not be corrected by ablation. Better results are obtained if uterine size is less than the equivalent of a 12 weeks gestation. The presence of submucous fibroids is not a contraindication to surgery and in this case ablation can be combined with hysteroscopic myomectomy with the loop.

The most important determinant of long-term success is the age of the patient. Younger women have a less successful outcome than older ones. Patients should be informed that the expected result of treatment is light or normal periods and that amenorrhoea only occurs in a minority of women.

The histology of the endometrium must be known because retrograde seeding of endometrial carcinoma may occur.[13] Women with atypical or adenomatous hyperplasia should not be treated, but cystic glandular hyperplasia without atypia is not a contraindication. Resection has the advantage that tissue is sent for histological examination to confirm the pre-operative assessment.

Pelvic inflammatory disease and endometriosis are relative contraindications. Similarly, dysmenorrhoea, which is mainly pre-menstrual, is not helped by ablation.[14] There is some evidence that the pre-menstrual syndrome is improved after surgery.[15]

Duration of treatment

Endometrial ablation is generally a quick procedure, certainly when compared to hysterectomy. Procedure time depends on a number of factors, of which uterine cavity size, endometrial thickness, the presence of myomas and not least the experience of the operator are the most important. To give an example, the mean operating time for endometrial resection was found to be significantly shorter than for laser ablation — 20 min vs 30 min in a study of 372 patients by Bhattacharya.[16]

Analgesic requirements

The procedure may be performed under general, regional and even local anaesthesia. If local anaesthesia is used, pre-medication of a benzodiazepine is given combined with per-operative sedation with intravenous midazolam. Local anaesthetic block is provided by intracervical, paracervical and intrauterine lignocaine with adrenaline and additional analgesia is obtained by small intravenous doses of an opiod such as fentanyl.[17]

Techniques

TCRE

The cervix is first dilated incrementally to a size 10 Hegar dilator. A blended cutting and coagulation current is used to produce cutting with haemostasis (e.g. 100–120 W set at blend 1). Any submucous fibroids are usually resected first, particularly if they obscure parts of the uterine cavity. The uterine fundus is treated next, either using a forward angled loop to resect the endometrium or a rollerball to ablate it. The rest of the uterus is resected with the conventional loop in a systematic manner down to the internal os. It is essential only to activate the loop while cutting towards the cervix as resecting towards the fundus risks perforation. The depth of resection is judged by the appearance of the circular myometrial fibres and it is important not to cut too deep as this could lead to haemorrhage and ultimately uterine perforation.

The resected tissue chips can be pushed towards the fundus to enable visualisation of the unresected part of the endometrial cavity and removed at the end of the procedure using a flushing curette. This is our preferred technique but, when the endometrium is thick, it is sometimes easier to cut full length chips which are removed from the uterine cavity with each pass of the resectoscope. At the end of the procedure, the uterus is re-inspected to ensure the resection is complete and that there are no bleeding vessels. Any obvious bleeding points can be cauterised using 60 W of coagulation current (or the same cutting current as for resection, providing the loop electrode is in contact with the tissue). Generalised bleeding can be staunched by inflating the 30 ml balloon of a urinary catheter inside the uterine cavity to cause tamponade but this is rarely needed.

Rollerball

This is a technique which is commoner in the United States and Australia than in Europe and relies on the modified urological resectoscope fitted with a ball electrode. This is moved across the endometrial surface whilst a blended cutting current is used to cause tissue blanching and destruction. The key to success is to move the rollerball *slowly* across the endometrial surface to ensure that tissue destruction is deep enough. Increasing the power setting on the electrosurgical generator has a much lesser effect.[18] For optimum results, it is important to ensure that the endometrial thickness is no more than 3–4 mm at the time of surgery and this can be achieved by pre-treatment with a GnRH analogue or by curettage.

Results

Without exception, all published series of endometrial resection or rollerball ablation have shown favourable outcomes for the majority of patients, both in terms of reduced menstrual bleeding and dysmenorrhoea. Objective measures of menstrual blood loss have confirmed these subjective findings.[19] While the initial reports included relatively few patients and/or a short follow-up period,[5,20] there are now several larger studies with longer-term follow-up periods which have confirmed that these procedures can be effective in the medium to long term as well.[21–24]

One issue which has only recently been resolved, is the correct method to summarise the success rate of surgery. First, it has become apparent that treatment failures can occur at variable times after the initial surgery. Any analysis which fails to take account of the duration of follow-up, particularly if the follow-up time is relatively short, is therefore likely to over-estimate the success of the procedure. Secondly, indexes such as amenorrhoea or patient satisfaction are difficult to assess as they can fluctuate with time. Instead, the optimum statistical technique, to assess the success of procedures such as endometrial ablation, is survival analysis using the need for further surgery, for instance, as the definite end-point.

O'Connor and Magos in 1996 reported on the follow-up, using life-table analysis for up to 5 years,[21] of 525 patients undergoing endometrial resection

- 26–40% of women reported amenorrhoea,
- 71–80% noted an absence or amelioration of their dysmenorrhoea,
- 79–87% were satisfied with their treatment,
- 3% of women were given medical therapy for recurrent symptoms,
- 16% required further surgery.

Most of the surgeries were done within 3 years of the initial resection, a finding that is similar with rollerball ablation.[22] Ultimately, 9% of women underwent hysterectomy for heavy, painful periods or pelvic pain. Life-table analysis showed that 80% of women avoided further surgery and 91% avoided hysterectomy during the 5 years of their surgery. Using these results as the bench-mark, electrosurgical endometrial ablation, particularly endometrial resection, appears to have a higher success rate than laser ablation.[25]

There have been several comparative trials of endometrial ablation and hysterectomy. Although the trials differed in their size and follow-up period (several have updated their results) and some reported relatively poor outcomes after hysteroscopic surgery. They essentially all came to the same conclusion — operative complications and recovery were inferior with hysterectomy but patient satisfaction was better with the more major operation. However, psychological and social testing showed no significant differences. Despite the need for re-treatment for some of the women treated hysteroscopically, hysterectomy remained a more costly treatment option than endometrial ablation.[26–28] It should not be assumed that only women treated by endometrial ablation are at risk of needing additional surgery. In our trial, for instance, 9% of those randomised to hysterectomy required further surgical intervention during the follow-up period.[29]

As the efficacy and low risk of endometrial ablation became established, other comparative trials were set up against established medical treatments. In one trial, hysteroscopic surgery was compared with a variety of standard medical treatments:

1. progestogens,
2. combined contraceptive pill,
3. tranexamic acid,
4. danazol,
5. hormone replacement therapy with a non-steroidal anti-inflammatory.

Patients allocated to hysteroscopic surgery were significantly more satisfied with their allocated treatment and indeed almost two-thirds of those randomised to medical therapy had undergone surgery within 2 years.[30] This lead the authors to suggest that endometrial ablation should be offered as first line treatment instead of long-term medical therapy for patients with persistent menorrhagia.

Two trials have compared endometrial resection with the levonorgestrel intrauterine system.[28,31] They both came to the same conclusions, namely, that the reduction in menstrual bleeding and patient satisfaction was slightly greater after hysteroscopic surgery. Whether this small difference is clinically significant is doubtful. These studies show that it is reasonable to offer women the choice between these two modes of management.

Operative complications

Endometrial ablation may be a relatively minor procedure for the patient but is a major procedure as far as potential complications are concerned. Chief amongst the risks are uterine perforation with visceral or vascular intra-abdominal damage and fluid overload — both are potentially fatal. Other potential complications include haemorrhage and air or fluid embolism.

It is very important that fluid balance is strictly monitored per-operatively to avoid the complications of fluid overload which is associated with hyponatraemia and encephalopathy if glycine is used as the distension medium.[32,33] The use of electrosurgical instruments is more problematic in this regard than, for instance, with Nd:YAG laser, as the uterine distension medium has to be electrolyte-free unless a bipolar instrument is used. As a result, surgery should be stopped, intravenous diuretics administered, the patient catheterised and blood electrolytes checked if the fluid absorbed is greater than 1½ to 2l. Fluid overload is in fact totally preventable as long as surgery is stopped in time. Factors which decrease the operating time (e.g. the presence of thin endometrium, a uterine cavity which is not grossly enlarged by fibroids) also reduce the risk of fluid absorption problems, as does ensuring that the distension pressure within the uterus is not excessive (80–120 mmHg).

Uterine perforation is, in principle, also preventable by good technique (e.g. resecting towards, rather than away, from the cervix), but is a definite risk. If it is suspected, for instance, if there is sudden fluid absorption or uterine deflation, surgery should be stopped immediately and only continued if perforation has been excluded. This may mean having to perform a laparoscopy. If the uterus has been perforated while using an activated resectoscope, a laparoscopy and often a laparotomy must be done to exclude bowel or vascular injury. In some cases, the perforation can be repaired laparoscopically and the ablation continued.[34]

The literature contains numerous case reports, observational series and comparative data from randomised trials with hysterectomy but one of the largest and most detailed studies of complications associated with hysteroscopic electrosurgery comes from the MISTLETOE survey of the Royal College of Obstetricians and Gynaecologists in London, England.[35]

The operative records of over 10,000 endometrial ablation procedures performed in 1993/1994 were audited prospectively.[35] The results showed that immediate operative complications, such as perforation and haemorrhage, were relatively infrequent, ranging from 2.1% for rollerball ablation to 6.4% for endometrial resection. Fluid overload (defined as a fluid deficit >2l) was greatest with laser ablation — 5.1%. Endometrial thinning agents did not reduce the risk of complications. The presence of uterine leiomyoma increased the risk of haemorrhage.

Although the MISTLETOE survey had shortcomings, it confirmed that, even in the hands of non-experts, endometrial ablation was a relatively safe procedure. It is evident that uterine perforation can be avoided by experience and good technique. Fluid overload is totally preventable by careful measurement of fluid balance throughout surgery. Ethanol tagging of the distension medium has been suggested as an aid to accurate monitoring,[36] but this can give a false sense of security as it does not predict trans-peritoneal fluid absorption which can continue for several hours after the end of surgery.[37,38]

Post–operative complications

Endometritis, secondary haemorrhage, recurrence of symptoms, pelvic pain, haematometra and pregnancy are some of the commoner complications reported after endometrial ablation.[21] Tubo-ovarian abscess, haematosalpinx, uterine granulomata, pyometra, ectopic pregnancy and even endometrial malignancy have also been reported in isolated cases. Pelvic pain and recurrent menorrhagia are certainly the major reasons for treatment failure and the need for further surgery. Their incidence varies greatly in the literature and it seems that younger women and those with uterine fibroids are most likely to become symptomatic.[21]

Costs

Sculpher et al conducted a randomised trial comparing hysterectomy and TCRE, looking particularly at the difference in costs 2 years after surgery.[26] In their study of 196 women, 12% had a repeat resection and 16% had a subsequent hysterectomy.

At 1994 prices the initial cost at 4 months was £1059.73 ($1604.11 or €1684) for an abdominal hysterectomy and £560.05 ($847.75 or €890) for endometrial resection — a difference of £499.68 ($756.37 or €794). By 2 years of follow-up, the cost of further surgery in the ablation group had increased the average cost in this group to £790 ($1195.82 or €1255). Thus the mean total cost of resection was 53% that of hysterectomy at 4 months and 71% at 2.2 years.

The Aberdeen Endometrial Trials Group has published a series of 204 women followed up for over 4 years.[27] In the endometrial ablation arm, 38% received at least 1 additional surgical treatment for their menorrhagia. The initial costs in the endometrial ablation group were much lower (mean: £726 [$1099 or €1154] vs £1247 [$1888 or €1982]) but by 4 years the costs had risen to £1231 ($1863 or €1956) vs £1332 ($2016 or €2117) respectively (93% of the cost of hysterectomy).

Conclusions

Endometrial ablation by electrosurgery is a well-proven and effective treatment for menorrhagia. It compares well against drug therapy and hysterectomy with many advantages as well as some disadvantages. Procedures, such as endometrial resection, have become the 'gold standard' with which the newer, non-hysteroscopic techniques of endometrial ablation have to compare.

Advantages and disadvantages of endometrial ablation with hysterectomy

Advantages	Disadvantages
Endometrial ablation	
Minor surgery	Not suitable for some women
Can be performed without general anaesthetic	Risk of fluid absorption anaesthetic during surgery
No external scars	Risk of intra-operative complications leading to
Shorter hospital stay	major surgery
Faster convalescence	Need for future contraception
Uterus retained	Periods and period pains may continue as before
	Hysterectomy may prove necessary in the future
	Undetected fibroids may cause symptoms later
	Does not eliminate chance of endometrial or cervical cancer
Hysterectomy	
Periods and period pains will definitely cease	Involves major surgery
	Requires general anaesthetic
	Longer hospital stay
Suitable for any uterine size	Slower convalescence
	Possibly
No risk of uterine or cervical cancer	Abdominal scar
	Earlier menopause
No need for future contraception	Bowel symptoms
	Urinary symptoms

References

1. Goldrath MH, Fuller TA, Segal S. Laser photovaporization of endometrium for the treatment of menorrhagia. *Am J Obstet Gynecol* 1981; 140: 14–19.

2. DeCherney A, Polan ML. Hysteroscopic management of intrauterine lesions and intractable uterine bleeding. *Obstet Gynecol* 1983; 61: 392–397.

3. Perino A, Cittadini E, Colacurci N, De Placido G, Hamou J. Endometrial ablation: principles and technique. *Acta Europaea Fertilitatis* 1990; 21: 313–317.

4. Hallez JP, Netter A, Cartier R. Methodical intrauterine resection. *Am J Obstet Gynecol* 1987; 156: 1080–1084.

5. Vancaillie TG. Electrocoagulation of the endometrium with the ball-end resectoscope. *Obstet Gynecol* 1989; 74: 425–427.

6. Lin BL, Miyamoto M, Tomomatu M et al. The development of a new hysteroscopic resectoscope and its clinical applications on transcervical resection (TCR) and endometrial ablation (EA). *Jpn J Gynecol Obstet Endosc* 1988; 4: 56–61.

7. Vercellini P, Oldani S, De Giorgi O, Milesi M, Merlo D, Crosignani PG. Endometrial ablation with a vaporizing electrode. II Clinical outcome of a pilot study. *Acta Obstet Gynecol Scand* 1998; 77: 688–693.

8. Magos AL, Baumann R, Lockwood GM, Turnbull AC. Experience with the first 250 endometrial resections for menorrhagia. *Lancet* 1991; 337: 1074–1078.

9. Lefler HT Jr, Sullivan GH, Hulka JF. Modified endometrial ablation: electrocoagulation with vasopressin and suction curettage preparation. *Obstet Gynecol* 1991; 77: 949–953.

10. Duffy S, Reid PC, Sharp F. In-vivo studies of uterine electrosurgery. *Br J Obstet Gynaecol* 1992; 99: 579–582.

11. Townsend DE, Richart RM, Paskowitz RA, Woolfork RE. 'Rollerball' coagulation of the endometrium. *Obstet Gynecol* 1990; 76: 310–313.

12. Erian MM, Thomas IL, Buck RJ, Lewin MW, Coglan M, Battistutta D. The effects of danazol after endometrial resection — results of a randomised, placebo-controlled, double-blind study. *Aust New Zeal J Obstet Gynaecol* 1998; 38: 210–214.

13. Romano S, Shimoni V, Muralee D, Shalev E. Retrograde seeding of endometrial carcinoma during hysteroscopy. *Gynecol Oncol* 1992; 44: 116–118.

14. Molnar BG, Baumann R, Magos AL. Does endometrial resection help dysmenorrhoea? *Acta Obstet Gynecol Scand* 1997; 76: 261–265.

15. Lefler HT Jr. Premenstrual syndrome improvement after laser ablation of the endometrium for menorrhagia. *J Reprod Med* 1989; 34: 905–906.

16. Bhattacharya S et al. A pragmatic randomised comparison of transcervical resection of the endometrium with endometrial laser ablation for the treatment of menorrhagia. *Br J Obstet Gynaecol* 1997; 104: 601–607.

17. Lockwood GM, Baumann R, Turnbull AC, Magos AL. Extensive hysteroscopic surgery under local anaesthesia. *Gynaecol Endosc* 1992; 1: 15–21.

18. Duffy S. The tissue and thermal effects of electrosurgery in the uterine cavity. *Bail Clin Obstet Gynaecol* 1995; 9(2): 261–277.

19. Cooper MJW, Magos AL, Baumann R, Rees MCP. The effect of endometrial resection on menstrual blood loss. *Gynaecol Endosc* 1992; 1: 195–198.

20. Magos AL, Baumann R, Turnbull AC. Transcervical resection of endometrium in women with menorrhagia. *Br Med J* 1989; 298: 1209–1212.

21. O'Connor H, Magos A. Endometrial resection for the treatment of menorrhagia. *New Engl J Med* 1996; 335: 151–156.

22. Chullapram T, Song JY, Fraser IS. Medium-term follow-up of women with menorrhagia treated by rollerball endometrial ablation. *Obstet Gynecol* 1996; 88: 71–76.

23. Martyn P, Allan B. Long-term follow-up of endometrial ablation. *J Am Assoc Gynecol Laparosc* 1998; 5: 115–118.

24. Tsaltas J, Taylor N, Healey M. A 6-year review of the outcome of endometrial ablation. *Aust New Zeal J Obstet Gynaecol* 1998; 38: 69–72.

25. Phillips G, Chien PF, Garry R. Risk of hysterectomy after 1000 consecutive endometrial laser ablations. *Br J Obstet Gynaecol* 1998; 105: 897–903.

26. Sculpher JM, Dwyer N, Byford S, Stirrat GM. Randomised trial comparing hysterectomy and transcervical endometrial resection: effect on health related quality of life and costs two years after surgery. *Br J Obstet Gynaecol* 1996; 103: 142–149.

27. Aberdeen Endometrial Ablation Trials Group. A randomised trial of endometrial ablation versus hysterectomy for the treatment of dysfunctional uterine bleeding: outcome at four years. *Br J Obstet Gynaecol* 1999; 106: 360–366.

28. Crosignani PG, Vercellini P, Mosconi P, Oldani S, Cortesi I, DeGiorgi O. Levonorgestrel-releasing intra-uterine device versus hysteroscopic endometrial resection in the treatment of dysfunctional uterine bleeding. *Obstet Gynecol* 1997; 90: 257–263.

29. O'Connor H, Broadbent JA, Magos AL, McPherson K. Medical Research Council randomised trial of endometrial resection versus hysterectomy in management of menorrhagia. *Lancet* 1997; 349: 897–901.

30. Cooper KG, Parkin DE, Garratt AM, Grant AM. Two year follow-up of women randomised to medical management or transcervical resection of the endometrium for heavy menstrual loss: clinical and quality of life outcomes. *Br J Obstet Gynaecol* 1999; 106: 258–265.

31. Kittelsen N, Istre O. A randomised study comparing levonorgestrel intrauterine system (LNG IUS) and transcervical resection of the endometrium (TCRE) in the treatment of menorrhagia: preliminary results. *Gynaecol Endosc* 1998; 7: 61–66.

32. Baumann R, Magos AL, Kay JDS, Turnbull AC. Absorption of glycine irrigating solution during transcervical resection of the endometrium. *Br Med J* 1990; 300: 304–305.

33. Istre O, Bjoennes J, Naess R, Hornbaek K, Forman A. Post-operative cerebral oedema after transcervical endometrial resection and uterine irrigation with 15% glycine. *Lancet* 1995; 345: 1187–1189.

34. Broadbent JAM, Molnar BG, Cooper MJW, Magos AL. Endoscopic management of uterine perforation occurring during endometrial resection. *Br J Obstet Gynaecol* 1992; 99: 1018.

35. Overton C, Hargreaves J, Maresh M. A national survey of the complications of endometrial destruction for menstrual disorders: the MISTLETOE study. Minimally Invasive Surgical Techniques — Laser, EndoThermal or Endoresection. *Br J Obstet Gynaecol* 1997; 104: 1351–1359.

36. Olsson J, Hahn RG. Ethanol monitoring of irrigating fluid absorption in transcervical resection of the endometrium. *Acta Anaesth Scand* 1995; 39: 252–258.

37. Istre O, Skajaa, K, Schjoensby AP, Forman A. Changes in serum electrolytes after transcervical resection of endometrium and submucous fibroids with use of glycine 15% for uterine irrigation. *Obstet Gynecol* 1992; 80: 218–222.

38. Molnar BG, Magos AL, Kay J. Monitoring fluid absorption using 1% ethanol-tagged glycine during operative hysteroscopy. *J Am Assoc Gynecol Laparosc* 1997; 4: 357–362.

9

Uterine endometrial cryoablation with ultrasound visualisation

Martha C.S. Heppard and John D. Dobak

Introduction

Cryosurgical endometrial ablation is being evaluated as an alternative to hysteroscopic or balloon based endometrial ablation. Studies by Pitroff and Rutherford demonstrated the clinical feasibility of the technique.[1,2] Their studies indicate that cryosurgery has a number of potential advantages over hysteroscopic or balloon based techniques. These advantages include:

- Higher amenorrheic rates
- Lighter anaesthesia requirements
- Ability to use ultrasound monitoring to make the procedure visible
- The ability to treat submucosal myoma.

Utilising a novel mixed gas cryosurgical system, FIRST OPTION™ Uterine Cryoblation Therapy (CryoGen, Inc, San Diego, CA) specifically tailored for endometrial ablation, Dobak demonstrated the destructive capacity and safety profile of cryosurgical endometrial ablation *in vivo*.[3] This pivotal study was the basis for a clinical study in which 275 patients were randomised 2:1 (cryoablation to rollerball) and the clinical efficacy and safety of this technique was demonstrated.[4]

Description of instrumentation

The CryoGen Inc FIRST OPTION™ System is compressor driven and utilises a novel mixed gas coolant to generate temperatures of $-90°C$ to $-100°C$. A Cryoprobe which generates the cold temperatures is attached by flexible hoses to the compressor system. The Cryoprobe requires the use of a sterile, disposable control unit. The control unit has a metallic tip with an electrical heater and thermocouple which aligns with the freezing tip of the Cryoprobe. A thermally conductive silicon grease is applied to the inside of the control unit tip prior to use and then slid over the Cryoprobe. A catheter shaft, which extends from the control unit tip has a saline flush port. The system offers greater power, safety and convenience over existing cryosurgical systems. If necessary, the endocervical canal was dilated to accommodate the FIRST OPTION™ cryosurgical probe (5.5 mm). Trans-abdominal ultrasound is performed concurrently with the FIRST OPTION™ cryoablation.

Ultrasound allows monitoring of the freezing process.[2,5] Resolution of the ice front is sufficient to allow cryosurgical treatment of liver and prostate tumours percutaneously with excellent safety and efficacy.[6,7] In studies comparing iceball diameter as measured by ultrasound with iceball diameter as measured by callipers, less than 1 mm discrepancy is observed for iceballs less than 55 mm in diameter.[8] During freezing, the leading edge of the ice front reflects a significant fraction of the incident acoustic waves resulting in a hyperechoic or white line. The body of the iceball is very homogeneous and does not produce differential reflections. This, in combination with the ice front reflection, produces a post-acoustic shadow.[5] By tracking the position of the ice front relative to the serosal surface, the physician can maintain a safety margin. It should be noted, however, that the leading edge of the ice front is non-destructive.[9] Tissue is destroyed at $-15°C$ to $-20°C$ and the leading edge of the ice front, as seen on ultrasound, is only $-1°C$ to $-2°C$.[6,7,9,10] Destructive temperatures are found 3–5 mm behind the leading edge (data submitted for publication). Thus, even if the ice front reached the serosal surface, it is unlikely that tissue necrosis would occur. It should be noted that although the ultrasound only monitors one side of the iceball, the opposite side is essentially a mirror image. Size and shape of the iceball, as seen on one side, can be conferred to the opposite side. Tissue necrosis was similarly symmetrical.

Practical aspects of treatment

Patients who had completed childbearing and were between 30 and 50 years of age with a uterine sound less than 10 cm, normal pap smear, endometrial biopsy and negative pregnancy test were included in the pivotal trial. Patients with active PID, a history of gynaecological malignancy within the post 5 years, clotting defects/bleeding disorders, septate uterus and who had undergone a previous uterine surgery were excluded from the study. Of note, since the completion of the study, patients with septate, bicornuate and uterine didelphus have been treated without difficulty. All patients in the clinical study received pre-operative pregnancy tests, smears, endometrial biopsies and pelvic ultrasounds. Lupron 3.75 mg was administered IM approximately 28 days before the planned endometrial ablation. After initiation and completion of the first phase (as described in 'Description of instrumentation') the probe tip was thawed which allowed disengagement of the probe from the tissue (1–2 min). The probe was then positioned to the opposite cornua by withdrawing the probe into the endocervical canal, angling toward the cornua and inserting. In some cases it was necessary to wait for several minutes for the first iceball to partially melt, before the probe could be advanced. In addition, it was learned that flushing with 15 ml of saline, prior to withdrawal of the probe from the first iceball, facilitated repositioning by helping to melt the first iceball. Probe placement to the fundus was confirmed on ultrasound. After repositioning, 5 ml of saline was instilled into the cavity to thermally couple the probe to the tissue. The second freeze was initiated and continued for 6 min. Serial ultrasound and temperature measurements were taken as in the first freeze.

To minimise this problem, the first freeze was limited to 4 min. This resulted in a slightly smaller iceball and less chance of internal os obstruction. In addition, flushing with 15 ml of normal saline is believed to help melt the proximal portion of the iceball. The outlet for the saline flush port of the system's control unit is aligned with the proximal portion of the iceball. Thus, the heat load provided by the saline is concentrated in this area. It is important to note that, regardless of what techniques are employed to minimise internal os obstruction, the blockage is only temporary as the iceball will eventually melt, thus patience will always allow for probe angling.

The second procedural issue worth noting is the importance of inserting the probe tip to the fundus on both freezes. The extension of the iceball from the tip of the probe is limited which is a benefit since we are angling the tip toward the cornu. This is a fine point, but an important one, because the cornu is thinner than other areas of the uterus. Once the probe was angled toward the cornu and visualised here on ultrasound, it was pulled back about 2 mm. Probe positioning should be confirmed utilising ultrasound. During angling, the probe can be observed moving along side the first iceball in the transverse or sagittal planes.

In our initial study, general anaesthesia was utilised. Since that time, it has become evident that only a minimal amount of anaesthetic is necessary (thought due to the natural anaesthetic properties of cold). Most patients are very comfortable during the procedure when Toradol is administered IM 1 h before the procedure and a paracervical block is administered during the procedure.[11]

Results of *ex vivo* and *in vitro* studies

An extirpated uterine study was undertaken to evaluate the tissue effects of cryosurgical endometrial ablation in women just prior to hysterectomy. In addition, the use of ultrasound to monitor freezing was characterised. The feasibility of a novel probe angling procedure was evaluated and the safety profile was assessed by monitoring serosal surface temperatures.

Abdominal ultrasound provided adequate monitoring of the freezing. Iceball diameters measured 24–34 mm after the first freeze and 28–37 mm after the second freeze. Predictably, the distance between the two points narrows from 10.8 mm at 1 min to 4.8 mm at 6 min. However, it never reached less than 3 mm.

There was no visualisation of ice penetration to the serosal surface and there was no indication on ultrasound of ice penetration to serosal surface. Further, the average uterine thickness in the AP direction was greater than the average iceball diameter (52 mm vs 34 mm respectively). The average probe surface temperatures were 72°C for the first freeze and −82°C for the second freeze during the study.

Tetrazolium staining for tissue destruction indicated that all necrosis occurred within the boundary of the iceball. The average maximum iceball diameter was 34 mm while the average maximum diameter of non-viable tissue as determined by Tetrazolium staining was 24 mm. Depth of necrosis as measured by Tetrazolium staining and electron microscopy measured 9–12 mm. Tissue destruction as determined by Tetrazolium staining and tissue destruction as determined by electron microscopy correlated very well. Complete coverage of the endometrial cavity could be obtained through angled freezes.

This study demonstrated the safety and feasibility of cryosurgical endometrial ablation *in vivo*. From a procedural standpoint, two important issues should be highlighted.

1. Probe angling toward each cornua is essential and can be accomplished. Difficulty with repositioning likely occurs when part of the first iceball obstructs the internal os.

2. Due to the triangular shape of the cavity, obstruction is unlikely toward the fundus.

Subsequently a pre-hysterectomy study was performed. The study findings demonstrated that, of the patients included:

1. The average endometrial width was 2.6 cm and the average endometrial length was 3.9 cm.

2. Total endometrial destruction was achieved.

3. The depth of penetration of cell damage exceeded the expected level of the basal cells.

4. The presence of fibroids did not alter iceball growth or tissue destruction.

5. Ultrasound provided excellent visualisation.

6. Heating allowed rapid tissue thawing to 4.5 mm without charring.

Results of treatment

The pivotal clinical trial, including 275 cases, has been completed and as of the time of this writing (February 2000) is very close to having adequate 12 months follow-up prior to PMA submission. The study protocol was as detailed in the first paragraph of Practical Aspects of Treatment. To be included in the study, the patient's Pictorial Blood Assessment Chart (PBAC) needed to be greater than or equal to 150. Patients with intramural fibroids greater than or equal to 2 cm, submucosal myomas, intrauterine polyps and pedunculated fibroids were excluded. The study endpoints included success as defined as a PBAC score less than or equal to 75. Quality of Life Scores as measured by Dartmouth COOP chart and safety evaluation based on analysis of unanticipated adverse effects.

The uterine measurements, recorded pre-treatment, demonstrated a mean uterine sound depth of 8.2 cm (range 6.5 mm to 10 cm) and width of endometrial stripe 2.7 cm (range 1.6–6.4 cm). Demographic data by race was similar in the patients randomised to both arms of the study. The position of the uterus at pre-treatment was also similar in both study arms.

Preliminary comparison of post-operative effectiveness comparisons for Cryoablation, and Rollerball (based on PBAC diary feedback at 12 months) demonstrates success in 87% of Cryoablation patients, 80% of Rollerball patients; and normal bleeding (less than or equal to PBAC of 100), 92% in Cryoablation patients, 87% Rollerball patients (Table 9.1).

The pre-treatment menstrual diary scores based on PBAC for Cryoablation demonstrated a mean of 588 (range 150–2913) and Rollerball demonstrated a mean of 468 (range 150–1880). A large reduction was noted in the post-treatment PRAC scores. Cryoablation demonstrated a mean of 30 (range 0–162), and Rollerball demonstrated a mean of 36 (range 0–460).

The study participants in both Cryoablation and Rollerball were similar in there pre-treatment scores for severe cramping, severe PMS, hematocrit and FSH. Post-treatment values showed similar improvements in hematocrit (pre-treatment 38.4%, post-treatment

Table 9.1 — The preliminary comparison of post-operative effectiveness comparison data in percentage at 12 months based on PBAC diary feedback

Measurement	Cryoblation (*n* = 58)	Rollerball (*n* = 23)
Amenorrhoea (0)	43	61
Amenorrhoea and spotting (0–15)	57	74
Hypomenorrhoea (16–75)	34	13
Eumenorrhoea (76–100)	2	0
Menorrhagia (100+)	7	13

40.7%) and FSH values. However, the post-treatment evaluation demonstrated two differences between the Cryoablation and Rollerball patients:

1. Significant reduction in severe menstrual pain/cramping in the Cryoablation patients (pre-treatment) 47%, post-treatment 2%), versus Rollerball patients (pre-treatment 43%, post-treatment 15%).

2. Significant reduction in severe PMS symptoms in the Cryoablation patients (pre-treatment 35%, post-treatment 3%), versus Rollerball patients (pre-treatment 34%, post-treatment 12%).

In summary, the clinical study has demonstrated a total procedure time (from set-up to completion) of 20 min. The procedure can be performed in an office or outpatient environment, no significant complications to date. Preliminary data indicates endometrial Cryoablation is safe and effective.

Complications and rate of adverse incidences

Two uterine perforations have occurred in the Cryoablation study (both during dilation and thus the procedures were not performed).

Costs

	US	ECU
First Option™ Console	$20,000	
Disposable Control Unit™	$650	

Conclusions

In summary, the clinical study has demonstrated a total procedure time (from set-up to completion) of 20 min. The procedure can be performed in an office or outpatient environment. No significant complications to date. Preliminary data indicates endometrial Cryoablation is safe and effective.

Advantages and disadvantages

Advantages	Disadvantages
Minimal anaesthesia required	Although it is FDA approved for destruction
No or minimal dilation required	of endometrial lining, it does not have the technical
May be used with distorted uterine	term 'endometrial ablation' attached to it. It is hoped
Cavity shape	this will be obtained
Time of procedure is 20 min	when the PMA is complete this year (2000)
May be used in an outpatient or office setting	

References

1. Pittrof P, Majid S, Murray A. Transcervical endometrial cryoablation (ECA) for menorrhagia. *Int J Gynaecol Obstet* 1994; 47(2): 135–140.

2. Rutherford TJ, Zreik TG, Troiano RN et al. Endometrial cryoablation, a minimally invasive procedure for abnormal uterine bleeding. *J Am Assoc Gynaecol Loparosc* 1998; 5(1): 23–28.

3. Dobak JD, Williams J, Howard R et al. *In vivo* uterine endometrial cryoablation with ultrasound visualisation (submitted for publication).

4. Indman PD. First Option cryoablation therapy. Presented at the *International Symposium of Diagnostic and Operative Hysteroscopy*. Free Communications Session II, February 25–27, 2000.

5. Onik G, Cooper C, Goldberg HI et al. Ultrasonic characteristics of frozen liver. *Cryobiology* 1984; 21: 321–328.

6. Onik GM, Cohen JK, Reyes GD et al. Transrectal ultrasound-guided percutaneous radical cryosurgical ablation of the prostate. *Cancer* 1993; 72(4): 1291–1299.

7. Onik GM, Atkinson D, Zemel R et al. Cryosurgery of liver cancer. *Semin Surg Oncol* 1993; 9(4): 309–317.

8. Lam C, Shimi S, Cuschieri A. Ultrasonic characterisation of hepatic cryolesions. *Arch Surg* 1995; 130: 1068–1072.

9. Smith JJ, Fraser J. An estimation of tissue damage and thermal history in the cryolesion. *Cryobiology* 1974; 11(2): 139–147.

10. Orpwood R. Biophysical and engineering aspects of cryosurgery. *Phys Med Biol* 1981; 26(4): 555–575.

11. Heppard M, Duleba A, Isaacson KB et al. Anaesthesia requirements — data from a multi-centre study using CryoGen First Option uterine cryoablation therapy in women with AVB. Syllabus for the *International Symposium of Diagnostic and Operative Hysteroscopy*. Free Communications — Session II, February 25–27, 2000.

10

Endometrial cryoablation

C. Kremer, J.F. Bodle and S.R.G. Duffy

Introduction

Endometrial ablation with a cryoprobe was one of the first methods of endometrial ablation to be described. In 1964, Cahan reported three patients who underwent hysterectomy shortly after endometrial ablation.[1] A further *in vivo* study by Droegenmuller showed that the endometrium could be entirely destroyed after a short freezing sequence without substantially damaging the myometrium.[2,3] The clinical application of this technique ceased temporarily after the publication of several reports on pelvic abscesses after cryosurgery.[4,5]

Cryoinjury is caused initially by the osmotic changes that follow the formation of extra-cellular ice.[6,7] The resulting damage is compounded by the effects of intra-cellular ice when freezing occurs rapidly.[8,9] Re-crystallisation during the thawing phase further aggravates physical disruption by allowing the development of large ice crystals.[6,10] Ultimately ischaemic changes complete the injury process.[11–13]

Until recently there was a significant lack of *in vitro* data relative to endometrial cryoablation. Little or no data on tissue temperatures had been obtained in early studies on endometrial cryoablation even though cell death can be seen in a wide range of temperatures when parameters are altered such as[14,15]

1. the number of freezes,
2. freezing rates,
3. thawing rates,
4. duration of freezing.

The extent of tissue damage obtained with cryosurgery was questioned by Waldron in 1981.[16] He postulated that only 0.5 mm of endometrial tissue could be destroyed by a probe with a tip temperature of −40°C to −50°C using a single freeze thaw sequence. This assumption was based on temperature readings in uteri perfused with near physiological fluid and the widely held theory that only tissue temperatures below −20°C are associated with cell death. However, no histological observations were provided to support this assumption and the thermometric evidence relied upon to make such extrapolations has been disputed.[17–20]

Tissue studies indicate that tissue destruction of at least 3 mm depth is required to ensure comprehensive destruction of the deep endometrial glands responsible for endometrial regeneration.[21] To produce this depth of tissue death a cryoprobe would have to form an ice ball where the temperature at 4 mm was sufficient to produce cell death whilst that at 10 mm (90th centile of endometrial and myometrial thickness)[22] would be

high enough so that adjacent structures were protected. The Endocryo™ system is designed to fulfil these criteria and to provide an application that is not only effective but also eminently safe.

Description

The Endocryo™

The Endocryo™ system (Spembly Medical Andover, UK) consists of three principal assemblies:

1. the service module,
2. the console with controls,
3. status indicators and the cryoprobe.

The service module (Fig. 10.1), measures 91 cm × 57 cm × 48 cm and houses three liquid withdrawal carbon dioxide (CO_2) cylinders together with a vaporiser. Carbon dioxide vapour is boiled off in the vaporiser (this achieves maximum endurance and probe performance) then supplied to the probe. The vaporised CO_2

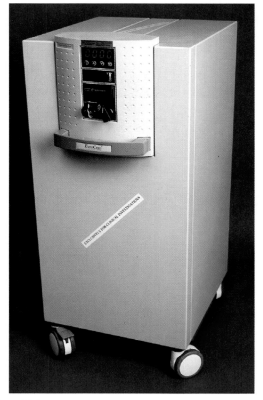

Figure 10.1

is regulated to 711 psi by a regulator and supplied to the probe via the gas socket.

The console provides a system capable of monitoring the probe temperature and controlling the CO_2 supply. Temperature is measured by a thermocouple situated in the probe tip. The display panel indicates tip temperature, freeze time and status of the unit (level of regulated pressure, thermocouple connection and possible probe fault).

The Endocryo™ probe (Fig. 10.2) consists of a 159 mm long stainless steel cylinder of 9 mm diameter with the tip of the probe curved similar to a Hegar dilator. Freezing occurs in the distal 6 cm, the inactive proximal part of the probe is insulated by an internal vacuum jacket to prevent injury to the vagina and cervix. The probe handle incorporates the freeze/defrost control.

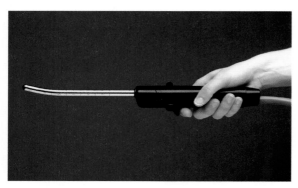

Figure 10.2

During freezing carbon dioxide vapour, under pressure, is forced through a minute orifice within the tip of the probe and expands. This expansion causes freezing of the probe (Joule Thompson principle) producing tip temperatures between −50°C and −55°C. Exhausted gas is vented through the probe connection and out of the system by means of a barbed connector situated at the rear of the service module. By activating the defrost mechanism the exhaust path is blocked and the pressure equalises either side of the Joule Thomson orifice to the regulated pressure of 711 psi. Consequently, there is no rapid expansion of gas into the tip chamber and the probe tip warms to body temperature. A syringe can be attached to the Luer lock at the rear of the handle to inject saline through the probe into the uterine cavity.

Practical aspects of treatment

The Endocryo™ is designed to perform optimally within uteri of normal size and shape. With its un-insulated distal end measuring 6 cm treatment of a cavity larger than 10 cm in length would result in a substantial area of endometrium being under treated. Also, it is not designed to treat endometrial polyps or submucous fibroids (although the latter is currently under investigation) therefore a patient with this type of endometrial lesion would be precluded from receiving cryoablation using the Endocryo™. Patients should be selected after outpatient diagnostic hysteroscopy,

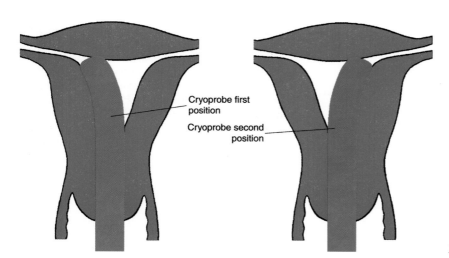

Cryoprobe first position

Cryoprobe second position

Figure 10.3

to rule out any intrauterine lesions and endometrial biopsy, to exclude endometrial pathology.

Treatment cycles are designed to produce adequate depth of endometrial and myometrial freezing without causing damage to adjacent structures. To facilitate this it is important to either prepare the endometrium with an appropriate thinning agent or time the procedure post menstruation.[23]

The Endocryo™ is simple and easy to use. It does not require the acquisition of complex hand eye co-ordination necessary to perform laser endometrial ablation. After dilatation of the cervix to Hegar number 9, the probe is inserted so that its tip is positioned in one cornua (Fig. 10.3). A single freeze thaw sequence is then applied. Once detached, the probe is withdrawn and the freeze thaw sequence repeated with the tip in the other cornua, thereby treating the whole uterine cavity. The optimal treatment cycles for the Endocryo™ are currently under investigation, however, we estimate treatment time will be in the region of 15–20 min.

In vitro and *in vivo* assessment of the Endocryo™

Results of in vitro *tissue studies*

Pittrof, using crude histological features of cell death, observed that in 5 out of 14 uteri there was incomplete destruction of the endometrium using an early prototype of the Endocryo™ (without CO_2 vaporiser) despite the injection of saline into the uterine cavity to enhance the contact between the probe and the endometrium.[24] Thermometric data relevant to these experiments has not been published. A single 5 min freeze thaw sequence was used.

Recently the cryolesion found in human uterine tissue has been described and quantified in a controlled laboratory setting. Using the Endocryo™, it has been determined which freezing and thawing parameters are important in producing an effective cryolesion *in vitro*. The impact of a distension medium in the development of a cryolesion has also been assessed.

Tissue injury

Initial experiments were performed in a purpose built jig on blocks of freshly excised uterine tissue from hysterectomy specimens. The Endocryo™ produces consistent tissue effects *in vitro*, a typical cryolesion comprising three distinct areas. At the endometrial end the tissue is necrosed and at the myometrial end it is entirely live. Between these two zones, there appears to be an area of sublethal damage.

The Endocryo™ produced 5 mm (SD 1.2) of cell death with a single 5 min freeze thaw cycle. Multiple freeze thaw cycles did not cause a significant increase in depth of cell death unless four cycles were repeated. The depth of cell death was not affected by the thawing rate.

The absence of direct contact between probe and endometrium had a pronounced effect on tissue temperatures during freezing and depth of cell death. An air gap of 1 mm between probe and endometrium resulted in no freezing temperature on the endometrial surface and no tissue damage. Using a distension medium, such as saline, between probe and endometrium could overcome a gap of 2 mm but no more. Morphometric studies of the uterine cavity showed, that whilst there is good contact between probe and endometrium at the internal ostium and lower 3 cm of the cavity, contact at the uterine cornu and central fundus is generally poor.

Thermometric studies

The mean temperature which produced cell death was $-16.1°C$ (SD 5.9, range $-2.4°C$ to $-30.8°C$). Factors that correlated with increasing depth of cell death were increased freezing rates ($p < 0.05$, $r = +0.35$), the minimum temperature reached ($p < 0.01$) and the length of time that tissue was subjected to that minimum temperature ($p < 0.01$, $r > +0.35$).

Summary

In summary, tissue damage is reproducible *in vitro* and can be increased by increasing the duration of freezing or by using 4 or more freeze thaw cycles. However, the latter is probably not clinically useful. An area of sublethal damage develops between the necrotic area and the live tissue. A mean tissue temperature of $-16°C$ will cause cell death in tissue blocks *in vitro*, however a temperature of $-30°C$ is required to ensure cell death. The presence of air between probe and endometrium renders the probe ineffective but can be overcome by the use of a distension medium in areas where this does not exceed 2 mm.

Results of in vivo *studies*

Pre-hysterectomy studies have been carried out in patients with a uterus of normal size and shape undergoing hysterectomy for dysfunctional uterine bleeding. No endometrial thinning agent was used. A 5 min freeze thaw sequence was applied to both sides of the uterus, as described above under 'practical aspects'.

Tissue injury

The mean depth of cell death produced by the Endocryo™ was 2.3 mm (SD 0.26) in the uterine body. The depth of tissue necrosis was not consistent throughout the uterine body, cornua and fundal regions due to varying degrees of contact between probe and endometrium.

Thermometric studies

The mean temperature which produced cell death was −7.14°C (SD 1.43, range −5.4°C to −9.8°C). The temperature at the cornual serosa and in the uterovesical pouch never dropped below +18°C.

Summary

In summary, the results of in vivo studies did not reflect those of in vitro experiments. Temperatures during the 5 min freeze thaw protocol were higher due to the ambient temperature of the uterus in vivo and the warming effect of circulating blood. Also, the temperatures required to produce cell death in vivo were not as low as those in vitro: −16.1°C (5.9) vs −7.14°C (1.43). Depth of cell death was less than that predicted by in vitro investigation. It appears that the Endocryo™ in its current form is unable to produce clinically effective endometrial ablation in vivo using a 5 min freeze thaw protocol.

Results of in vitro perfusion experiments

Results of in vivo testing demonstrated the need for a better in vitro model to enable development of clinically effective cryoablation. An in vitro uterine perfusion model was designed and built to do this. The aims were to simulate as closely as possible, in vivo temperature conditions including blood circulation.

The model consisted of a thermostatically controlled chamber warmed to 37°C in which the uterus was placed. After cannulation the uterus was perfused with warmed culture medium (also at 37°C) via a non-pulsatile pump, thereby mimicking the heat exchange properties of the uterine circulation.

Tissue injury

The Endocryo™ produced 1.57 mm (SD 1.0) of cell death in the uterine body with a single 5 min freeze thaw cycle. No cell death was seen in the cornual areas. Data from the Kamolocoff Smirnoff statistical test, when applied to in vivo and in vitro perfusion showed the depth of cell death to be the same.

Thermometric studies

The mean temperature which produced cell death was −7.43°C (SD 6.23, range −19°C to +3.6°C). The Kamolocoff Smirnoff statistical test when applied to in vivo and in vitro perfusion, showed the temperature data during freezing to be the same.

Summary

The uterine perfusion model described appears to be a good representation of in vivo conditions in terms of temperatures during freezing and the temperatures required to produce cell death. Depth of cell death was not significantly different from in vivo experiments. This model is currently being used to develop a clinical treatment protocol for the Endocryo™. There are also wider applications for its use in the development of other endometrial ablative devices.

Results of clinical studies

Sixty-seven women have been treated for menorrhagia with the Endocryo™.[25,26] A 5 min freeze thaw sequence was applied to each side of the uterus, as described above under 'practical aspects of treatment'. Normal saline was instilled into the uterus prior to each freeze cycle to improve contact between probe and endometrium. All patients had endometrial preparation with a thinning agent.

There were no surgical complications and operative blood loss was less than 5 ml. The only post-operative complications were transient urinary frequency, urgency and moderate pelvic pain. All but two patients were discharged within 24 h of surgery (they had undergone concomitant surgery: mini-laparotomy and pelvic floor repair). The main side effect was vaginal discharge due to endometrial sloughing which lasted up to 2 weeks.

Follow-up at 3 months found 64% of women were satisfied with the improvement in their menstrual loss, however none was amenorrhoeic. All patients had returned to normal social and sexual activities and there were no long term complications. Failure rates assessed by the hysterectomy rate at three to eighteen months follow-up were 32.8%. Results at 2 year follow-up indicated a disappointing 25% success rate (unpublished communication).

Costs

Capital costs are low with an initial set up, comprising one service module and three cryoprobes, in the region of £6000. Once purchased maintenance requirements and servicing are minimal. With a life span of around 10 years the Endocryo™ becomes a very cost effective capital investment. The major running cost of this equipment is the purchase of carbon dioxide gas cylinders. To undertake five procedures per week would require a change of gas cylinders approximately every 2 weeks costing around £2000 per year. The cryoprobes themselves are reusable and sterilisation between procedures using Cidex™, or a similar liquid, would incur minimal additional costs as most theatre complexes already have this capacity for other equipment.

If five patients were treated every week for 10 years, the cost per patient procedure would be £4 excluding sterilisation costs.

Conclusions

The Endocryo™ has reproducible tissue effects *in vitro* that theoretically would prevent endometrial regeneration clinically, however, these effects *in vivo* have been more difficult to reproduce. Initial *in vitro* testing did not take into account *in vivo* ambient temperatures or the blood circulation within the uterine wall, which would account, in part, for discrepancies between early *in vitro* and *in vivo* experimentation. The development of an *in vitro* perfusion model has largely overcome these problems and will allow an effective freeze thaw sequence to be established. However, poor contact between probe and endometrium in parts of the upper uterine body, cornua and mid fundus resulting in insufficient depth of cell death, remains a problem. The use of a distension medium may improve this in areas where the gap does not exceed 2 mm.

Despite these hurdles the uterus seems naturally suited for cryosurgical procedures. Its thick, vascular myometrium, theoretically, affords effective insulation against the excessive advance of freezing, thereby providing a margin of safety against inadvertent damage to neighbouring structures. Temperatures recorded at the fundal serosa, cornual serosa and uterovesical pouch during *in vivo* testing showed that cryoablation of the endometrium with the Endocryo™ is safe with a 5 min freezing sequence. Within the cervix there was tissue destruction right to the level of the external ostium. Although without risk (tissue necrosis did not exceed 5 mm) such an affect is unwanted because it would add significant discharge per vaginum in clinical practice.

The system itself is simple to use with little more than an on/off switch on the control panel and no complicated dials or readouts to interpret. The cryoprobe design has a familiar feel and shape and the procedure of cryoablation is no more difficult to perform than a dilatation and curettage. The low capital and maintenance costs of the Endocryo™ make the cost per procedure attractive from an economic viewpoint.

Although still under investigation, with the correct freeze thaw sequence, the Endocryo™ should produce amenorrhoea and patient satisfaction rates comparable with other second generation ablative devices. With the development of smaller diameter cryoprobes, this technique also has the potential for surgical treatment of menorrhagia in the outpatient setting. Perhaps its place will be that of a cheap first line surgical option for women with menorrhagia where its relative inability to produce amenorrhoea is offset by its cost, ease of performance and low complication rates.

Advantages and disadvantages of cryoablation

Advantages	Disadvantages
Low capital outlay maintenance and running costs	Only suitable for normal uteri
Familiar shape of device	Low amenorrhoea rates
Easy to perform	Destroys endometrium therefore no histological specimen
Good safety data	
Low complication rates in clinical trial	

Acknowledgements

The Endocryo™ is manufactured by Spembly Medical Ltd (an Integra company) who has sponsored our research.

References

1. Cahan WG. Cryosurgery of the uterus: description of technique and potential application. *Am J Obstet Gynecol* 1964; 88(3): 410–414.

2. Droegenmueller W, Greer BE, Makowski EL. Preliminary observations of cryocoagulation of the endometrium. *Am J Obstet Gynecol* 1970; 107(6): 958–961.

3. Droegenmueller W, Makowski EL, Macsalka R. Destruction of the endometrium by cryosurgery. *Am J Obstet Gynecol* 1971; 110(4): 467–469.

4. Burke L, Rubin HW, Kim I. Uterine abscess formation secondary to endometrial cryosurgery. *Obstet Gynecol Surv* 1972; 41(2): 224–226.

5. Cahan WG, Brockunier A. Cryosurgery of the uterine cavity. *Am J Obstet Gynecol* 1967; 99: 138–153.

6. Mazur P. Freezing of living cells: mechanisms and implications. *Am J Physiol* 1984; 247(3): 125–142.

7. Mazur P. Cryobiology: the freezing of biological systems. *Science* 1970; 168: 939–949.

8. Meryman HT, Platt WT. Mechanics of freezing in living cells and tissues. *Science* 1956; 124: 515–521.

9. Mazur P. A role of intracellular freezing in the death of cells cooled at supraoptimal rates. *Cryobiology* 1977; 14: 251–272.

10. Farrant J, Walter CA, Lee H, McGann LE. The use of two-step cooling procedures to examine factors influencing cell survival following freezing and thawing. *Cryobiology* 1977; 14: 273–286.

11. Albrektsson B, Branemark PI. Early micro vascular reactions to slow and rapid thawing of frozen tissue. *Adv Microcircul* 1969; 2: 37–68.

12. Kulka JP. Cold injury of the skin. The pathogenic rate of microcirculatory impairment. *Arch Environ Health* 1965; 11: 484–497.

13. Rubinsky B, Lee CY, Bastacky J, Onik G. The process of freezing and the mechanism of damage during hepatic cryosurgery. *Cryobiology* 1990; 27: 85–97.

14. Gage AA, Guest K, Montes M, Whalen DA, Caruana JA. Effect of varying freezing and thawing rates in experimental cryosurgery. *Cryobiology* 1985; 22(2): 175–182.

15. Neel H, DeSanto L. Cryosurgical control of cancer: effects of freeze rates, tumour temperatures and ischemia. *Ann Otol Rhinol Larygol* 1973; 82: 716–723.

16. Waldron HA. Investigation into the temperature field produced during endometrial cryosurgery of the perfused human uterus. *Phys Med Biol* 1980; 25: 323–331.

17. Gage AA. Experimental cryogenic injury of the palate: observations pertinent to cryosurgical destruction of tumours. *Cryobiology* 1978; 15: 415–425.

18. Gill W, Long W. A critical look at cryosurgery. *Int Surg* 1971; 56: 344–351.

19. Jacob G, Kurzer MN, Fuller BJ. An assessment of tumour cell viability after *in vitro* freezing. *Cryobiology* 1985; 22(417): 426.

20. Gage AA, Greene G, Neiders M, Emmings F. Freezing bone without excision: an experimental study of bone-cell destruction and manner of re-growth in dogs. *J Am Med Assoc* 1966; 196: 770–774.

21. Reid PCR. Nd:YAG laser ablation: *in vitro* and *in vivo* studies of laser–tissue interaction and therapeutic application. University of Manchester, 1989.

22. Duffy SRG. A study of the safety and application of electrosurgery in the treatment of refractory dysfunctional uterine bleeding. University College Cork, pp 124–148, 1993.

23. Sutton CJG, Ewen SP. Thinning of the endometrium prior to ablation: is it worthwhile? *Br J Obstet Gynecol* 1994; 101: 10–12.

24. Pittrof R, Majid S. Endometrial cryoablation using 0.9% saline as a uterine distension medium: a feasibility study. *Minimally Invasiv Ther* 1992; 1: 283–286.

25. Pittrof R, Majid S, Murray A. Initial experience with transcervical endometrial cryoablation of the endometrium using saline as a uterine distension medium. *Minimally Invasiv Ther* 1993; 337: 1074.

26. Pittrof R, Majid S, Murray A. Transcervical endometrial cryoablation (ECA) for menorrhagia. *Int J Gynecol Obstet* 1994; 47(2): 135–140.

11

ThermaChoice™ I: Balloon ablation

S.R. Watermeyer and N. Amso

Introduction

Uterine balloon ablation therapy provides a safe and simple alternative to hysterectomy or hysteroscopic techniques for the treatment of menorrhagia. There are essentially two uterine balloon ablative techniques described. These include devices utilising heated fluid within a balloon (ThermaChoice™, Gynecare, Ethicon Ltd., USA and Cavaterm™, Wallsten Medical SA, Switzerland) or electrodes mounted on the surface of the balloon (Vesta™, Valleylab, Colorado, USA). Within the confines of this chapter we will deal with ThermaChoice™.

ThermaChoice™ ablation system

The ThermaChoice™ uterine balloon ablation system was first described by Neuwirth et al.[1] It consists of a 16 cm long by 4.5 mm wide catheter with a latex balloon at its distal end that houses the heater element. Prior to the balloon catheter being primed and inserted, the patient who is placed in the lithotomy position is cleaned and draped. The uterus is sounded to gauge its depth and position. If the cervical os is very tight, then one can dilate to no more than Hegar 5. To do so would reduce the efficiency of the procedure since the possibility of the balloon herniating through the os is then increased. The catheter is then connected to a control unit that monitors, displays and controls pre-set intrauterine balloon pressure, temperature and duration of treatment. The balloon catheter is then primed by expelling all the air from the balloon itself by turning the tip of the catheter downwards and repeatedly injecting 5% dextrose into the balloon and aspirating air and fluid, whilst at the same time checking for any leaks within the system. It is very important to ensure that the catheter is connected to the control unit and that the control unit is turned on prior to priming. Failure to do this will result in abnormal pressure readings during the treatment cycle. At this point the catheter is ready for insertion. The catheter tip is lubricated with some normal saline and inserted through the cervix. The catheter is introduced into the uterus to the depth already determined by the uterine sound and then withdrawn by 0.5 cm to ensure that the heating element has no direct contact with the uterine wall.

When the balloon catheter has been correctly positioned, sterile 5% dextrose water is injected into the balloon until the intrauterine pressure stabilises between 160 and 180 mmHg. The fluid within the balloon is heated to approximately 87°C and the treatment automatically continues at that temperature for 8 min. For safety, the device automatically deactivates if the pressure or the temperature fluctuate below or above pre-set values. Once the treatment cycle is completed as indicated by the control unit, the balloon is deflated by aspirating the 5% dextrose. The catheter is then withdrawn from the uterine cavity.

Practical aspects of treatment

Inclusion criteria used in the authors' hospital for uterine endometrial ablation include women who have been diagnosed as a candidate for endometrial ablation or hysterectomy due to uncontrolled, excessive uterine bleeding related to benign endometrial pathology determined by endometrial biopsy taken within 6 months prior to the procedure. The patient must have an anatomically normal uterine cavity as determined by a transvaginal ultrasound scan (TVS) or hysteroscopy within 6 months of the procedure. The cavity depth must also sound to at least 4 cm but not greater than 10 cm. The woman must have had a normal smear within the previous 3 years. Finally, the patient must realise that her fertility is likely to be impaired but that endometrial ablation is not a method of contraception and she will require some method of birth control until the menopause. Exclusion criteria would include any patient with a pathology distorting the uterine cavity, with atypical endometrial hyperplasia, suspected genital infection or malignancy or a desire for preservation of fertility.

The method of pre-operative endometrial preparation remains undetermined. Some studies suggest a higher rate of amenorrhoea when a gonadotrophin release hormone analogue (GnRh-a) is used for endometrial thinning[2–4] whilst others[5] do not. It is hypothesised that the use of GnRh-a leads to a reduction in the vascular flow of the uterus, endometrial/myometrial atrophy and thus diminished regeneration post-operatively. Various studies are still ongoing including one by the author. Alternatively, the operation can be timed to coincide with the early part of the menstrual cycle after shedding of the endometrium. Various other endometrial preparation protocols have been tried with varying success, in particular dilatation and curettage, just prior to uterine balloon ablation that appears not to be helpful except to rule out occult malignancy. In fact, in one study,[2] women who had pre-operative dilatation and curettage experienced more treatment failures. It would therefore seem sensible to avoid this for the time being.

ThermaChoice™ balloon ablation therapy can be carried out either under general anaesthetic or local anaesthetic with or without sedation. Increasingly, the procedure is being carried out under local anaesthesia or conscious sedation.[2,6–9] Careful pre-operative assessment to determine the patient's tolerance of pain is essential. Pre-medication with non-steroid anti-inflammatory drugs given either orally or rectally to alleviate uterine pain is obligatory. Further non-steroidal anti-inflammatory drug should also routinely be given post-operatively. Intra-operative medication may include local injection of 1% lidocaine or bupivicane with or without epinephrine 1:100,000 and/or a combination of a rapid, short-acting opioid such as fentanyl and a benzodiazepine such as midazolam. The combination is given intravenously shortly before the operation to provide the required sedation and amnesiac effects of the former and the analgesic effects of the latter. A dedicated nurse should be available at the patient's bedside throughout the operation to reduce their anxiety and provide the necessary feedback to the clinician. The operation is usually well tolerated by the majority of patients and with a high satisfaction rate after 24 h.[7,9]

Concept, device development and safety

Measurement of serosal temperatures and depth of thermal injury generated by the ThermaChoice™ system was studied both in *ex vivo* and *in vivo* uteri.[10,11] *In vivo* serosal temperatures from 12 anatomic locations did not exceed 39.9°C with a mean of 36.1°C. Histological examination revealed deep endometrial and superficial myometrial damage to all areas. The greatest depth of myometrial injury occurred in the midfundus (3.4 mm).[11] By electron microscopy, no thermal effect could be demonstrated in the myometrium beyond 15 mm from the endometrial surface following up to 16 min of therapy.[11]

It would appear that the uterine balloon pressure used influences the outcome of treatment. In one study[12] 116 patients underwent uterine balloon ablation. The starting pressure was 80–140 mmHg in the first 13 women, and greater than 140 mmHg in all the rest. At 6 months follow-up persistent menorrhagia was reported by 38% of patients treated with pressures less than 140 mmHg and 12% by women treated with pressures greater than 140 mmHg. Furthermore, the

same study analysed outcome results between women treated for 8 min and women treated for 12 min. They reported no difference and concluded that uterine balloon therapy is a safe and effective treatment for menorrhagia at uterine pressures of 150–180 mmHg and of 8 min duration.

Follow-up is usually undertaken at 3, 6 and 12 months post-uterine balloon ablation. It is probably important to monitor outcome for up to 1 year to ensure no regeneration of endometrial tissue. Follow-up undertaken should include status not only with regard to menorrhagia, eumenorrhoea, and amenorrhoea but also patient satisfaction and dysmenorrhoea if applicable. A number of studies have reported on the outcome following this treatment.[2,6,13] In a large observational multi-centre study,[2] treatment led to a significant reduction in the severity and duration of menstrual flow and dysmenorrhoea with 15% amenorrhoea at 12 months. Overall, it was successful in 88% of women who reverted to eumenorrhoea or less. Increasing age, higher balloon pressure, smaller uterine cavity and a lesser degree of pre-procedure menorrhagia were associated with significantly improved results.

In a randomised study comparing ThermaChoice™ endometrial ablation with rollerball ablation,[6] no operative complications occurred with balloon therapy whilst two cases of fluid overload, one uterine perforation and one case of cervical laceration occurred in the rollerball group (3.2% of cases). One-year follow-up data did not show any significant difference between the two groups in:

1. percentage of women whose diary score decreased by 90% or less;
2. patients highly satisfied (balloon 85.6% vs rollerball 86.7%);
3. impact of treatment on quality of life;
4. dysmenorrhoea scores.

However, a greater percentage of women in the rollerball were amenorrhoeic at 12 months (27% vs 15%, $p < 0.05$). In the balloon group more procedures were carried out under sedation or local anaesthesia (47% vs 16%) and the mean operating time was significantly shorter in the balloon group (27.4 vs 39.6 min). In 71% of cases the procedure was completed in 30 min, or less, compared with 28.6% in the rollerball group ($p < 0.05$). In another recent study,[14] 147 women were treated by two experienced gynaecological surgeons. One performed 73 thermal balloon ablations and the other 74 endometrial resections between November 1994 and April 1998. The inclusion criteria were the same in both groups. When the balloon technique was utilised the operating time was significantly reduced. There were no intra-operative complications in either group and the morbidity, post-operatively, was not statistically different between the two techniques and was minimal. The overall success rate did not differ significantly between the two groups 83 ± 5% for balloon ablation and 76 ± 6% for endometrial resection. Certainly balloon ablation appeared much easier to use and therefore more widely applicable and safer. The requirement for further surgery, whether this constitutes a repeat ablation procedure or hysterectomy, appears to vary from about 10% to 20% depending on the study quoted.

Complications of uterine balloon ablation

It would appear from the published data that the incidence of intra-operative complications appears to be very low and compares favourably to hysteroscopic techniques of endometrial ablation or hysterectomy. The procedure of uterine balloon ablation may pose some rare, but possible, safety risks including blood loss, heat or electrical burns of the internal organs, perforation or rupture of the wall of the uterus, or leakage of heated fluid from the balloon into the cervix or vagina. In addition, the collection of blood or tissue in the uterus, and/ or fallopian tubes, during the months post-procedure is also possible and may require an outpatient procedure to correct the problem. As with any type of uterine procedure, there may also be the risk of infection, usually easily managed with oral antibiotic therapy. Post-operative and intra-operative morbidity appears to be minimal. In a large observational multi-centre study[2] involving 296 procedures, no intra-operative complications were reported and there was minimal post-operative morbidity. One woman developed a post-operative cystitis, six others developed febrile morbidity of unproven aetiology that were treated empirically as endometritis and resolved with a standard course of antibiotics. Two women had haematometra that was successfully treated with uterine sounding. Finally, one woman was hospitalised for pain which responded well to analgesics and resolved within 24 h. Therefore overall, there were no major complications and a minor complication rate of 3%. In another large study,[6] there was again no intra-operative complications with uterine balloon ablation as compared to a 3.2% rate of complications in patients undergoing hysteroscopic rollerball surgery. Post-operative complications can include cystitis (0.8%), endometritis (2.6%), haematometra (1.7%) seen in a group of 116 patients undergoing balloon ablation in a Canadian study.[12] Probably the most common post-operative complication is pelvic cramp-like discomfort that usually settles with a simple analgesic. In addition, women may experience a profuse watery discharge for anything up to 2-week post-ablation.

Factors influencing efficacy

As already mentioned some studies suggest a higher rate of amenorrhoea when a GnRh-a is used for endometrial thinning prior to conventional endometrial resection[3] or balloon endometrial ablation.[2,4] Improved efficacy is also achieved using greater balloon pressures as previously demonstrated by Vilos et al[12] where pressure values suggested a minimum of 140 mmHg were required for success. It is accepted that older women generally have better results from all types of endometrial ablation and this appears to be true for uterine balloon ablation.[2,13] Reduced outcome success was associated with larger uterine cavity volumes, greater levels of pre-procedure pain and bleeding, and, finally, dilatation and curettage just prior to the procedure.[2] Although some studies have suggested that uterine position has no effect on outcome,[13] others have suggested an association between anteverted uteri and higher success rates.[2] The senior author of this chapter has carried out intra- and post-operative ultrasound scans on women having uterine balloon therapy. During the balloon ablation, a transvaginal ultrasound probe was placed transrectally and images recorded on a Panasonic VCR. In the case of the retroverted uterus, the catheter's position may be much closer to the anterior wall and exposure of the posterior uterine wall does not appear as marked.

Subsequent 6-month follow-up of the same patient showed a thickened endometrium on the posterior uterine wall measuring 12 mm and an extremely thin endometrium on the anterior wall. This clearly demonstrates the effect of the proximity of the heater element to either wall on the eventual effect and this clearly has implications for the treatment of women with a retroverted uterus.

Relative costs

At the present time NHS budgets are being heavily scrutinised. Health Service Managers as well as organisations such as 'The National Institute for Clinical Excellence' (NICE) are trying to ensure cost effectiveness and value for money with regard to various treatment options offered by the NHS. It is, therefore, entirely appropriate to consider any financial implications of this relatively new treatment. The initial outlay for the ThermaChoice™ control unit is £4000 inclusive of VAT. The catheters, which are disposable, cost at present £325 each inclusive of VAT. ThermaChoice™ uterine balloon ablation can be carried out either as an outpatient or as a day case procedure. We have estimated that after taking into account various theatre costs such as consumables, equipment, staff costs, anaesthetics and overheads, ThermaChoice™ costs approximately £500–550 per patient depending whether it is carried out as an outpatient or as a day case procedure. It has been estimated[15] that the mean cost of transcervical endometrial resection is £560 although this figure did include hotel costs for 2 days. The inpatient hotel costs were estimated at £113 per day. This study was published in 1993 and, in most cases, the present-day practice is to carry out endometrial resection as a day case therefore reducing the overall amount to approximately £330. Although this appears to be significantly cheaper than balloon ablation, the latter is much easier to learn and can, therefore, be carried out by more junior staff. Additionally, complications including perforation and fluid overload are unheard of with balloon ablation. The cost of treatment of complications, therefore, also needs to be taken into account. The same study[15] also estimated the mean cost of Abdominal Hysterectomy (AH) at £1059, the major component of which was the 'hotel' inpatient component. Whilst this appears expensive, one must also remember that 10–20% of ablation procedures will have an unsuccessful outcome and this means that the procedure either needs to be repeated or the patient will require a hysterectomy. Hence in some cases, the more expensive option in the short term may in fact be cheaper in the longer term. Finally, it is important to remember that one needs to consider more than just health care costs. Balloon ablation or endometrial resection enables women to return to normal functioning, be it occupational or social, more rapidly than with a hysterectomy. The economic and social consequences of this are impossible to measure.

Conclusion

By the age of 55 years, 20% of British women would have had a hysterectomy with menorrhagia being the indication in 35–64% of cases.[16] Menorrhagia represents an enormous challenge to the medical establishment, not to mention a considerable drain on financial resources. Pharmacological treatment of this condition is limited and dilatation and curettage often provides relief for only the first few subsequent cycles. Surgical options include hysterectomy and various forms of endometrial ablation. Current research demonstrates that thermal uterine balloon ablation is the safest of these options and has resulted in successful reduction in menstrual flow in 70–90% of patients treated.[17] Furthermore, not only does it have a favourable efficacy and complication profile, it is also cost effective, can be done as an outpatient procedure and is a very simple operation to teach and learn.

References

1. Neuwirth RS, Duran AA, Singer A, Macdonald R, Buldoc L. The endometrial ablator: a new instrument. *Obstet Gynecol* 1994; 83: 792–796.

2. Amso NN, Stabinsky SA, McFaul P, Blanc B, Pendley L, Neuwirth R. Uterine thermal balloon therapy for the treatment of menorrhagia: the first 300 patients from a multi-centre study. International Collaborative Uterine Thermal Balloon Working Group. *Br J Obstet Gynaecol* 1998; 105: 517–523.

3. Donnez J, Vilos G, Gannon MJ, Stampe-Sorensen S, Klinte I, Miller RM. Goserelin acetate (Zoladex) plus endometrial ablation for dysfunctional uterine bleeding: a large randomised, double-blind study. *Fertil Steril* 1997; 68(1): 29–36.

4. Schaffer M. Endometrial ablation with a thermal balloon system for the treatment of menstrual disorders. Presented at the *6th Annual Congress of the European Society for Gynaecological Endoscopy*, Birmingham, UK, 7–10 December 1997.

5. Lissak A, Fruchter O, Mashiach S, Brandes-Klein O, Sharon A, Kogan O, Abramobici H. Immediate versus delayed treatment of perimenopausal bleeding due to benign causes by balloon thermal ablation. *J Am Assoc Gynecol Laparosc* 1999; 6(2): 145–150.

6. Meyer WR, Walsh BW, Grainger DA, Peacock LM, Loffer FD, Steege JF. Thermal balloon and rollerball ablation to treat menorrhagia: a multicentre comparison. *Obstet Gynecol* 1998; 92(1): 98–103.

7. Fortin C, McColl MB. Gynecare UBT system under local anaesthesia. *Am Assoc Gynecol Laparosc* 1996; 3(Suppl 4): S13.

8. Fernandez H, Capella S, Audibert F. Uterine Thermal balloon therapy under local anaesthesia for the treatment of menorrhagia: a pilot study. *Hum Reprod* 1997; 12(11): 2511–2514.

9. Amso NN, Abramovich, Cullimore J, Parker M, Stabinsky S. Uterine balloon therapy under local analgesia: a feasibility study. Presented at *7th Annual Meeting of the International Society of Gynaecologic Endoscopy*, Sun City, South Africa, 15–18 March 1998.

10. Shah AA, Stabinsky SA, Klusak T, Bradley KR, Steege JF, Grainger DA. Measurement of serosal temperatures and depth of thermal injury generated by thermal balloon endometrial ablation in *ex vivo* and *in vivo* models. *Fertil Steril* 1998; 70: 692–697.

11. Anderson LF, Meinert L, Rygaard C, Junge J, Prento P, Ottesen BS. Thermal balloon endometrial ablation: safety aspects evaluated by serosal temperature, light microscopy and electron microscopy. *Eur J Obstet Gynecol Reprod Biol* 1998; 79: 63–68.

12. Vilos GA, Fortin C, Sanders B, Pendley L, McColl M. Uterine balloon therapy for the treatment of menorrhagia. *J Am Assoc Gynecol Laparosc* 1996; 3(Suppl 4): S54.

13. Vilos GA, Fortin CA, Sanders BA, Pendley L, Stabinsky SA. Clinical trial of the uterine thermal balloon for the treatment of menorrhagia. *J Am Assoc Gynecol Laparosc* 1997; 3(3): 383–387.

14. Gervaise A, Fernandez H, Capella-Allouc S, Taylor S, Vieille SL, Hamou J, Gomel V. Thermal balloon ablation versus endometrial resection for the treatment of abnormal uterine bleeding. *Hum Reprod* 1999; 14(11): 2743–2747.

15. Sculpher MJ, Bryan S, Dwyer N, Hutton J, Stirrat GM. An economic evaluation of transcervical endometrial resection versus abdominal hysterectomy for the treatment of menorrhagia. *Br J Obstet Gynaecol* 1993; 100: 244–252.

16. Vessey MP, Villard-Mackintosh L, McPherson K, Coulter A, Yates D. The epidemiology of hysterectomy: findings in a large cohort study. *Br J Obstet Gynaecol* 1992; 99: 402–407.

17. Barrow C. Balloon endometrial ablation as a safe alternative to hysterectomy. *AORN J* 1999; 70(1): 80, 83–86, 89–90.

12

ThermaChoice™ II: Balloon ablation

George A. Vilos and David A. Grainger

Introduction

Dysfunctional uterine bleeding (DUB) is defined as endometrial bleeding unrelated to anatomic lesions in the pelvis or systemic diseases and can be due to both ovulatory and anovulatory abnormalities. The consequences of DUB are excessive menstrual blood loss (menorrhagia, polymenorrhea) which is often a serious, embarrassing and debilitating condition for many women and together with uterine fibroids account for up to 75% of all hysterectomies performed worldwide.[1,2]

Hysterectomy is the most frequently performed major gynaecologic operation.[1,2] It is a major surgical procedure associated with a mortality rate of 0.6–1.1 per 1000 and morbidity of up to 40%.[3,4] The financial loss to the patient, the employer and the health care systems can only be estimated. Although self-reported outcomes of hysterectomy have revealed high levels of patient satisfaction, comparisons to alternative therapies have not been reported.[5]

In order to address the high and variable hysterectomy rates, alternative therapies for menorrhagia have been introduced including medical treatment and endometrial ablation procedures.

Endometrial ablation is the destruction or elimination of the endometrium by coagulation, freezing or resection and offered as an alternative to hysterectomy to those patients with DUB and benign pathology who are unable or unwilling to tolerate traditional therapies.

Although hysteroscopic endometrial ablation has been shown to be effective,[6–9] it is associated with reduced morbidity, mortality, hospitalisation and convalescence and health care costs compared with hysterectomy.[10,11] It requires additional training and surgical expertise, excessive non-physiologic solutions to distend the uterus, and energy sources with their inherent hazards and complications.[12] Its general application has, therefore, been reluctantly accepted because many surgeons find the procedure and the energy sources intimidating.

ThermaChoice I (Non-circulating Fluid, Latex Balloon, Gynecare, Menlo Park, CA)

To overcome these potential risks and complications, the hot water balloon endometrial ablation was developed and introduced by Dr Neuwirth in 1994.[13]

Preliminary results on 18 patients were published in 1994 by Singer et al[14] and the first pilot study on 30 patients was performed in June/July 1994 when the pressure and time of treatment were established by Vilos et al.[15]

The results from a Canadian Clinical Trial,[16] an International Clinical Trial[17] and a Food and Drug Administration (FDA) approved United States study comparing the ThermaChoice versus Rollerball[18,19] are consistent. The efficacy of the ThermaChoice is equivalent to the rollerball hysteroscopic endometrial ablation with an overall success rate of 85%. The ThermaChoice balloon catheter requires skills equivalent to those of inserting an intrauterine device. It is simple, safe and effective with no serious complications in over 40,000 procedures performed worldwide to date.[20–24]

During the initial pilot study, it was observed that the energy distribution within the balloon and the uterine cavity was non-uniform and gravity dependent. Using thermographic pictures in vitro and real time ultrasonic scanning during treatment in vivo, it was shown that heat tended to concentrate in the uppermost section of the uterine cavity. It was confirmed hysteroscopically post-balloon ablation that the uppermost areas of the uterus was better coagulated than the bottom ones. It was thought that this non-uniform distribution of the heat energy within the uterine cavity may have been responsible for the low amenorrhea rate following the ThermaChoice I balloon therapy.

ThermaChoice II (Circulating Fluid Silicon Balloons, Gynecare, Menlo Park, CA)

The ThermaChoice II system also consists of a 16 cm long by 5 mm diameter catheter with a tear-shaped silicon balloon attached to its distal end housing the heating element, temperature sensors and impeller fan raising the temperature to 87°C (186°F) and evenly circulating fluid within the silicon balloon. The other end of the catheter allows for inflation of the balloon and connects to a controller unit and monitors and controls preset intraballoon temperature, pressure and duration of treatment. In addition, the catheter contains a wire which is connected to a motor system within the controller that turns the impeller inside the balloon (Fig. 12.1).

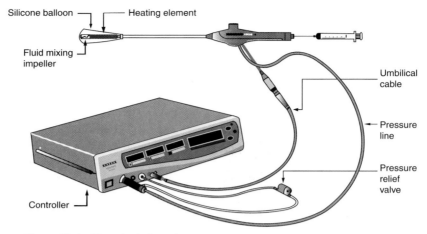

Figure 12.1 — Gynecare ThermaChoice II: uterine balloon therapy system.

The balloon catheter is first tested for leaks and the system is primed by inflating it with 30 ml of five dextrose in water (D5W) and deflating it to 180 mmHg negative pressure to remove any air. Subsequently, the balloon is inserted transcervically without hysteroscopic visualisation. The balloon is inflated with D5W slowly to a pressure of 180 mmHg. Once the pressure is confirmed to be stable, by waiting for a few seconds, the heating element and the impeller are activated which circulate and maintain the intraballoon D5W solution at 87° ± 5°. An effective therapy has been determined to be 8 min. The heating element automatically deactivates if preset parameters are exceeded. Safety features are built into the device to deflate the balloon if the temperature rises too high or to cool the liquid if the pressure exceeds a threshold of 200 mmHg. When the controller signals that treatment is completed, the balloon is deflated and the catheter is withdrawn and discarded.

Validation of ThermaChoice II

In vitro studies

Thermographic pictures confirmed uniform distribution of the heat energy within the silicon balloon compared to latex balloon which showed cold areas at the bottom of the fluid.

Studies on extirpated uteri

Grainger et al demonstrated in extirpated human uteri that the depth of tissue necrosis was consistent to a depth of 4 mm of myometrium except the cornua which extended only for 1 cm into the myometrium. Figure 12.2 indicated that the endomyometrial necrosis

was uniform throughout the uterine cavity with the ThermaChoice II (V2.0) compared to ThermaChoice I (V1.2).

Clinical trial

Vilos et al initiated a pilot clinical trial in June of 1998 to evaluate two endometrial thinning modalities prior to the treatment with the new ThermaChoice II uterine balloon therapy system.

The primary objectives were to compare the reduction of menstrual blood loss in two groups of premenopausal women with DUB randomised into endometrial thinning via either pre-operative suction curettage or a gonadotrophin releasing analogue (GnRHa, goserelin 3.6 mg sc, Zeneca Pharma) approximately 4 weeks prior to surgery.

The secondary objective was to compare the rate of menstrual bleeding to ThermaChoice I from previous studies (historical control).

Patient study design

After informed consent and IRB approval, 105 patients who met inclusion and exclusion criteria were randomised into suction curettage or GnRHa pre-treatment. Inclusion criteria required a patient's Higham menstrual score of >150, 1–2 months prior to surgery. Higham diary scores were validated pre- and post-procedure at 3, 6 and 12 months. The patient entry characteristics included the average age (41.0 years) and mean baseline Higham scores (407.5) in the GnRHa group and 40.5 years and 450.7 in the suction curettage group.

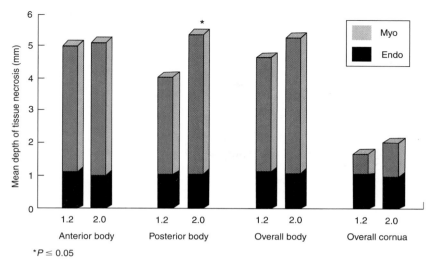

*P ≤ 0.05

Figure 12.2 — Depth of tissue necrosis results, mean overall depth of tissue necrosis comprised of endometrial and myometrial necrosis. (David A. Grainger, MD; Thomas R. Kluzak, MD; George A. Vilos, MD; Scott Ciarrocca and Thomas A. Barbolt, PhD; Thermal efficacy of V2.0 ThermaChoice II uterine balloon therapy catheter in extirpated human uteri.)

ThermaChoice II treatment was performed in 102 patients. Preliminary post-operative Higham scores at 3, 6 and 12 months consistently showed a reduction of menstrual blood loss up to 90% with mean Higham scores of 25 vs 32 in the GnRH and suction curettage groups, respectively. Patient satisfaction was reported to be up to 95% in both groups.

Compared to historical control, the post-operative Higham score of ThermaChoice I was 65 and reduction of menstrual bleeding was 84%.

Conclusions

The *in vitro* studies by Grainger et al demonstrated that fluid circulation within the silicone balloon provide more uniform and greater tissue necrosis compared to ThermaChoice I.

The preliminary clinical results indicate a substantial reduction in menstrual bleeding (up to 90%) compared to pre-procedure levels.

Summary

Advantages

The ThermaChoice II UBT is quick, simple and easy to use requiring similar skills to those of inserting an intrauterine device. The cannula is small and flexible

requiring no cervical dilatation and minimal analgesia/anaesthesia. It can be performed outside an operating room in an office/clinic setting. Silicon balloon material minimises the risk of adverse reactions for patients with latex sensitivity.

References

1. Bachmann GA. Hysterectomy. A critical review. *J Reprod Med* 1990; 35: 839–862.

2. Carlson KJ, Nichols DH, Schiff I. Indication for hysterectomy. *N Eng J Med* 1993; 83: 792–796.

3. Wingo PA, Huezocm, Rubin GL, Ory HW, Peterson HB. The mortality risk associated with hysterectomy. *Am J Obstet Gynecol* 1985; 152: 803–808.

4. Boyd ME, Groome PA. The morbidity of abdominal hysterectomy. *Can J Surg* 1993; 36: 155–59.

5. Dicker RC, Greenspan JR, Strauss CT et al. Complications of abdominal and vaginal hysterectomy among women of reproductive age in the United States. *Am J Obstet Gynecol* 1982; 144: 841–848.

6. Garry R, Shelley-Jones D, Mooney P, Phillips G. Six hundred endometrial laser ablations. *Obstet Gynecol* 1995; 85: 24–29.

7. Baggish MS, Eddie HM. Endometrial ablation. A series of 568 patients treated over an 11 year period. *Am J Obstet Gynecol* 1996; 174: 908–913.

8. O'Connor H, Magos A. Endometrial resection for the treatment of menorrhagia. *N Eng J Med* 1996; 335: 151–156.

9. Martyn P, Allan B. Long-term follow up of endometrial ablation. *J Am Assoc Gynecol Laparosc* 1998; 5: 115–118.

10. Vilos GA, Vilos EC, King JH. Experience with 800 hysteroscopic endometrial ablations. *J Am Assoc Gynecol Laparosc* 1996; 4: 33–38.

11. Vilos GA, Pispidikis JA, Botz CK. Economic evaluation of hysteroscopic endometrial ablation versus vaginal hysterectomy for menorrhagia. *Obstet Gynecol* 1996; 88: 241–245.

12. Vilos GA, Brown S, Graham G, McCulloch S, Borg P. Genital tract electrical burns during hysteroscopic endometrial ablation: Report of 13 cases in the United States and Canada. *J Am Assoc Gynecol Laparosc* 2000; 7: 141–147.

13. Neuwirth RS, Duran M, Singer et al. The endometrial ablator: a new instrument. *Obstet Gynecol* 1994; 83: 792–796.

14. Singer A, Almanza R, Gutienrez A et al. Preliminary clinical experience with a thermal balloon endometrial ablation method to treat menorrhagia. *Obstet Gynecol* 1994; 83: 732–734.

15. Vilos GA, Vilos EC, Pendley L. Endometrial ablation with a thermal balloon for the treatment of menorrhagia. *J Am Assoc Gynecol Laparosc* 1996; 3: 383–387.

16. Vilos GA, Fortin CA, Sanders B, Pendley L, Stabinsky SA. Clinical trial of the uterine thermal balloon for treatment of menorrhagia. *J Am Assoc Gynecol Laparosc* 1997; 4: 559–565.

17. Amso NN, Stabinsky SA, McFaul P, Blanc B, Pendley L, Neuwirth R. Uterine thermal ballon therapy for the treatment of menorrhagia. The first 300 patients from a multicentre study. International collaborative uterine thermal balloon working group. *Br J Obstet Gynecol* 1998; 105: 517–523.

18. Meyer WR, Walsh BW, Grainger DA, Peacock LM, Loffer F, Steege JF. Thermal balloon and rollerball ablation to treat menorrhagia. A multicentre comparison. *Obstet Gynecol* 1998; 92: 98–103.

19. Grainger DA, Tjaden BL, Meyer WR et al. Thermal balloon and rollerball ablation to treat menorrhagia: two-year results from a multicentre prospective randomized clinical trial. *J Am Assoc Gynecol Laparosc* (accepted).

20. Fernandez H, Capella S, Audibert F. Uterine thermal balloon therapy under local anesthesia for the treatment of menorrhagia: a pilot study. *Hum Reprod* 1997; 12: 2511–2514.

21. Lissak A, Fruchter O, Mashiach S et al. Immediate versus delayed treatment of perimenopausal bleeding due to benign causes by balloon thermal ablation. *J Am Assoc Gynecol Laparosc* 1999; 6: 145–150.

22. London R, Holzman M, Rubin D, Moffitt B. Payer costs savings with endometrial ablation therapy. *Am J Managed Care* 1999; 5: 889–897.

23. Aletebi FA, Vilos GA, Eskandar MA. Thermal balloon endometrial ablation to treat menorrhagia in high risk surgical candidates. *J Am Assoc Gynecol Laparsc* 1999; 4: 435–439.

24. Aletebi FA, Vilos GA, Eskandar MA. Endometrial thermal balloon ablation (ThermaChoice) to treat menorrhagia: effects of intrauterine pressure and duration of treatment. *J Am Assoc Gynecol Laparosc* (accepted, July 2000).

13

Cavaterm™ thermal balloon ablation

Jed Hawe, Jason Abbott and Ray Garry

Summary

Dysfunctional uterine bleeding is one of the commonest reasons for referral to gynaecology departments. Treatment options include hysterectomy and more recently endometrial ablation and resection techniques. These are associated with a lengthy learning curve and are not without risks. Newer techniques are now available which aim to reduce the learning curve and associated risks without compromising the clinical effect. One of these second-generation devices is the Cavaterm™ thermal balloon system which has been in clinical use since May 1993. We would like to, through this chapter, describe the system, its clinical use and provide a review of the available literature.

Introduction

Menorrhagia is one of the most common clinical problems encountered by gynaecologists. Five percent of women between the ages of 34 and 49 years consult their GP with this problem, and it represents 12% of all gynaecological referrals.[1] When medical therapy fails, women have traditionally undergone hysterectomy. Since the mid-1980s, endometrial ablation and resection techniques have been introduced and have gained popularity for their ability to successfully treat menstrual problems without the need for hysterectomy.[2-3] These techniques have been carefully evaluated with:

- large observational studies,
- long-term follow-up,
- randomised controlled trials,[4-6]
- a national audit.[7]

These confirm the safety and efficacy of these techniques. Despite this well-documented efficacy, 50% of the 70,000 hysterectomies performed each year in the UK are still performed for menorrhagia.

Data from the MISTLETOE study indicated that most doctors who performed hysteroscopic surgery for menorrhagia only did so infrequently. Sixty per cent of the 690 doctors who took part in the study performed less than 10 cases in the 18-month data collection period.[7] Primarily, to meet the needs of this large group of infrequent hysteroscopists, there are now a number of second-generation ablation devices being developed.

One such system is the Cavaterm™ thermal balloon. Hans Wallsten, a Swedish engineer and inventor developed the Cavaterm™ thermal balloon ablation system in the late 1980s. Prior to developing the Cavaterm™ system, Hans Wallsten was known in the medical field for the development of the Wallstent™ and UroLume™, which are medical stents for use in the coronary arteries, biliary tree, prostate and oesophagus.

The aim of the Cavaterm™ system was to simplify endometrial ablation without compromising clinical effect, thereby making endometrial ablation more widely available to both gynaecologists and patients alike. The first procedures were performed on extirpated uteri in 1992. The first clinical application was performed in Sweden in May 1993. The first 60 patients were treated for 30 min. Since 1995, all patients have been treated for 15 min, with two-thirds being performed under general anaesthetic.

Currently, more than 300 hospitals in Europe are using the Cavaterm™ system with more than 10,000 patients being treated. Despite these large numbers, there remains a paucity of publications in peer review journals evaluating the ease of use, efficacy and safety of the device. Most of the available data is in abstract form following presentations at International meetings. The aim of this chapter is to describe the system, its safety features, clinical applications and results from the literature available.

The Cavaterm™ system

The system comprises of two major components; a central computerised unit (Fig. 13.1) and a disposable catheter (Fig. 13.2). Neuwith et al described the first balloon system (ThermaChoice™) in the literature in 1994.[8] The Cavaterm™ system differs from this system in a number of ways; a battery powered central unit, heating system within the balloon catheter, a silicone rather than latex balloon, an adjustable balloon and a circulation system.

The central unit has four main functions: power supply, fluid circulation, operator's keyboard and treatment monitoring. The unit measures $420 \times 320 \times 95$ mm and weighs 6 kg without batteries. The power supply to the heating elements comes from a 24 V-lead/acid-gel battery source. This form of battery is reliable, can be recharged at any time and used for numerous treatment cycles. Each battery lasts for a maximum of 3 h at normal treatment and takes 4–5 h to recharge. There is also an internal 12 V battery that protects the data stored in the central unit, should the battery run flat during a case. The battery can be changed in these situations without loss of treatment data. There is a current

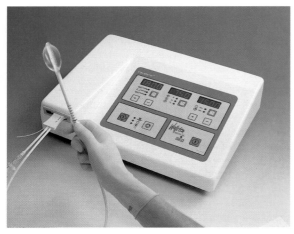

Figure 13.1 — Central computerised unit.

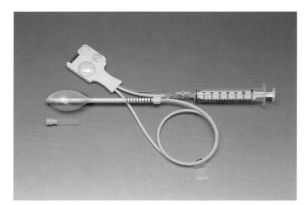

Figure 13.2 — Disposable catheter.

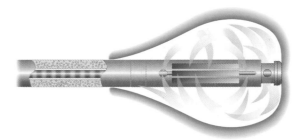

Figure 13.3 — Circulation of fluid and heat distribution within the balloon.

limiter set to 4 A which allows a maximum heating power of 100 W to enable fast heating of the fluid within the balloon, and ensures safety. The central unit also allows the operator to monitor time, temperature and balloon pressure throughout the case.

The central unit generates pulses through the liquid in the generator, which with the help of a back-valve system, leads to a vigorous circulation of the fluid within the balloon. Circulation is required to ensure a flow of fluid from the heating elements in the centre of the balloon and provide a uniform heat distribution on the balloon surface. The heating element operates at 80°C, but the balloon surface temperature is 75°C indicating a thermal gradient of 5°C despite fluid circulation (Fig. 13.3). Experiments have shown that

in the absence of circulation, this gradient may be as much as 18°C, which could lead to areas of sub-optimal treatment.[9]

The disposable catheter is 8 mm in diameter with the balloon made of silicone. Silicone was chosen as it has the ability to conform to the shape of the cavity and remains flexible and strong even when heated. The other advantage is that silicone is hypoallergenic. The unique feature of this balloon system is that it is adjustable in length, which ensures that the balloon can adapt to individual cavity sizes and at the same time protects the cervical canal from heat damage (Fig. 13.4). It can be used to treat inter-cavity (total length minus cervical length) lengths of 4–10 cm. The system uses 1.5% glycine to distend the balloon. The maximum volume that can be used is 30 ml and the volume required is pressure dependent. The eruptive volume of the balloon is 300 ml. A second-generation catheter has recently been developed and is undergoing evaluation in the clinical setting. The measuring device for the balloon length has been simplified and the shape of the balloon is now 'heart-shaped' rather than oval when filled with glycine, the aim of which is to improve treatment in the cornual areas (Fig. 13.5).

The catheter also contains the heating elements. This consists of thin lamellae of a special conductive ceramic material with self-regulating properties. The design of the lamellae provides a large surface area leading to rapid heating of the fluid. The electrical resistance of the ceramic material is very high and is fixed at the time of manufacture below a reference point. Below this reference point, the heating capability of the element is very high, but as the reference point is approached the conductivity of the material rapidly decreases, thereby reducing the heating effect. This provides an important safety feature, ensuring that the heating power of the element will automatically decrease if the temperature of the element

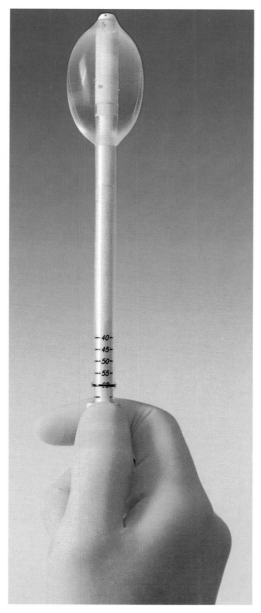

Figure 13.4 — Adjustable balloon length.

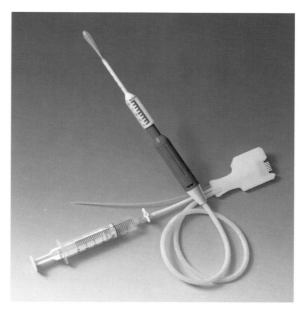

Figure 13.5 — New balloon catheter.

exceeds 75°C by 7°C. The aim of the system is to produce a steady state, whereby the heating power and the cooling effect are the same. The temperature at the balloon surface will differ slightly from patient to patient due to differences in fluid volume, blood circulation and state of the endometrial lining.

The other safety feature of the unit is the ability to monitor continuously the balloon pressure. The optimal pressure for treatment is 200 mmHg ± 20. At this pressure, there is tamponade of the superficial myometrial blood flow, which reduces the heat-sink effect of blood flow enabling adequate superficial myometrial temperatures to be reached to cause cell death. The pressure can fluctuate during a case, and the system allows further glycine to be added to the balloon during the procedure to keep the pressures to optimal treatment levels. If the pressure exceeds 250 mmHg, an alarm will sound to alert the surgeon and a mechanical valve will open and release fluid in order to return to the normal operating pressure.

Procedure

Pre-operative

The Cavaterm™ system can be considered for the treatment of menorrhagia in patients with a normal uterine cavity. All patients prior to treatment should have a normal cervical smear, endometrial biopsy, combined with either outpatient or inpatient hysteroscopy or ultra-sound scan to confirm the absence of fibroids, septae or endometrial pathology.

Contraindications

- Undiagnosed uterine bleeding.
- Any endometrial or cervical histology with atypical cells.
- Uterine abnormalities such as submucous myomas, uterine septae that would prevent the balloon from making uniform contact with the endometrium.
- Suspicion of uterine wall weakness.
- Patients with an anterior–posterior diameter of <4 cm and/or uterine wall thickness of <18 mm should not have hormonal pre-treatment. Patients who have had two or more caesarean sections should have the anterior uterine wall thickness estimated to avoid thermal injury to the bladder in cases where the anterior wall is thin (18 mm).
- Pregnancy or desire for future pregnancy.
- Uterine cavity length (internal os to fundus) <4 cm or >10 cm.
- Active infection.

The type of endometrial preparation is surgeon dependent. It can be

- hormonal preparation,
- timed to the menstrual cycle,
- immediate pre-treatment curettage (recommended by company).

If hormonal preparation is to be used, it is recommended that patients should have an ultra-sound scan to ensure that the uterine thickness is appropriate pre-preparation (AP diameter >4 cm or uterine wall thickness >18 mm) to prevent the potential risk of thermal transmission in cases where the uterine wall is very thin. Previous work using the traditional methods of ablation (laser, rollerball) reported a thinner pre-operative endometrial thickness and higher amenorrhoea rates in patients undergoing hormonal preparation with GnRHa to placebo and menstrually timed treatments.[10] Hawe et al found no difference in the amenorrhoea rate in patients using different methods of endometrial preparation, however, those patients undergoing curettage had the shorter follow-up.[11] There is no randomised data using the Cavaterm™ system comparing hormonal pre-treatment to immediate pre-operative curettage as recommended by the company.

Operative procedure

The procedure can be performed under GA or IV sedation with para-cervical block. At present, there is no published data comparing patient acceptability for outpatient to inpatient, or different methods for anaesthesia. In one study, 72% were performed under GA with 28% being performed using IV anaesthesia and para-cervical block.[11]

The patient is placed in the lithotomy position. The total length of the uterus is measured with a uterine sound and the cavity length calculated by subtracting the cervical length. The balloon length is then adjusted to the measured cavity length. In our unit, we perform a para-cervical block using 0.5% plain bupivicaine (Astra, Kings Langley, Herts.) to aid intra-operative and post-operative analgesia. The supplied syringe is filled with 30 ml of 1.5% glycine and attached via the three-way tap to the balloon, which is held vertically upwards. Air is purged from the system, the balloon deflated by retracting the syringe plunger, and the system is now primed and ready for use. The syringe is refilled to 30 ml with 1.5% glycine.

The cervix is dilated to Hegar 8 and the catheter inserted until the fundus is reached. In our unit, especially in training cases, we recommend that a hysteroscopy be performed prior to catheter insertion to exclude a false passage or perforation with the dilator. Once in position, the balloon is inflated until a stable pressure of 200 (±20) mmHg is obtained. The pump circulates the glycine within the balloon and checks for leaks in the system. Heating commences up to the pre-set temperature of 75°C, which is self-regulated and stable. The pressure may vary during the procedure but usually stabilises in the early treatment phase. The pressure is maintained by adding glycine during the procedure. The catheter has a drain tube which automatically drains excess glycine if the set pressure is exceeded and a maximum of 30 ml can be used per case. If greater than 30 ml is required, the operator should be alert to the possibility of uterine perforation or balloon rupture. Heating will continue until the treatment time, 15 min, has elapsed. On pressing the stop button, the pump will be deactivated. The balloon is then deflated and removed from the uterus.

In our unit, at the end of the procedure, the patient is given rectal diclofenac sodium 100 mg for post-operative analgesia unless there are any contraindications. Compared to endometrial ablation using the Nd-YAG laser, we have found Cavaterm™ thermal balloon ablation to be associated with more post-operative pain. In a RCT comparing the two techniques, we found higher pain scores using visual analogue scores (62.5 vs 43, levels 0–100) and semantic differential techniques (1.2 vs 0.4, levels −3 to 3) but neither of these levels reached statistical significance (unpublished data).

In vitro and *in vivo* studies

The first extirpated uteri studies were performed in 1992. Friberg et al published data in 1996 demonstrating that endometrial destruction by hyperthermia using the Cavaterm balloon was a potential treatment of menorrhagia.[12] Eight cases, five post- and three pre-hysterectomy, Cavaterm procedures were described using a treatment time of 30 min at 75°C at a balloon pressure of 180 mmHg. Histological examination revealed myometrial damage up to a maximum depth of 8 mm (range 2–8 mm). In none of the cases was a rise in serosal temperature >1°C seen. The first clinical cases were performed in 1993. The initial treatment time of 30 min was used for the first 60 patients but, since 1995, the treatment time has been reduced to 15 min. We repeated the post- and pre-hysterectomy studies in 1999 for treatment times of 15, 10 and 7 min using a diaphorase staining technique to detect immediate cell death (Fig. 13.6). The mean depth of immediate myometrial cell death was 4, 3 and 2 mm at 15, 10 and 7 min respectively, with no significant increases in serosal temperature seen (unpublished data). The areas most likely to have residual untreated endometrium in both studies were the cornua. Concern over the potential for inadequate cornual treatment led to the development of a second-generation catheter, where the balloon is more 'heart-shaped' compared to the oval shape of the first balloon (Fig. 13.5). At present, there is a clinical study ongoing comparing the efficacy of 10- vs 15-min treatment times.

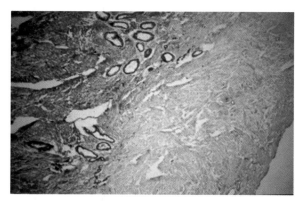

Figure 13.6 — Diaphorase staining to demonstrate cell (pink stain = cell death), magnification 2.5×.

Clinical studies

There are few published studies using the Cavaterm™ system. There has been a total of 12 publications, seven in the English language and five non-English. Of the six in English, only three are clinical studies,[11,13,14] the others are pre-clinical studies to confirm safety and likely efficacy.[9,12,15,16] There is one published RCT in German comparing the Cavaterm™ system to rollerball.[17]

Friberg et al in 1998, published data on the first 36 patients treated with the Cavaterm™ system in their department.[13] They followed the cohort for 18–24 months. Early in the use of the equipment they concluded that the system is only suitable for use in normal shaped cavities. Four patients, who underwent hysterectomy, were excluded from the data analysis due to the finding of intrauterine pathology at hysterectomy (2 myomas, 1 septum, 1 pre-malignant curettings). Friberg et al, have recently published data from 117 women followed-up for a maximum of 4 years (mean 25 months).[14] Success rates were quoted at 94%, with 30% amenorrhoea and 37.3% spotting or hypomenorrhoea. There were 10 hysterectomies, four secondary to myomata and one secondary to a septum. These occurred early in the series when patient selection had not yet been defined. Using life table analysis, 85% of women would have avoided a hysterectomy at 50 months.

Hawe et al in 1999, published data from a prospective, two centre pilot study. Fifty patients were included, with a mean follow-up time of 14.4 months (range 6–24).[11] Regarding the menstrual status and satisfaction rates there were two failures in this series. One patient underwent an endometrial laser ablation for persistent menorrhagia with a successful outcome; the other had a vaginal hysterectomy for persistent bleeding, discharge and pain. This patient's post-operative course had been complicated by endometritis treated as an outpatient with antibiotics and the histology revealed adenomyosis. Survival curve analysis revealed that 93% (95% CI 84–100) of those recruited would avoid any further surgery (hysterectomy or endometrial ablation) for failed Cavaterm™ ablation. The main conclusion of this study was that the system was simple to use, well designed, efficacious and safe. The authors felt that larger series with longer follow-up was required, together with results from RCTs comparing Cavaterm™ to traditional endometrial ablation/resection techniques. There are several RCTs currently being performed using the Cavaterm™

system, comparing it to traditional techniques and other second-generation devices. The results are awaited with interest.

The majority of data using the Cavaterm™ system is available in abstract form from presentations of personal series at International meetings. This data has been summarised in a chapter published in 2000.[18] The largest study is ongoing in Switzerland and Sweden (Genolet et al, Friberg et al respectively). This study commenced in 1993, with 280 patients treated and greater than 12-month follow-up in 156 patients. Out of the first 156 patients, 12 (7.6%) underwent a hysterectomy. There have been three other small prospective and retrospective studies presented (Alailey, UK; Halvorsen, DK; Kleine-Gunk, GER). The number of patients ranges from 21 to 42, with a follow-up of 3–17 months. 'Success rates' are quoted as 96–98%, with amenorrhoea rates between 29% and 43% and combined amenorrhoea and spotting rates between 56% and 72%.

Complications

The Cavaterm™ system has been designed to reduce the potential complication rates of ablation without reducing efficacy. Due to its design, intra-operative fluid absorption is impossible and the risk of haemorrhage should be virtually eliminated as the technique relies on thermal conductivity. Potential complications include false passage formation or complete uterine perforation with the risk of thermal injury to surrounding structures. A full thickness uterine perforation should be identified, as it should be impossible to reach the treatment pressure with the maximum 30 ml glycine allowed. It may, however, be more difficult to identify a false passage, where the treatment pressure may be achievable. We would recommend that in any case of difficult dilatation, that a hysteroscopy or ultrasound scan should be performed immediately pre-treatment. The three published clinical studies in the English language are too small to make statistically significant conclusions about the incidence of complications. Hawe et al,[11] described two cases (4%) of post-operative endometritis treated as an outpatient with the appropriate antibiotics. One patient required an overnight stay and investigations for unexplained right iliac fossa pain immediately post-treatment which settled with conservative management. There were no intra-operative complications in either studies.

The fact that potential complications of fluid overload and intra-operative haemorrhage should be avoided,

means that this system may be suitable to treat patients with renal or cardiac problems, bleeding disorders, and anti-coagulation therapy. Hawe et al,[11] treated two patients with chronic renal failure and three with clotting disturbances in their series with good results and no increase in morbidity. However, care has to be taken in these patients because even though the technical surgical risk is reduced, they remain a high operative risk for other reasons and this has to be taken into account when discussing the benefits and risks of surgery to the patient.

Until larger RCTs are available, the data for complications using this system are limited. The occurrence of major complications with endometrial ablation techniques are so rare, that it is unlikely that any RCT in the future will have sufficient power to compare the complication rates of individual techniques.

Cost

The initial cost of the central unit is $6000 (6000 ECU) and for the single use catheters, $600 (600 ECU). Studies comparing endometrial laser ablation, rollerball and endometrial resection to hysterectomy have shown a cost saving in favour of the hysteroscopic techniques, even when re-treatment rates are accounted for.[19,20] This cost saving should continue with the Cavaterm™ system, even when the disposables are accounted for, but there are no published studies comparing the cost of Cavaterm™ to alternative treatments.

Conclusion

The Cavaterm™ thermal balloon ablation system is simple and easy to use. It has some excellent design features, including fluid circulation, unique heating element within the balloon and adjustable balloon length, which distinguish it from its competitors. The device is suitable to treat any patient complaining of menorrhagia with a normal uterine cavity and endometrial biopsy. One criticism of the majority of second-generation devices is their ability to only treat normal uterine cavities. However, even if restricted to use on normal uterine cavities, the procedure would still be suitable for 66–79% of procedures based on results from previously reported studies.[20]

In this modern era of evidence-based medicine, Class A evidence is needed to ensure proper evaluation before recommending any new treatment. For the

Cavaterm™ system, there is currently only Class C available in the form of three small prospective studies with short- to medium-term follow-up. To date, it would appear that the Cavaterm™ system is simple to use, reliable and associated with success rates at least as good as the traditional techniques for short- and medium-term follow-up. The studies are too small to comment on safety, but no increase in perforation rates or thermal injuries to surrounding structures has yet been observed. Such a problem is a concern to some people with the blind second-generation techniques. RCTs comparing the device to traditional techniques, other second-generation techniques, and looking at shorter treatment times, are nearing completion. The results are awaited with interest. They are likely to confirm the results from prospective studies and show that the system will become a useful treatment option in the modern day management of dysfunctional uterine bleeding.

Advantages	Disadvantages
Simple to use and reliable system	Only suitable for normal uterine cavities
Adjustable balloon length for different size cavities	Disposable cost
Fluid in circulation — more reliable balloon surface temperature leading to a uniform and reproducible ablation	Lack of publications in peer review journals
	Lack of Class A evidence
No risk of fluid absorption	
Reduced risk intra-operative bleeding	
Success and patient satisfaction rates >90%	

References

1. *The management of menorrhagia. Effective health care.* Leeds: University of Leeds, 1995: 9: 1–14.

2. Phillips AG, Chien PFW, Garry R. Risk of having a hysterectomy after endometrial laser ablation — analysis on 1000 consecutive cases. *Br J Obstet Gynaecol* 1998; 105: 897–903.

3. O'Connor H, Magos AL. Endometrial resection for menorrhagia: evaluation of results at 5 years. *New Engl J Med* 1996; 335: 151–156.

4. Dwyer N, Hutton J, Stirrat GM. Randomised controlled trial comparing endometrial resection with abdominal hysterectomy for the surgical treatment of menorrhagia. *Br J Obstet Gynaecol* 1993; 100: 237–243.

5. Pinion SB, Parkin DE, Abramovich DR et al. Randomised trial of hysterectomy, endometrial laser ablation, transcervical endometrial resection for dysfunctional uterine bleeding. *Br Med J* 1994; 309: 379–383.

6. O'Connor H, Broadbent JAM, Magos AL, McPherson K. Medical Research Council trial of endometrial resection versus hysterectomy in the management of menorrhagia. *Lancet* 1997; 349: 897–901.

7. Overton C, Hargreaves J, Maresh M. A national survey of the complications of endometrial destruction for menstrual disorders: the MISTLETOE study. *Br J Obstet Gynaecol* 1997; 104: 1351–1359.

8. Neuwith RS, Duran AA, Singer A, MacDonald R, Bolduc L. The endometrial ablator: a new instrument. *Obstet Gynaecol* 1994; 83(5 pt. 1): 792–796.

9. Friberg B, Wallsten H, Henrikkson P, Personn BRR, Petterson F, Willen R. A new, simple, safe and efficient device for the treatment of menorrhagia. *J Gynaecol Tech* 1996; 2: 103–108.

10. Donnez J, Vilos G, Gannon MJ, Stampe-Sorenson S, Klinte I, Miller RM. Goserelin acetate (Zoladex) plus endometrial ablation for dysfunctional uterine bleeding: a large randomised study, double-blind study. *Fertil Steril* 1997; 68(1): 29–36.

11. Hawe JA, Phillips AG, Erian J, Garry R. Cavaterm™ thermal balloon ablation for the treatment of menorrhagia. *Br J Obstet Gynaecol* 1999; 106: 1143–1148.

12. Friberg B, Persson BRR, Willen R, Ahlgren M. Endometrial destruction by hyperthermia — a possible treatment of menorrhagia. *Acta Obstet Gynaecol Scand* 1996; 75: 330–335.

13. Friberg B, Ahlgren M. Thermal balloon endometrial destruction: the outcome of treatment of 117 women followed up for a maximum period of 4 years. *Gynaecol Endosc* 2000; 9(6): 389–396.

14. Friberg B, Persson BRR, Willen R, Ahlgren M. Endometrial destruction by thermal coagulation: evaluation of a new form of treatment for menorrhagia. *Gynaecol Endosc* 1998; 7: 73–78.

15. Friberg B, Joergensen A, Ahlgren M. Endometrial thermal coagulation — degree of uterine fibrosis predicts treatment outcome. *Gynaecol Obstet Invest* 1998; 45(1): 54–57.

16. Olsrud J, Friberg B, Ahlgren M, Persson BRR. Thermal conductivity of uterine tissue *in vitro. Phys Med Biol* 1998; 43(8): 2397–2406.

17. Romer T. Die therapie rezidivierender menorrhagien — Cavaterm-ballon koagulation versus roller-ball endometrium koagulation — eine prospektive randomiserte vergleichstudie. *Zentralblatt fur Gynakologie* 1998; 120: 511–514.

18. De Grandi P, El-Din A. Endometrial ablation for the treatment of dysfunctional uterine bleeding using balloon therapy. In: OR Kochli (Ed.) *Hysteroscopy: state of the art*, Vol. 20, pp 145–153, 2000. Contrib Gynaecol Obstet. Basel: Karger.

19. Sculpher M. The cost-effectiveness of preference based treatment allocation: the case of hysterectomy versus endometrial resection in the treatment of menorrhagia. *Health Econ* 1998; 7: 129–142.

20. Cameron IM, Mollison J, Pinion SB, Atherton-Naji A, Buckingham K, Torgerson D. A cost comparison of hysterectomy and hysteroscopic surgery for the treatment of menorrhagia. *Eur J Obstet Gynecol Reprod Biol* 1996; 70(1): 87–92.

14

The MenoTreat® balloon ablation

Arne Rådestad and Ulf Ulmsten

Women complaining of menorrhagia often seek surgical options when pharmacological treatment is insufficient. Most women with menorrhagia are in their late fertile age with no desire for future pregnancies and prefer to have a definitive treatment. Abdominal or vaginal hysterectomy are the major surgical options with a relative high risk for psychological and physical complications, and long recovery time.

Endometrial ablation via hysteroscopy offers a more rapid postoperative recovery. However, to be safe and effective the procedure requires a special skill in operative hysteroscopy. Serious short-comings are risks for fluid overload and uterine perforation.

Treatment of menorrhagia with thermal uterine balloons require less surgical training but can sometimes be less effective due to present intrauterine pathology, preventing adequate balloon contact with the uterine wall.

The MenoTreat® System for thermal endometrial balloon ablation consists of a disposable balloon set and system controller designed to work together. The balloon set comprises an inflatable silicone balloon catheter, configured as a closed system with no electric or electronic components to minimise patient risk. It has an oval cross section diameter of 7 mm and an angular shape to better fit the anatomy of the uterus. The procedure requires a dilation of the cervical canal to 8 mm and measurement of the uterine sound depth. The circulating sterile saline solution is heated in the system controller rather than in the uterus. The MenoTreat® System controller also contains a pump, a temperature and pressure sensor, a keyboard and a display for monitoring the entire procedure. A constant treatment pressure of 200 mmHg and a temperature of 85°C are maintained during a treatment period of 11 min, enough to destroy the endometrium and a few millimetres of the myometrium.

Several safety functions are integrated in the MenoTreat® System. The treatment stops automatically after 11 min and the treatment solution is reversed. Should a sudden change in temperature or pressure occur during treatment, the pump reverses automatically to empty all the heated saline from the balloon, thus, eliminating burns to the vaginal wall. The controller is also testing all functions of the system during the fully automatic testing phase.

A prospective multi-centre clinical study, including 51 women with menorrhagia treated with the first version of the MenoTreat® System, resulted in an overall success rate of 74–94% (95% confidence interval) based on changes in bleeding score. The main pain score during each menstrual cycle assessed by a visual analogue scale was more than 50% lower compared to the scoring prior to treatment. A significant improvement in the women's quality of life was rated parallel with the improvement seen in bleeding scores.

The treatment procedures in this clinical trial were all performed under general anaesthesia. However, in an ongoing study with the redesigned MenoTreat® System we have experienced that a paracervical block with light sedation during the procedure gives an acceptable anaesthesia in most women. The postoperative pain, which usually disappears after a few hours, occasionally needs additional treatment with morphine.

Preliminary results of the ongoing study with the presently marketed system show that amenorrhoea and spotting are achieved in approximately 60% of the women. Contraceptives are recommended to fertile women since sterility cannot be assured after treatment.

Conclusion

The MenoTreat® System is a safe and effective procedure for the treatment of menorrhagia in selected patients. The technique is easy to learn and can be considered as an ambulatory procedure performed under paracervical block and light sedation. The majority of the women can be discharged a few hours after treatment. Complications such as endometritis and haematometra are rare. No pre-endometrial thinning is needed. Instead, a suction curretage is used prior to treatment to remove part of the endometrium. This reduces the amount of necrotic debris in the uterine cavity and decreases the brownish and watery discharge commonly seen for 3–6 weeks after treatment.

The cost for the MenoTreat® System controller is USD or ECU 6000 and the MenoTreat® System balloon set is USD or ECU 350.

Advantages	Disadvantages
A high satisfaction rate among women with amenorrhoea	Amenorrhoea or sterility cannot be guaranteed
Easy to use	Should not be used when intrauterine pathology is present.
Complications rare	
Shorter hospitalisation	
Rapid recovery	
In-patients' and social costs reduced.	

Bibliography

1. Amso N, Stabinsky S, McFaul P, Blanc B, Pendley L, Neuwirth R. Uterine thermal balloon therapy for the treatment of menorrhagia: the first 300 patients from a multicentre study. *Br J Obstet Gynaecol* 1998; 105: 517–523.

2. Gervaise A, Fernandez H, Capella-Allouc S, Taylor S, la Vielle S, Hamou J, Gomel V. Thermal balloon ablation versus endometrial resection for the treatment of abnormal uterine bleeding. *Hum Reprod* 1999; 11: 2743–2747.

3. Aletebi F, Vilos G, Eskander M. Thermal balloon endometrial ablation to treat menorrhagia in high-risk surgical candidates. *J Am Gynecol Laparosc* 1999; 6: 435–439.

4. Duggan PM, Dodd J. Endometrial balloon ablation under local analgesia and intravenous sedation. *Aust NZ J Obstet Gynaecol* 199; 39: 123–126.

15

Vesta™: Distensible multi-electrode balloon endometrial ablation

K.D. Jones, L. Spangler and C.J.G. Sutton

Introduction

Electrosurgical endometrial ablation remains the gold standard minimal access technique for the treatment of abnormal uterine bleeding in the absence of demonstrable pathology. Therefore, the second-generation endometrial ablation devices must be compared to this procedure in order to assess their safety features, complication rates, cost-effectiveness and efficacy in clinical practice.

Success rates for hysteroscopic endometrial ablations vary. Typically, 30–50% of women report amenorrhoea and 35–65% experience significant reduction of bleeding.[1] Failures are attributed to incomplete ablation of endometrial tissue or to adenomyosis. There are several reasons for the inconsistent results. The procedure requires intensive training and therefore has a long learning curve. The surgeon must achieve an even distribution of tissue destruction >3 mm into the myometrium without perforating the uterine wall or leaving areas untreated.[2] This may be difficult if visualisation is hampered by floating debris, bleeding or inadequate distension. Some surgeons choose the coagulation waveform, whereas others use the cut waveform. Wattage ranges from 45 to over 100 W. Many surgeons prefer to resect the endometrium. Others use roller electrodes, which are inconsistent in size and surface area. Adding to these confounding factors are the different methods of preparing the endometrium pre-operatively.

The Vesta™ System (Valleylab, Boulder, CO) was developed to reduce these variables and to provide consistent, cost-effective and predictable results in the outpatient setting.

Instrumentation and ancillary devices

The Vesta™ System consists of

1. a Valleylab Force 2™ electrosurgical generator set to supply 'pure cut' mode (undampened) current at 45–50 W,

2. a disposable handset for the introduction of an electrode carrier,

3. a cable connecting the handset to the generator,

4. a patient return electrode pad,

5. a controller to monitor and distribute the electrical energy.

The silicone inflatable electrode carrier has an inverted triangle shape that unfurls when its insertion sheath is withdrawn.

A through-tube traverses the centre for access to the uterine cavity whilst the carrier is in place to check for potential perforation or residual space. There are six ventral and six dorsal flexible electrode plates covering the surface of the carrier, each with its own thermistor. The controller functions in two phases, warm-up and treatment. It monitors generator output as well as the temperature and impedance of the 12 electrodes throughout both phases.

If the impedance for any one electrode is too high, indicating poor tissue contact, the controller will not permit treatment to begin. Each electrode is monitored three times per second and the generator will energise the electrode which is farthest below its set point temperature each cycle. Warm-up is programmed to occur within 3 min. The controller automatically shifts to a 4-min treatment phase as soon as all electrodes have reached their set points and ends the procedure when treatment is completed.

Safety features

- The electrode balloon expands to fit the uterine cavity ensuring a uniform depth of desiccation.
- If the silicone balloon is properly positioned and the uterine wall is intact, the through-tube should not accept air.
- A stationary electrode system reduces the risk of uterine perforation while the electrode is activated.
- Electrosurgical energy moves throughout the endometrium for a pre-set duration allowing the minimum amount of power required to be used.
- The system provides continuous and automatic monitoring of temperature (measured three times per second), electrical power and electrode–tissue impedance.

Practical aspects of treatment

Technique

The cervical canal is dilated to 9–10 mm. The handset (the sheath containing the electrode balloon) is introduced into the uterine cavity and advanced until its tip reaches the fundus. The sheath is withdrawn; this deploys the silicone balloon which is then inflated with 8–12 ml of air. This brings the 12 electrodes into contact with the uterine wall. An attempt is then made to introduce air into the through-tube. If the carrier is properly positioned and the uterine wall is intact, the through-tube should not accept air. The controller is turned on and indicates a 'ready' condition when it has checked the generator output and all connections. Warm-up is initiated by pressing a 'start' button. The operator has to maintain pressure on the syringe plunger attached to the carrier inflation port, throughout the warm-up and treatment phases. The electrosurgical generator is set at 40–45 W in an undampened waveform. The warm-up time lasts approximately 1 min and this is followed by a 4-min therapeutic phase. Radiofrequency (RF) energy is supplied to the electrodes by the generator. The electrodes apply the RF to the tissue which is then returned to the generator by the patient return electrode pad. The RF current heats the uterine tissue performing the endometrial ablation.

Because the myometrium near the tubal ostia is relatively thin, the four cornual electrodes have set temperatures of 72°C, whereas the remaining eight electrodes have set temperatures of 75°C. Automated maintenance of these temperatures for 4 min, with constant distension of the carrier lumen to keep the electrodes in intimate surface contact, produces uniform thermal destruction to a depth of 4–5 mm into the myometrium. When the controller ends treatment, the silicone balloon is deflated and the handset is withdrawn without re-sheathing the carrier.

Endometrial preparation

In clinical evaluation studies conducted in Europe and the USA, investigators were free to use timing alone, oral contraceptive cycling, depot progestogens or gonadotrophin-releasing hormone (GnRH) agonists.[3] In studies carried out in Mexico and the US, oral contraceptives were taken for at least 2 weeks, then discontinued 1 week before the procedure to allow for endometrial sloughing.[4,5]

Analgesic requirements

In the clinical studies carried out to evaluate the Vesta™ System[3,5] general anaesthesia was used five times as commonly as paracervical block with conscious sedation. Where a paracervical block was used it was commonly supplemented with topical mepivacaine injected into the electrode carrier through-tube before inflation. During the randomised controlled

trial (RCT), general or epidural anaesthesia was used in only 16.7% of Vesta™ procedures; 20% of rollerball resection group (R/R) procedures were done with paracervical block and intravenous sedation. No difference in result was noted in either case as a function of anaesthesia employed.

Ex vivo/in vitro studies

Laboratory and initial clinical testing

To establish safety parameters prior to in vivo studies, laboratory tests were conducted on animal tissue and extirpated uteri.[4] Once the safety parameters had been established, in vivo studies were performed. These studies took place in Mexico, the UK and the Netherlands in 30 women scheduled for hysterectomy. Uterine serosal temperatures were monitored in 17 women during the procedure. Treatment variables ranged from 30 to 45 W, 90 to 240 s duration and 65°C to 75°C. After hysterectomy, the uterus was dissected into sections to determine depth of necrosis, with six alternate sections analysed histochemically. The extent and depth of tissue necrosis were measured to establish the optimum pre-selected temperature, time and power.

Initial findings

No significant serosal temperature increases were reported and no complications occurred as a result of the procedures. The extent of necrosis varied depending on the treatment variables and the degree to which the electrode balloon conformed to the uterine cavity. Residual necrotic endometrium measured approximately 0.2 mm. The depth of myometrial necrosis varied from 1.0 to 6.0 mm with 88% of the sections averaging from 2 to 4 mm. An intermediate layer of cells between the viable and non-viable tissue was evident. This intermediate layer of cells has been excluded from measurements of depth of necrosis and would be expected to slough.

In vivo studies

Inclusion and exclusion criteria used in the clinical evaluation studies

All the patients in the initial in vivo studies were screened by pre-operative hysteroscopy or ultrasound and endometrial biopsy to rule out abnormal uterine cavities and unexpected malignancy or atypical hyperplasia.[4]

Following this, a multicentre, single armed evaluation study was conducted.[3] The patients were admitted to the study if they had failed to respond to medical therapy and they had no systemic or local cause for their excessive bleeding. All the patients were booked to undergo a hysterectomy. Patients were generally excluded if they had distorted uterine cavities or a sounding length >10 cm but 12 women with 3 cm or smaller submucous leiomyomata were selected to have laser myomectomies immediately preceding their ablations.

A multicentre, prospective, RCT was then carried out.[5] Women between the ages of 30 and 49 were recruited. All the patients had completed their families and were using non-hormonal contraception or one of the partners had been sterilised. Women with FSH levels >40 mIU/ml were excluded from the study group. A previously validated pictorial blood loss assessment chart was used to quantitate monthly menstrual blood loss. The women used the same brand of sanitary pad or tampon (New Freedom Super or Tampax Super). After 3 months of completing a menstrual diary, if the scores were >150, the patients were then evaluated with hysteroscopy or ultrasonography. Patients with distorted uterine cavities, myoma or polyps or a cavity in excess of 9.75 cm were excluded from the study. Other exclusion criteria included:

- significant systematic medical diseases,
- pregnancy,
- pelvic inflammatory disease,
- carcinoma,
- clotting defects,

- previous unsuccessful endometrial ablation,
- myomectomy,
- uterine reconstruction and/or long-acting hormonal therapy within 3 months of enrolment.

All patients had endometrial sampling performed and the finding of any hyperplasia was cause for exclusion.

Results

Therapeutic studies

Follow-up data for 3–24 months is available on 246 patients recruited into the multicentre, single armed evaluation study conducted in Europe and Mexico.[3] Stability data from the study has been analysed on the same 117 patients at 6, 12, 18 and 24 months and this is shown in Figure 15.1. At each time interval the classification of blood loss has been checked by menstrual diary sampling. During the 24-month follow-up period, the proportion of patients who reported amenorrhoea, hypomenorrhoea and eumenorrhoea has remained constant. In particular, the amenorrhoea rate has remained between 40% and 45%.

During the randomisation process for the trial carried out in the USA,[5] 126 patients were allocated to endometrial resection and coagulation, with 150 randomised to Vesta™ ablation. This is shown in Figure 15.2. In the Vesta™ group, 144 patients reached the point of anaesthesia and 132 patients were treated according to the study protocol. Of these, 122 have had 12-month follow-up. In the R/R group, 123 patients were treated according to the study protocol and of these, 112 have had 12-month follow-up.

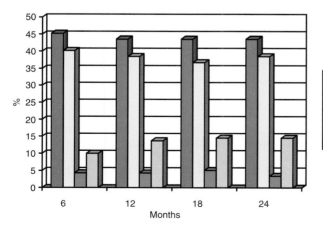

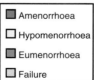

Figure 15.1 — Stability of 117 patients with 24 months of follow-up.

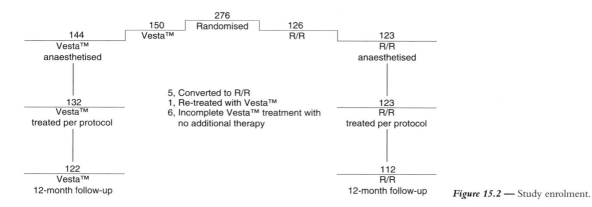

Figure 15.2 — Study enrolment.

Table 15.1 — US clinical study results

	Vesta™	**R/R**	*p* value
Pre-treatment PBAC	520 ± 600	447 ± 316	0.2272
Post-treatment PBAC	18 ± 37	28 ± 60	0.1281
All successfully treated patients	132	123	
Patient age at time of treatment	41.0 ± 4.19	40.1 ± 4.7	0.1122

Table 15.2 — US clinical study success

	Vesta™	**R/R**	*p* value
PBAC <75 at 12 months and no additional therapy required	86.9% (*n* = 122)	83.0% (*n* = 112)	0.465
Amenorrhoea at 12 months (PBAC — 0)	31.1% (*n* = 122)	34.8% (*n* = 112)	0.579

Table 15.1 shows the pre-treatment menstrual scores and the mean patient age in the Vesta™ treated group. These were similar to those in the R/R patients. In both groups the menstrual scores fell dramatically following treatment.

Table 15.2 shows the clinical success. In the Vesta™ treated group 87% of patients had menstrual scores <75 and did not require any additional treatment during the initial 12 months following treatment. Whereas, 83% of patients in the R/R group

had scores <75 at the 12-month follow-up visit. The amenorrhoea rate, defined as a menstrual score of 0, was 31% in the Vesta™ group and 35% in the R/R group.

The most recent results from the 305 cases carried out in Europe and the RCT carried out in the USA are summarised in Tables 15.3 and 15.4. The same information is shown in terms of life table analysis in Tables 15.5 and 15.6

Complications and rate of adverse incidences

During the single armed evaluation study[3] no perforations of the uterus occurred. Most patients experienced a serosanguineous discharge for 3–5 weeks following treatment, but no cases of endometritis occurred. There were eight device failures during the first 60 attempts at treatment. In these cases the warm-up phase could not be completed within 3 min or the controller detected too much variability in electrode temperatures and the controller would not permit conversion to the treatment phase. These situations were resolved by pre-calibration of the generators and by allowing a 5 W increment in generator output setting if warm-up cannot be achieved within 3 min at 45 W.

One patient experienced painful muscle twitching during treatment in the single armed evaluation study[3] and in 18 cases during the trial carried out in the USA.[5] In only one of these was it necessary to halt the procedure because of pain, the other patients were simply aware of it. RF current oscillates too rapidly for muscle to respond and, following these adverse events, sources of low-frequency transients were identified in

Table 15.3 — European Vesta™ trial data summary (total treated: 305)

	6 months	12 months	18 months	24 months
Fail	13 (5.42%)	18 (7.79%)	18 (8.91%)	19 (11.24%)
Eumenorrhoea	20 (8.33%)	16 (6.93%)	15 (7.43%)	6 (3.55%)
Hypomenorrhoea	120 (50.00%)	122 (52.81%)	100 (49.50%)	78 (46.15%)
Amenorrhoea	87 (36.25%)	75 (32.47%)	69 (34.16%)	66 (39.05%)
Total:	240	231	202	169

Failure: hysterectomies, 6; 2nd procedures, 6; menorrhagia, 7.

Table 15.4 — US clinical trial data summary (total treated: Vesta™, 132; R/R, 123)

Outcome	6 months		12 months	
	Vesta™	R/R	Vesta™	R/R
Fail	19 (14.80%)	17 (15.00%)	16 (13.10%)	19 (17.00%)
Success (PBAC < 75)	109 (84.40%)	98 (85.00%)	106 (86.90%)	93 (83.00%)
Amenorrhoea	37 (28.90%)	45 (39.10%)	38 (31.10%)	39 (34.80%)

Amenorrhoea patients include 'Success' row as well.

some controllers and then eliminated by more restrictive testing. However, as with all electrosurgical procedures performed in the absence of pharmacological neuromuscular blockade, minor fasciculations can still occasionally occur, typically in the thigh muscles on the side where the dispersive pad is applied.

In addition to the two patients who had hysterectomies for hematometra listed as failures, two other patients developed cervical stenosis and minimal menstrual blood retention that responded to a single cervical dilation. They both continue to be hypomenorrhoeic.

During the trial carried out in the USA[5] there was a total of 16 device failures in 12 of the 144 treatments. The inflatable tip of the Vesta™ device failed to fully deploy and the electrodes failed to come to satisfactory operating temperatures. One Vesta™ procedure was halted because the balloon entered what appeared to be a weak caesarean section scar.

There were six adverse events during the electrosurgical procedures in the same trial. There were two cases of cervical lacerations, one case each of a hematometra, a fluid deficit of 1300 ml without electrolyte disturbance, one of myometritis and one small fundal perforation.

Cost analysis (Tyco Healthcare cost analysis)

The Vesta™ system has never been sold in the USA so the cost was never set in North America. In the UK the cost of the Vesta™ DUB treatment system is calculated to be £593 per patient. This is equivalent to the amount spent per patient for an electrosurgical ablation of the endometrium (£602–£898) or 35% of the cost of a hysterectomy (£1641).

Discussion

The data presented in this chapter demonstrates that thermoregulated RF endometrial ablation produces comparable results to those reported for hysteroscopically directed laser and electrosurgical ablation, when patients are followed up for at least 2 years.[1,6–9]

Each electrode 'tile' treats the surface with which it has direct contact and also the surface between it and adjacent electrodes because of thermal spread and edge current density concentration. This preferentially directs current to the electrodes' edges.[10] Thermal destruction also extends well into the myometrium. The consistent

Table 15.5 — Life table analysis of European Vesta™ trial

Interval (months) from Vesta™ treatment	No. of patients	Lost/ withdrawn	Patients with menorrhagia	Probability		Cumulative probability	
				Developing menorrhagia	Not developing menorrhagia	No menorrhagia	Menorrhagia
0–3	305	60	8	0.029	0.971	0.971	0.029
4–6	237	5	6	0.026	0.974	0.946	0.054
7–12	226	8	7	0.032	0.968	0.916	0.084
13–18	211	18	1	0.005	0.995	0.911	0.089
19–24	192	32	1	0.006	0.994	0.906	0.094

Table 15.6 — Life table analysis of US' Vesta™ trial

Interval (months) from Vesta™ treatment	No. of patients	Lost/ withdrawn	Patients with menorrhagia	Probability		Cumulative probability	
				Developing menorrhagia	Not developing menorrhagia	No menorrhagia	Menorrhagia
Vesta™							
0–3	132	2	22	0.168	0.832	0.832	0.168
4–6	108	3	5	0.047	0.953	0.793	0.207
7–12	100	4	3	0.031	0.969	0.769	0.231
R/R							
0–3	123	4	21	0.174	0.826	0.826	0.174
4–6	98	5	5	0.052	0.948	0.783	0.217
7–12	88	2	2	0.023	0.977	0.765	0.235

nature of the treatment results from precise regional control of the 12 individual electrodes. Calculations of joules delivered to individual electrodes indicate considerable variability in the energy required for electrodes in one area versus those in another and from one patient to another. The system is able to accommodate the different heat sink patterns which reflect variations in intramural uterine blood flow.

The Vesta™ System stands apart from all the other second-generation ablation techniques because it is able to provide precise regional feed back control.

Summary

The Vesta™ System is designed to provide highly predictable, repeatable endometrial ablation. It uses 12 temperature-controlled electrodes to treat all the areas of endometrial lining simultaneously. Each of the electrodes is independently controlled to adapt to differences in perfusion within the individual uteri and conventional electrosurgery is used to heat the endometrium for a pre-set duration.

The advantages and disadvantages of technique are set out in Table 15.7.

Two international multicentre clinical trials have been carried out. A single arm evaluation study and an RCT comparing the Vesta™ treatment system with electrosurgical ablation.

In Europe, 305 patients have been treated and 169 have been followed up for 24 months. The amenorrhoea rate is 39% and if the hypomenorrhoea rate is included the success rate (menstrual score <75) is 85.2%. The failure rate at 24 months is 11%. In the USA, patients have been followed up for 12 months and in the Vesta™ group (n = 132) the average menstrual score fell from a pre-operative value of 529 to a post-operative value of 24. The average score reduction was 94% and the amenorrhoea rate was 31%. In the resection group (n = 123) the average menstrual score fell from a pre-operative value of 425 to a post-operative value of 28. The average score reduction was 91%, and the amenorrhoea rate was 34.8%.

Conclusion

The Vesta™ treatment system has been shown to achieve impressive control of menorrhagia and it is an excellent alternative to electrosurgical endometrial ablation.

References

1. Baggish MS, Sze EHM. Endometrial ablation: a series of 568 patients treated over an 11 year period. *Am J Obstet Gynecol* 1996; 174: 908–913.

2. Indman PD, Soderstrom RM. Depth of endometrial coagulation with the urologic resectoscope. *J Reprod Med* 1990; 35: 633–635.

3. Desquesne J, Gallinat A, Garza-Leal, Sutton CJG, Van der Pas HFM, Wemsteker K, Chandler JG. Thermoregulated radiofrequency endometrial ablation. *Int J Fert* 1997; 42: 311–318.

4. Sonderstrom RM, Brooks PG, Corson SL et al. Endometrial ablation using a distensible multi-electrode balloon. *J Am Assoc Gynecol Laparosc* 1996; 3: 403–407.

5. Corson SL, Brill AI, Brooks PG, Cooper JM, Indman PD, Liu JH, Soderstrom RM, Vancaillie TG. Interim results of the American Vesta™ trial of endometrial ablation. *J Am Assoc Gynecol Laparosc* 1999; 6(1): 45–49.

6. O'Connor H, Magos A. Endometrial resection for the treatment of menorrhagia. *N Engl J Med* 1996; 335: 151–156.

7. Unger JB, Meeks GR. Hysterectomy after endometrial ablation. *Am J Obstet Gynecol* 1996; 175: 1432–1437.

8. Erian J. Endometrial ablation in the treatment of menorrhagia. *Br J Obstet Gynaecol* 1994; 101: 19–22.

9. Garry R, Shelley-Jones D, Mooney P et al. Six hundred endometrial laser ablations. *Obstet Gynecol* 1995; 85: 24–29.

10. Pearce JA. *Electrosurgery*, pp 148–153, 1986. London: Chapman and Hall.

Table 15.7 — Advantages and disadvantages of technique

Advantages	Disadvantages
Consistent, predictable results	Not recommended for distorted uterine cavities
Easy to learn	Not recommended for uterine cavities measuring <5 cm or >10 cm by uterine sound
Short procedure time	
No risk of fluid overload	
Sophisticated safety monitoring system	Uses disposable components
Potentially an out patient procedure	Blind rather than a hysteroscopically controlled procedure
Uses existing electrosurgical generator	

16

NovaSure™ endometrial ablation

Jason Abbott, Jed Hawe and Ray Garry

Summary

Traditional methods of endometrial ablation and resection have been carefully evaluated over the last decade. Considerable class A, B and C evidence is available to guide their use. Based on this evidence, the Cochrane collaboration[1] concluded that endometrial laser ablation and transcervical resection of the endometrium should be offered as a treatment option to all women needing surgical management of dysfunctional uterine bleeding. Based on the results of the MISTLETOE study,[2] it is very unlikely that all women are being offered this option due to difficulties in training and mastering the traditional techniques. There are now new second-generation methods of ablation being promoted, very strongly, by the manufacturers for the treatment of dysfunctional uterine bleeding, of which, the NovaSure™ system is just one. The concept of the use of bipolar technology to perform global ablation is interesting and appears scientifically sound. This is the newest of the devices and is still undergoing careful evaluation and as yet is not commercially available. The amount of data available is, therefore, very limited. Early data suggests that the NovaSure™ system may prove to be a very useful method in the treatment of dysfunctional uterine bleeding, but it is important that prior to its introduction, it undergoes rigorous evaluation in the form of randomised trials, comparing it to proven techniques and with data from reliable large series with long-term follow-up.

Introduction

Since the mid-1980s, endometrial ablation and resection techniques have been utilised to successfully treat menstrual problems without the need for hysterectomy. These techniques have been carefully evaluated, but despite this well-documented efficacy, 50% of the 70,000 hysterectomies performed each year in the UK are still performed for menorrhagia.

The MISTLETOE study revealed that most doctors who performed hysteroscopic surgery for menorrhagia only performed them infrequently[2] also, a large number of surgeons do not offer hysteroscopic surgery as a treatment option for menorrhagia at all, due to deficiencies in current training. A number of second-generation ablation devices have been developed to meet the needs of this large group of infrequent hysteroscopists and also surgeons not trained in hysteroscopic surgery. The aim of these second-generation devices was to reduce

the surgical skills necessary to perform a successful endometrial ablation, thereby making ablation more widely available to clinicians and patients alike. There are now more than 10 such second-generation devices available. These use a variety of different energy sources including:

1. thermal balloons,
2. hot water,
3. monopolar and bipolar electrosurgery,
4. radio-frequency energy,
5. microwave energy,
6. laser energy and cryotherapy.

The NovaSure™ endometrial ablation system is one of the newest of the global ablation techniques. A company called Novacept, based in California, USA, designed it in 1995. It introduces the concept of using bipolar electrosurgical energy to ablate the endometrium. Like other second-generation devices, the NovaSure™ system aims to produce a reproducible, controlled depth of ablation with a minimum of surgical skill. The other aim of the system was to develop a device that was quicker than the other devices available and by utilising a narrow diameter catheter, make global endometrial ablation a more acceptable outpatient or office procedure compared to its competitors. It has undergone *in vitro, in vivo,* Phase I clinical studies to assess the devices safety and efficacy. At present, there are randomised trials ongoing comparing the device to traditional methods of endometrial ablation and to other second-generation devices. At present, there are no publications in peer review journals detailing the NovaSure™ device. The only data available is in the form of personal communications and abstracts from International meetings. A number of features of the device are also awaiting patent and, therefore, cannot be fully described until these are available.

The aim of this chapter is to describe the system, its safety features, clinical applications and results from the data available.

The NovaSure™ system

The system comprises of two major components:

1. A modified electrosurgical generator.
2. A disposable catheter — NovaSure™ endometrial ablation device (NEAD) (Fig. 16.1).

The main function of the generator is to provide the power for the ablation process, perforation detection,

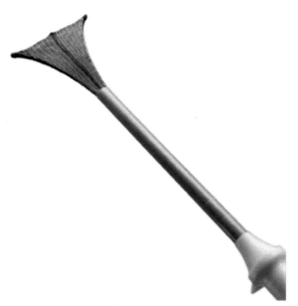

Figure 16.1 — The NovaSure™ bipolar endometrial ablation device.

moisture transfer and suction. The NovaSure™ generator is a modified electrosurgical generator that allows a maximal energy delivery of 180 W at 500 KHz. It measures: height 14 in., width 9.5 in., length 14.5 in. and weighs 23 lb. The power output of the generator is higher than that usually seen for other techniques of endometrial ablation and resection using electrosurgery. This is because the surface area of the NEAD within the cavity of the uterus is greater than, e.g. rollerball or electrosurgical loops and the current density at the electrode surface is, therefore, low. The power provided by the generator to produce the global ablation is determined by the uterine dimensions. The intercornual distance and the cavity length (total uterine length minus the cervical length) are entered into the generator. The generator then determines the power required to ablate the cavity. It will only deliver energy to tissues between tissue impedance ranges of 0.5–50 Ω. Compared to the traditional techniques, this is a very low level of impedance and this is a function of the large surface area of the NEAD. The ablation process is self-limiting. Once tissue impedance reaches 50 Ω or a treatment time of 120 s is reached, the treatment is terminated. The generator constantly monitors the tissue impedance at all areas on the mesh during the treatment.

The other functions of the generator are to exclude uterine perforation pre- and during treatment and to monitor the suction capability throughout the procedure. After the NEAD is deployed, the generator performs a pre-treatment safety check. The first check is perforation detection that utilises carbon dioxide pumped into the uterine cavity. The pressure within the cavity is monitored and if there is maintenance of this pressure, then the generator determines that there is no uterine perforation and will allow the procedure to proceed. Throughout the procedure, a second safety check is performed on the Moisture Transfer™ system. Suction is delivered through the handle of the NEAD and monitored by the generator. This has three actions — the first is to remove steam, endometrial effluent and blood from the cavity. This allows a uniform and controlled ablation of the entire cavity. The second action is to ensure that a close contact is maintained between the endometrium and the mesh electrodes of the NEAD. The last action of the suction system is to monitor the pressure within the cavity during the procedure and act as a safety check for perforations that may occur during the procedure. Should the pressure drop as determined by low suction, an alarm will sound and the procedure will terminate until a cause is determined. Similarly, should the pressure rise too high, e.g. due to a blockage in the suction device, the procedure will terminate. The removal of steam is important for the safety of the device. The device works by desiccating tissue. Desiccation is where temperature rises rapidly to 90°C causing the cells to dehydrate but preserve architecture. Tissues with high water content are very conductive and offer little resistance to the current flow. As the deeper tissues desiccate, that is dry out, their impedance or resistance to flow of current increases. When a level of 50 Ω is reached in a particular area the current, due to the design of the generator, ceases to flow. The only way to make current flow through the tissue would be to increase the voltage, that is, the force at which the current is driven through the desiccated tissue. If the moisture generated by the process was not removed, the presence of the moisture would allow the current to continue to flow in an uncontrolled manner, possibly leading to a greater and non-uniform depth of ablation.

The NEAD is a single-use instrument that device measures: length 483 mm, diameter 6.9 mm. It can only be used in conjunction with the NovaSure™ generator and is connected to the generator via a cable, which contains the radio-frequency cable and electrosurgical connections, suction tubing and vacuum monitoring tubing. The active component of the device comprises a single use, gold-plated bipolar electrode mesh which is mounted on an expendable and

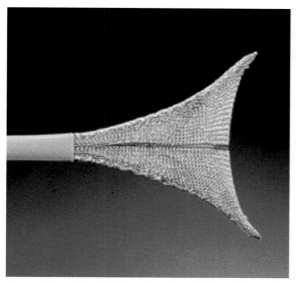

Figure 16.2 — The NEAD consists of a gold-plated bipolar electrode mesh that is mounted on an expendable and flexible frame.

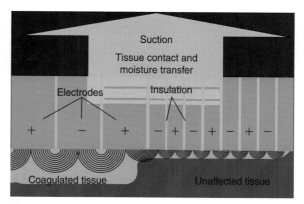

Figure 16.3 — Variation in the centre–centre electrode distance determines the depth of destruction. The greater the distance, the deeper the ablation. This configuration leads to a tapered ablation at the areas where the uterus is thinnest, namely the cornua and the isthmus.

flexible frame (Fig. 16.2). There are two electrodes on the front surface (positive and negative) and the same on the back in the opposite configuration. It is this arrangement of electrodes that allows flow of electrons between the poles of the device and cause cellular destruction of the endometrium. There is a 3 mm gap between the anterior and the posterior surface of the mesh. This gap allows the removal of steam and blood, and also allows the suction to draw the endometrial surface onto the mesh. Due to its flexibility, the frame can conform to the shape of the uterine cavity. The size of the mesh can also be adjusted to allow for variations in the length of the uterine cavity. The triangular shape of the mesh means that at the level of the cornua and at the internal os, the flow of electrons from positive to negative surfaces is shallower — hence the zone of thermal effect in these areas is more superficial. This occurs because the inter-electrode distance of the mesh is narrower at the angles of the triangle compared to its sides. It is the variation in the centre–centre electrode distance that determines the depth of the destruction (Fig. 16.3). This design ensures that the zone of thermal damage is less in the area where the myometrial thickness is reduced, that is, the cornua and the uterine isthmus.

Within the NEAD is the intrauterine measuring device used to determine the cornu-to-cornu distance. During the seating procedure, this distance is measured and displayed on a 'bobbin' on the handle which is then entered into the generator. The minimum intercornual distance that can be treated by the device is 2.0 cm. Sounding the uterus prior to the procedure and subtracting the cervical length from this measurement determines the endometrial cavity length. Uteri between 6 and 12 cm (fundus to external os) can be treated with this device.

Procedure

Inclusion and exclusion criteria

Since this device is not commercially available at this time, there are no guidelines as to inclusion and exclusion criteria. However, there are a number of trials currently underway in the USA and Europe and the criteria for inclusion into these trials are given below:

- A normal uterine cavity between 6 and 12 cm as assessed by hysteroscopy or ultrasonography.
- Normal endometrial biopsy.
- A normal cervical smear.
- Heavy menstrual loss as measured by objective means (menstrual diary).

Exclusion criteria

- Current pregnancy.
- Desire for fertility.
- Either confirmed or suspected gynaecological malignancy.

- Intra-cavity pathology.
- Active gynaecological or systemic infection.
- Chronic gynaecologic condition such as endo-metriosis or pelvic inflammatory disease.
- Congenital malformation of the uterine cavity (including septate of bicomuate uterus).
- Full thickness myometrial surgery (with the exception of lower segment caesarean section).

Endometrial preparation

At this time, the only results available are from abstracts presented at international meetings and include patients in whom endometrial preparation has been undertaken with the use of GnRH analogues and also patients in whom no endometrial preparation has occurred. Currently, it is not recommended to use endometrial preparation though there is no published data to support this recommendation at this time.

Operative procedure

The procedure can be performed under GA or IV sedation with para-cervical block. At present, there is no published data comparing patient acceptability for out-patient to inpatient or different methods for anaesthesia.

The patient is placed in the lithotomy position. The total length of the uterus is measured with a uterine sound and the cavity length calculated by subtracting the cervical length. The mesh length is then adjusted to the measured cavity length. In our unit, we perform a para-cervical block using 0.5% plain bupivicaine (Astra, Kings Langley, Herts.) to aid intra-operative and post-operative analgesia. The cervix is dilated to Hegar 7–8 and the NEAD inserted until the fundus is reached (Fig. 16.4). The device is then retracted slightly to allow the mesh to be opened by drawing back on the handle. As the mesh opens to fit the cornual areas, a strain gauge measures the inter-comual distance. The device then has to be moved slightly in a vertical, horizontal and rotational plane to 'seat' the device within the cavity. When the device is properly deployed, a green light is displayed on the RF generator. The system then performs its safety checks to exclude perforation and check the function of the moisture transfer system and the suction capability of the device. Power is then delivered until the tissue impedance reaches $50\,\Omega$ or the treatment time reaches 120 s, which ever is first. The mesh is then closed and the device removed from the cavity. If a post-operative hysteroscopy is performed, it demonstrates a uniform ablation of the whole cavity including the cornual areas

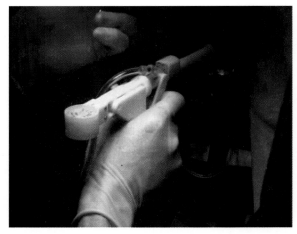

Figure 16.4 — The device is inserted until the fundus is reached. The mesh is then opened by puffing back on the handle, after retracting the device by about 1 cm.

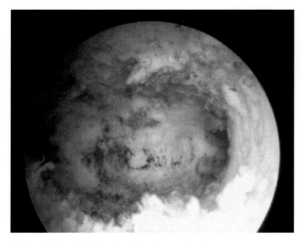

Figure 16.5 — Post-treatment hysteroscopic view.

(Fig. 16.5), with a striking demarcation line of ablated and untreated tissue at the level of the internal os.

At the end of the procedure, we administer rectal diclofenac sodium 100 mg for post-operative analgesia unless there are any contraindications. Using visual analogue scores at 4 h, we have found the NovaSure™ device to be associated with the lowest post-operative pain, with laser second and balloon ablation third (62.5 vs 43 vs 24, levels 0–100). The device also proved to be highly acceptable to patients as assessed by a semantic differential technique (unpublished data).

Table 16.1 — Zone of thermal necrosis as measured by diaphorase immuno-histochemical staining techniques, treatment times and maximum serosal temperatures

Study	n	Temperature (°C)	ZTN (mm)				Time (s) (range)
			Cornua	High-body	Mid-body	Lower-body	
In vitro	10	37.5	2.5	4.1	3.6	3.0	78 (44–120)
In vivo	21	38.5	2.3	4.1	3.7	2.8	60 (17–108)

ZTN = zone of thermal necrosis (unpublished data, personal communication).

In vitro and *in vivo* studies

The first extirpated uteri studies were performed in Hungary and as yet the data remains unpublished. The first aim of these studies was to assess the zone of thermal necrosis using validated tissue staining techniques to assess cell death (the diaphorase technique). The second aim was to confirm that the technique could be used without the fear of thermal transmission through the uterine wall, thereby preventing thermal injury to surrounding structures during the procedure. The maximum measured serosal temperature was 37.5°C. The depth of thermal damage and mean treatment time can be seen in Table 16.1.

Twenty-one *in vivo* cases were performed. Eleven cases were pre-treated with GnRH analogues, five with immediate pre-treatment curettage and five with no pre-treatment at all. The type of pre-treatment had no effect on the depth of thermal ablation, only the treatment time increased. The results are shown in Table 16.1.

Based on the results of the *in vitro* and *in vivo* work, Phase I clinical studies commenced in Europe.

Clinical studies

There are no published clinical studies using the NovaSure™ system. Again the only data available is in the form of personal communications from International meetings. Dr Tomas Fulop in Hungary performed the first Phase I study. He treated 21 patients, with a mean age of 45 years (range 37–52), for dysfunctional uterine bleeding. All the patients were treated with GnRH analogues. The mean treatment time was 64 s (range 42–103). There were no intra-operative complications and only one post-operative complication which was a case of endometritis treated

Table 16.2 — Summarised demographic, pre-operative PBLAC scores and operative data[3]

Demographics	Mean	Range
Age	41	34–39
Number of pregnancies	3.35	1–6
Pre-operative PBLAC	598	150–4449
Uterine sound measurement (cm)	8.8	6–10
Cornu–cornu distance (cm)	3.8	2.5–4.7
Uterine cavity length (cm)	5.4	4–7
Treatment time (s)	90	40–120
Post-operative recovery (min)	116	7–332

as an outpatient with antibiotics. The amenorrhoea rate at 6–9 months was 85% (personal communication).

A prospective trial began in 1998 to evaluate the NovaSure™ device. It involves 14 centres worldwide and the following data represent the results to date. There are over 300 patients treated to date, with 6-month or more follow-up available on 140 of these patients. The primary aim of the study was to evaluate the clinical efficacy of the NovaSure™ device as measured by pictorial blood loss chart (PBLAC). Secondary outcome measures include amenorrhoea rates, procedure times and overall patient satisfaction rates. Table 16.2 shows the demographic data, pre-operative PBLAC scores and operative data for patients in this study.

Analgesic use amongst centres was varied. Figure 16.6 shows the proportion of patients in each analgesic category in this trial.

Clinical outcomes for 6-month and 12-month follow-up are presented in the Figure 16.7. Overall, there is a 92.2% success rate as measured by PBLAC scores at 6 months. The mean PBLAC for the post-operative group was 25 (range 0–246), compared with a pre-operative average of 598.

In the post-operative period, one patient was excluded from study as she received progestogens for the treatment of endometriosis. Thus far, one patient has had a hysterectomy and was found to have adenomyosis and endometriosis histologically.

Brill et al have also presented preliminary data. The results from this preliminary trial, involving six centres in Northern America, are shown in Table 16.3.

This treatment is currently being investigated by a multi-centre study in the United States, Phase II trial and in several Phase III trials, comparing the device to other fonts of endometrial ablation, though no results are available at this time.

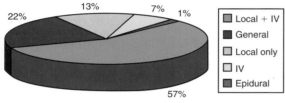

Figure 16.6 — Summary of analgesic regimens for patients undergoing NovaSure™ treatment.[3]

Complications

The NovaSure™ system has been designed to reduce the potential complication rates of ablation without reducing efficacy. The system does not require the use of distension media, thereby erasing the risk of intra-operative fluid absorption. The risk of haemorrhage should also be reduced as there is no surgical trauma to the sub-endometrial vasculature. The risk of false passage formation or complete uterine perforation with the risk of thermal injury to surrounding structures still exists. However, safety features have been designed to detect such an event, before treatment is commenced, therefore, potentially, eliminating the risk of thermal injury to surrounding structures. We would recommend in any case of difficult dilatation, that a hysteroscopy or ultrasound scan should be performed immediately pre-treatment to exclude such an event.

With the small number of patients treated, there are few reported complications. The most common complication appears to be endometritis. In the series presented by Abbott,[3] there were seven complications noted. These include five cases of endometritis (3.5%) which were effectively treated with oral antibiotics, one

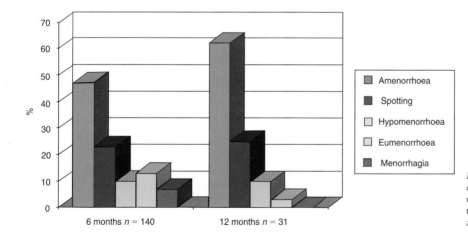

Figure 16.7 — Summary of clinical outcomes for patients undergoing NovaSure™ treatment[3] (results expressed as per cent).

Table 16.3 — Preliminary data from a large prospective study in the USA

Time	n	Amenorrhoea	Spotting	Hypomenorrhoea	Eumenorrhoea	Success
6/12	100	66	17	7.	8	98
12/12	44	85	7	3	5	100

Results expressed as percent; Personal communication.[4]

haematometra which resolved after cervical dilatation and one cervical burn that healed spontaneously without the need for further treatment. There is not enough published data or follow-up to assess the long-term efficacy or need for further surgery including hysterectomy.

Cost

The system is still undergoing rigorous evaluation in the form of clinical studies. The device is not yet commercially available and, therefore, costings are unavailable.

Conclusion

The NovaSure™ system appears to be simple and easy to use. It has sound scientific design features including a novel bipolar mesh which is adjustable in length and width for different sized cavities, a depth of destruction which is determined by tissue impedance and is self-limiting, rapid treatment times and important inbuilt safety features. The device is suitable to treat any patient complaining of menorrhagia with a normal uterine cavity and endometrial biopsy.

Whilst the technology behind the NEAD has many theoretical advantages it has yet to be evaluated either by large scale longitudinal trials with long follow-up or by evaluation in double blind trials comparing the device to existing technologies. In this modern era of evidence-based medicine, until these results are published, judgement must be reserved about the value, efficacy and safety of this device.

Advantages	Disadvantages
Adjustable device length for different size cavities	Only suitable for normal uterine cavities
No risk of fluid absorption	Disposable cost
Reduced risk intra-operative bleeding	Data only available for short-term follow-up
Rapid treatment times	NO publications in peer review journals
No endometrial preparation required	
? suitable for outpatient setting	
High amenorrhoea rates with short-term follow-up (>60%)	
Success and patient satisfaction rates >90% in the short-term	

References

1. Lethaby A, Shepperd S, Cooke 1, Farquhar C. Endometrial resection and ablation versus hysterectomy for heavy menstrual bleeding. In: *The Cochrane Library* Issue 4, 1999. Oxford: Update Software.

2. Overton C, Hargreaves J, Maresh M. A national survey of the complications of endometrial destruction for menstrual disorders: the MISTLETOE study. *Br J Obstet Gynaecol* 1997; 104: 1351–1359.

3. Abbott JA. The Novasure™ global ablation technique: results of a prospective multicentre trial. Presented at the 9th Annual Congress of the International Society for Gynaecologic Endoscopy. Gold Coast Australia April 2000.

4. Brill A. The Novasure™ endometrial ablator: preliminary results. Presented at the International Symposium for Operative hysteroscopy. Miami USA February 2000.

17

MEA: Microwave endometrial ablation

N. Sharp

Introduction

Microwave endometrial ablation (MEA™) utilises the heating effect of microwave energy to achieve endometrial coagulation. The advantage of using microwave energy is the precision with which the depth of heating is controlled.

All electromagnetic energy has the ability to penetrate tissue — the depth being a function of its wavelength.

Various regions of the electromagnetic spectrum have been explored in the past in an attempt to treat the endometrium.

Electrodiathermy (resection and rollerball) and radio-frequency utilise the MHz waveband (27.12 MHz). Laser light lies in the nanometre waveband and frequencies above this include ionising radiation which has been employed in former times (radium menopause).

Microwave energy, lying between the MHz waveband and visible light, has a tissue penetration that is very sensitive to frequency change.

Having established the first of three parameters for the microwave research, a penetration depth limited to 6 mm, experimentation confirmed the theoretical prediction of 9.2 GHz being required. Domestic microwave ovens use 2.3 GHz — the lower frequency and longer wavelength ensuring deeper penetration of microwave energy to ensure full even heating of food. The higher frequency and shorter wavelength at 9.2 GHz limits tissue penetration to the 6 mm required for safe endometrial ablation.

Having chosen the frequency, it was clear that wave-guide technology would be required to solve the problem of delivery to the uterine cavity. An air-filled wave-guide would be approximately 3 cm diameter — clearly unsuitable. Using a ceramic dielectric to fill the wave-guide, the microwaves are effectively compressed and can then be transmitted up the narrower 8 mm wave-guide. This forms the basis of the microwave applicator (Fig. 17.1) and fulfilled the second design requirement (should be less than 10 mm and preferably 8 mm).

The third design requirement was a treatment that should take no more than 10 min. MEA™ has superseded this requirement with an average treatment time of only 3 min. This is despite a very low power (22 W radiated power) and is due to the well-known property of microwaves: rapid and vigorous heating.

Activation of the applicator with the tip immersed in egg white gives a good visual representation of the energy zone around the applicator tip demonstrated by the ball of coagulated albumin. This ball forms rapidly, but as the power is maintained it does not continue to expand — the core simply desiccates further and gets hotter, and the desiccation and protein denaturation self-limits the microwave penetration which depends on tissue moisture. This feature gives it an inherent safety.

The surgeon is therefore provided with a 2 cm wide (6 mm + 8 mm + 6 mm) energy source to treat the endometrial surface. Since the average uterus has a cavity about 4 cm long from internal os to fundus and 3.5 cm from cornu to cornu, it is clear that a 2 cm 'brush' will rapidly cover the area to be treated. A thermocouple built into the applicator tip guides the surgeon with continuously displayed thermometry, so whilst being a non-visual technique it is therefore not 'blind'.

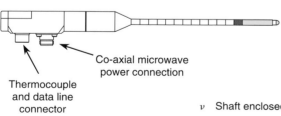

Thermocouple and data line connector

Co-axial microwave power connection

ν Shaft enclosed in permanent coating
ν Sterilisation in autoclave or Cidex
ν Connects to control unit via two cables
   λ Microwave cable
   λ Data cable
ν Can be used for 30 treatments

Figure 17.1 — MEA™ applicator.

Results of *ex vivo* and *in vivo* studies

Laboratory studies on a variety of animal tissues have shown a consistent 5–6 mm depth of thermal necrosis around the applicator tip and this penetration is due to the high water content of tissues. Animal liver is now used routinely for most bench tests and is a good tissue substitute for trialing system modifications.

Ex vivo organ testing was conducted initially with four excised uteri. During these tests there was no rise in serosal temperature despite high endometrial cavity temperatures.

To ensure that uterine blood flow would not reduce the effect of treatment by a coolant effect it was necessary to repeat the studies with perfused excised uteri. There were eight perfusion tests. Again there were no serosal temperature rises at any point and endometrial destruction was not adversely affected. During all excised organ tests measurements confirmed that no microwave leakage occurred, demonstrating complete absorption of the microwaves by the endometrial tissue.

In vivo testing was performed on 17 women at hysterectomy. Care was taken to pack the bowel away and serosal thermocouples were placed at various points to confirm absence of serosal heating during an MEA. Leakage studies were also performed confirming the *ex vivo* findings.

After MEA™ treatment, the uterus was removed and sent unfixed for immediate histochemical and histological examination. Histochemical analysis with nitro-blue tetrazolium[2] shows the effect of MEA™ quite clearly, with vital viable tissue staining a deep blue, but non-viable tissue remains unstained and pale. These tests show a consistent depth of cell death to 5–6 mm with a 1 mm transition zone of cell necrosis, confirming a very localised heating effect.

After the initial programme of research, clinical trials started at the Royal United Hospital in Bath in October 1994. Over 500 patients have now been treated over this 5-year period and over 2000 worldwide.

Equipment

The microwave treatment system (Fig. 17.2) comprises:

- magnetron microwave source, soon to be replaced with solid-state microwave generation;
- data acquisition system;

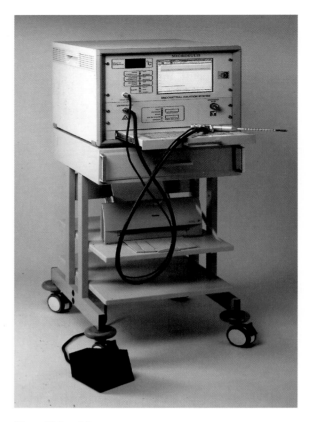

Figure 17.2 — Microwave treatment system.

- cabling;
- microwave applicator;
- foot-switch.

The microwave generation and data acquisition are housed in a cabinet (dimensions: 468 mm × 544 mm × 636 mm, weight: 52.8 kg). On the front of the cabinet are

1. digital temperature display;
2. safety system warning lights;
3. LCD computer screen to assist data entry and to display temperature profile during treatment.

A retractable keyboard is housed in the cabinet base. The data acquisition is via keyboard entry for patient details:

Name
Date of birth
Unit number
Uterine cavity length
Endometrial thickness (optional)

Also the surgeons name is recorded. The patients name is deleted from the final data storage on SIM card for confidentiality. The remaining data for storage is the temperature profile of each treatment and any electrical events during treatment (e.g. temperature trip or other safety system actuation). All such data are periodically accessed for central logging by Microsulis Plc.

Safety features include:

1. Temperature warning if thermocouple exceeds 85°C.
2. Temperature trip if thermocouple exceeds 90°C.
3. Magnetron will only be enabled when thermocouple senses 30°C or greater and only when temperature differential between ambient and thermocouple is less than 10°C. These features ensure that an applicator will not be used that is still hot from autoclaving and that it will only be activated when warmed by external warmth, from body heat, above 30°C.
4. System trip if excess reflected power sensed (e.g. caused by inadvertent removal of applicator from uterus while still active).
5. The system will not activate if the applicator is not connected or the thermocouple is not sensed by the system.

The microwave applicator is reusable and can be autoclaved or soaked to sterilise. It is therefore a surgical tool rather than a 'device' (applicator weight 0.29 kg, length 325 mm, diameter handle 30 mm, diameter shaft 8.5 mm). It is connected to the unit via two cables — one delivering microwave energy via an armoured co-axial cable, the other cable connects via multipin plug for data acquisition.

In addition to the microwave system, a standard D&C set is required to perform MEA™, with the addition of a sterile steel rule to note accurate sounding measurements.

Patient selection

MEA™ is used to treat dysfunctional uterine bleeding and endometrial pathology should be excluded. Patients are screened in the outpatient clinic with vaginal ultrasound assessment of their uterus and adnexae and endometrial biopsy.

A menstrual score is determined by a menstrual questionnaire (Table 17.1).[1]

Table 17.1 — Menstrual score chart

	Score
Dysmenorrhoea	2
Days of bleeding	
7–10	1
>10	2
Average length of cycle	
>28	0
24–27	1
<24	2
Heavy days	
For each day	1
Sanitary protection	
If doubled	2
Frequency of changing	
If >2 hourly	1
If >hourly	2
Clots	1
Flooding	1
Housebound or time off work	2
Pre-operation	
Duration of problem >5 years	1
Post-operation	
Any menstrual loss	1

Fibroids

The presence of fibroids, even sizeable ones, is not a contraindication to treatment. The main factor requiring assessment in this group is cavity distortion. Provided the applicator tip can be applied to the entire cavity surface, then treatment may be given. Vaginal ultrasound alone may determine this but, in cases of multiple fibroids, it may be necessary to arrange hysteroscopy to fully assess suitability. Large cavities may be treated but, cavities with a sounding greater than 110 mm experience less benefit.

Caesarean section

All women with a history of Caesarean section must have transvaginal ultrasound assessment of the Caesarean section scar. If it measures less than 8 mm thickness, then MEA™ should not be performed. In most cases the scar will have healed well but, in a small number of cases, a defective scar will be identified and treatment in such cases represents a risk of bladder injury. This is a simple precaution and in practice very few women are excluded.

Contraindications to MEA™

- Abnormal endometrial histology.
- Other uterine or pelvic pathology which would make hysterectomy a better choice.
- Previous uterine surgery, e.g. myomectomy or previous endometrial resection (Caesarean section — *vide supra*).
- Continued fertility needs.

Special precautions for MEA™

- Uterine retroversion — care is required to ensure instrumentation of the cavity.
- Chronic steroid use — increased risk of uterine perforation.
- Connective tissue disorder, e.g. osteogenesis imperfecta, Ehlers–Danlos syndrome, etc. — increased risk of uterine perforation.
- Uterine abnormality, e.g. bicornuate uterus — recommend abdominal ultrasound control to ensure treatment of both uterine cavities.

Practical aspects of patient management

Endometrial preparation

Initially all subjects had pre-treatment to ensure endometrial thinning. Either a single injection of Goserelin 3.6 mg (Zeneca, Cheshire, UK) or Danazol 800 mg daily for 4 weeks prior to MEA™.

Immediately prior to MEA™, endometrial thickness was measured with transvaginal scan (TVS) in theatre. Of 22 women prescribed Danazol the mean total endometrial thickness was 2.9 mm (0.5–6.0) and of 20 women prescribed Goserelin it was 3.6 mm (0.5–15).[2] The larger range with Goserelin is due to its stimulatory effect if given in the follicular phase. It is therefore advisable to administer Goserelin 5 weeks before MEA™ to overcome this. This has been found to be optimum timing. A longer gap than 5 weeks carries the risk of cervical hardening which makes cervical dilatation more difficult and increases the risk of inadvertent uterine perforation whilst attempting to dilate the cervix.

Both Goserelin and Danazol have a significant side-effect profile which affects patient acceptability. This feature, in conjunction with difficulties ensuring correct administration timing and the observation that endometrial thickness prior to MEA™ did not correlate closely with outcome, led to a study of mechanical thinning.

A pilot study of 12 subjects was undertaken, with full ethical committee approval, using suction aspiration of the endometrium immediately prior to MEA™. A small pregnancy termination catheter was used for this study. Follow-up at 3 months revealed 100% patient satisfaction (12/12) and 50% amenorrhoea (6/12). These preliminary findings encouraged adoption of this technique for the majority of patients. Follow-up of this growing cohort continues to reveal high satisfaction levels.

Analgesia

Post-operative pain is not a major problem with MEA™, but a small number of women will experience quite severe pain for which there appears to be no predictive factors. To minimise the incidence of post-operative pain, the following approach is quite effective:

1. Pre-operatively — Diclofenac 100 mg (Voltarol, Ciba Geigy, Horsham, UK) is given P.R. 1 h before MEA™. Experience has shown that omission of this non-steroidal anti-inflammatory drug (NSAID), through oversight or contraindication, increases the likelihood of post-operative discomfort. For those patients with an allergy to aspirin or NSAID or where NSAID is contraindicated because of a risk of bronchospasm, the new cyclo-oxygenase inhibitor Rofecoxib (Vioxx Merck, Sharp and Dohme, Herts, UK) may have a role.

2. Per-operatively, it is now our usual custom to administer a local anaesthetic block using 20 ml of 0.25% Bupivacaine (Marcain, Astra, Kings Langley, Herts, UK) in a four quadrant intra-cervical block technique at completion of the MEA™. This is given to all patients whether they have had a general anaesthesia or local anaesthesia (*vide infra*).

3. Post-operatively, patients are encouraged to use their favourite analgesia. Those containing NSAID are recommended as being particularly effective. With this thorough approach to analgesia, the incidence of post-operative discomfort is minimal.

Local anaesthesia for MEA™

The mean treatment time for MEA™ is around 3 min which makes it very suitable for a local anaesthetic approach. The technique is a four quadrant block technique, using four ampoules of Prilocaine 3% with Felypressin (Citanest with Octapressin, Astra, Kings Langley, Herts, UK) in a dental syringe. Having exposed the cervix, a small amount of local anaesthetic is injected into the anterior lip. After a few moments the cervix can then be grasped at this point and, with gentle traction, full exposure can usually be achieved. One 2.2 ml ampoule of local anaesthetic is then injected deeply into each cervical quadrant, the aim being to achieve a ring block at the level of the internal os. The two most important quadrants are the two posterior quadrants where the attachment of the uterosacral ligaments with the main uterine nerve supply are the aiming marks.

With this technique painless cervical dilatation to 9 mm is routinely accomplished. Despite a good cervical block, a proportion of women will retain some sensitivity of the uterine fundus. It is therefore advisable to inform patients that during treatment some may experience heat, cramp or severe dysmenorrhoea type pain. They should try and 'breathe through' this as it is transient with the aid of a nitrous oxide/oxygen gas inhalation if required. Since uterine pain is familiar to most women and most are highly motivated and very positive about the treatment, it is uncommon for additional sedation to be given. If, despite the use of nitrous oxide and insertion of the 'post-treatment' additional bupivocaine block early and waiting longer it is still not possible to proceed, intravenous sedation with Midazolam 5 mg (Hypnoval, Roche, Welwyn Garden City, Herts, UK) and Afentanil 0.5 mg (Rapifen, Janssen, Wantage, UK) will enable treatment to be accomplished. Pulse oximetry and supplemental inspired oxygen is mandatory with the patient in a supine position for intravenous sedation as both drugs cause a degree of respiratory depression. It is strongly advised that experience with these potent drugs be gained with the company of an anaesthetist initially.

MEA™ — treatment technique

After establishing anaesthesia the uterine cavity is sounded and the sounding checked against a sterile steel rule. The cervix is dilated to 9 mm and the sounding again checked with the 9 mm dilator — it should be identical.

Having already entered the patient data, the microwave applicator is connected to its cables by an assistant, the magnetron is then activated and the treatment screen is brought up. The applicator is then inserted until the tip abuts the fundus. The sounding is noted on the applicator shaft and this should correspond to the previous measurements. This strict triple check ensures that there is no risk of unrecognised inadvertent perforation.

Once the thermocouple at the applicator tip is warmed beyond 30°C by body heat, the magnetron is enabled and treatment may start.

The power is switched on by the surgeon using a footswitch and the temperature will be seen to rapidly rise. Once it reaches 60°C the applicator is gently but steadily moved from side to side to evenly heat the fundal and cornual areas.

Once the temperature sensed across the uterine fundus is in the therapeutic band the fundal treatment is complete and the applicator is then slowly withdrawn in 3 mm decrements, maintaining the even side-to-side motions.

When the applicator tip is moved from a treated to an untreated area, the temperature is seen to fall and it is then held in that position momentarily to treat that area. The therapeutic temperature will be displayed and the applicator can then be moved on. In this way the temperature profile develops a 'saw tooth', waveform. Using this steady sweeping motion in conjunction with a slow withdrawal, the microwave energy is dispersed evenly into the endometrium from fundus to internal cervical os, guided by the temperature display.

When the active tip reaches the internal os, a yellow band on the shaft starts to appear at the external os and when this is fully exposed, the power is switched off and the applicator withdrawn.

Treatment time therefore depends on cavity size.

Results of treatment

Life table analysis shows that the chance of avoiding hysterectomy (or being listed for hysterectomy) is 82% at 4 years, with most treatment failures occurring within the first 18 months. The chance of avoiding further treatment is 78% (repeat MEA™ or hysterectomy, Fig. 17.3).

Amenorrhoea is achieved in a third of patients treated and this is maintained over the longer term (Fig. 17.4).

Satisfaction rates over 80% are also maintained. Re-treatment in selected patients increases these rates to 40% and 88% respectively.[2]

Dysmenorrhoea is also usefully improved (Fig. 17.5). Many patients presenting at the Menstrual Ablation Clinic with menorrhagia, also describe significant dysmenorrhoea. The incidence of this is greatly reduced after treatment.

The complication rate is very low (Table 17.2).

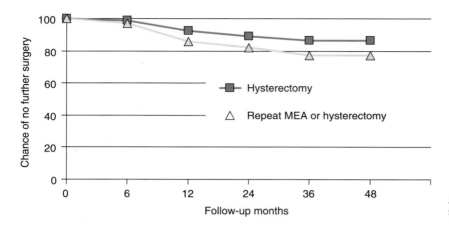

Figure 17.3 — Chance of avoiding further surgery after MEA™.

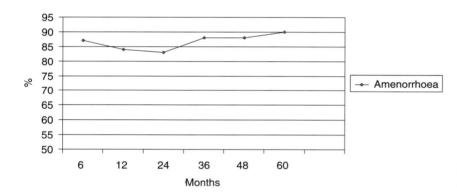

Figure 17.4 — Amenorrhoea and satisfaction rates after single MEA™ treatment.

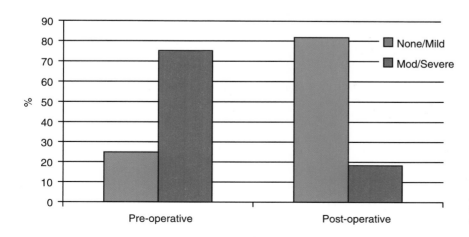

Figure 17.5 — Incidence of dysmenorrhoea pre- and post-operatively.

Table 17.2 — Complications of MEA™ treatment over 4 years (*n* = 304)

	Incidence
Operative	
Haemorrhage	Nil
Fluid overload	Nil
Admission to intensive care	Nil
Perforation with cervical dilator	1
Perforation with applicator	Nil
Emergency hysterectomy	Nil
Local anaesthetic converted to general anaesthetic	Nil
Bowel injury	Nil★
Bladder injury	Nil
Post-operative	
Re-admission with secondary infection	3★★
Haematometra resolved with D&C	2
Haematometra requiring hysterectomy	6
Development of cyclical dysmenorrhoea requiring hysterectomy	14★★★

★We are aware of one case in another centre, during a training list, in a patient who had a history of two previous Caesarean sections. Existing protocols are strongly reinforced to avoid a repetition of this complication.
★★Antibiotic prophylaxis (usually 5 days of Co-amoxiclav) is now routine post-operatively.
★★★Eight in the first year.

Randomised controlled trial of MEA™ and transcervical resection of the endometrium

MEA™ is the only new generation ablation technique to be compared in a randomised controlled trial (RCT) against the existing 'Gold Standard' of transcervical resection of the endometrium (TCRE).[3]

The trial contained 263 subjects treated under general anaesthesia after 5 weeks pre-treatment with Goserelin. Pre-treatment parameters were identical in both groups.

Menstrual outcomes were identical with amenorrhoea of 40% in both groups at 12 months. Satisfaction rates were similar: 77% for MEA™ and 75% for TCRE and about 90% found the treatments acceptable and would recommend them to others. Hysterectomy rates during 12-month follow-up were 7.8% for MEA™ (9/116) and 9.6% for TCRE (12/124).

MEA™ takes significantly less time compared to TCRE (11.4 against 15 min) in this study where the surgeons were highly skilled resectionists, but had only just learnt the MEA™ technique.

This operative time for MEA™ also includes additional gas hysteroscopy (part of their study protocol). There was no intra-operative haemorrhage during the MEA™ procedures compared to a 4% incidence during TCRE. One TCRE procedure had to be discontinued due to risk of fluid overload. Post-operative analgesia requirements were identical.

This RCT therefore confirms that excellent results and a high degree of safety are not operator dependent, but are inherent features of the technique itself.

Advantages	Disadvantages
Inherently safe	*Non-visual*
Microwave physics	'Flying by instruments'
Steady applicator withdrawal	*Applicator diameter 8.5 mm*
Continuous thermometry	'Ensures blunt broad brush'
Low power (22 W)	*Not portable*
Short treatment time	Light solid-state system in
Low energy	development
Uterine blood cooling unimportant	
No heated fluids	
No earthing risks	
Clean	
No bleeding or hysteroscopic fluids	
Quick	
3–4 min	
Simple	
Good outcomes are not operator dependent	
Interactive	
The surgeon is guided by the thermometry	
Display on screen	
Re-usable	
Surgical instrument not disposable	
No 'warm-up' phase	
Treatment commences with 'power on'	
Few exclusions	
Can treat large cavities	
Can treat irregular cavities	
Can treat bicornuate uteri	
Can treat subseptate uteri	
Can treat unicornuate uteri	

Costs

The MEA™ system costs from £195 per treatment ($310, €310).

For further details contact Microsulis Plc on telephone number +44(0)2392240011.

Conclusions

The MEA™ research was initially undertaken in an effort to find something that was quicker and simpler than TCRE for the treatment of DUB. The three basic design parameters were all fulfilled by the novel waveguide applicator. The third parameter — that it should take less than 10 min has been bettered with an average treatment time of less than 4 min.

An additional feature which was originally considered desirable was to have a device that could simply be inserted, switched on and then removed after a set period of time. Thoughts of microwaves diffusing out through some type of mesh covering or variable thickness fine metal coating remained unfulfilled. It therefore became necessary to devise a simple operative technique to move the microwave zone through the cavity to perform the treatment.

This has turned out to be an advantage for the surgeon as it requires an interactive approach to treatment, challenges the senses and induces a sense of pride at a treatment well done. Despite this it is not difficult to learn, has an established safety record as long as the established protocols are followed precisely and it is at least as effective as the more established technique of TCRE.

Long-term data has now accumulated that show good results are maintained and the attrition rates to hysterectomy, or other treatment, are as good or better than other published studies.[4–6]

During the time period of the MEA™ research and its clinical trial from 1992 onwards, other ablative techniques have emerged and are described elsewhere in this book. MEA™, with its solid safety record, substantial long-term data confirming its effectiveness and its ease and speed of use, compares favourably with all current third-generation ablative devices. The facility with which MEA™ can be performed under local anaesthesia in an outpatient setting not only offers real advantages to the patient as well as the surgeon, but must also be a genuine health benefit — providing high quality health care in a low cost environment.

Acknowledgements

The author would like to thank Professor Nigel Cronin at Bath University's School of Physics, Ian Feldberg, Technical and Clinical Research Manager of Microsulis Plc, Martyn Evans, Medical Physicist at the Royal United Hospital, Bath and my research fellows: David Hodgson, Michael Ellard and Trevor Hayes, as well as Microsulis Plc for their financial support.

I would also like to thank the women who took part in the study, especially in the early days when it was something of a leap into the unknown. Most of them seemed quite unafraid and even those with less than satisfactory outcomes often encouraged us to continue with the work — such is the motivation of women to seek a cure to this debilitating problem.

I have since met up with a number of our 'pioneers' and they have been aware of the increasing public interest in MEA™ and seem proud to have made their contribution.

References

1. Sharp NC, Cronin N, Feldberg I, Evans M, Hodgson DA, Ellis S. Microwaves for menorrhagia: a new fast technique for endometrial ablation. *Lancet* 1995; 346: 1003–1004.

2. Hodgson DA, Feldberg IB, Sharp N, Cronin N, Evans M, Hirschowitz L. Microwave endometrial ablation: development, clinical trials and outcomes at three years. *Br J Obstet Gynaecol* 1999; 106: 684–694.

3. Cooper KG, Bain C, Parkin DE. Comparison of microwave endometrial ablation and transcervical resection of the endometrium for treatment of heavy menstrual loss: a randomised trial. *Lancet* 1999; 354: 1859–1863.

4. Magos AL, Baumann R, Lockwood GM, Turnbull AC. Experience with the first 250 endometrial resections for menorrhagia. *Lancet* 1991; 337: 1074–1078.

5. Pinion SB, Parkin DE, Abramovich DR. Randomised trial of hysterectomy, endometrial laser ablation and transcervical endometrial resection for dysfunctional uterine bleeding. *Br Med J* 1994; 309: 979–983.

6. Cooper KG, Parkin DE, Garrath AM, Grant AM. Two year follow up of women randomised to medical management or transcervical resection of the endometrium for heavy menstrual loss: clinical and quality of life outcomes. *Br J Obstet Gynaecol* 1999; 106: 258–265.

18

ELITT: Endometrial laser intra-uterine thermal therapy

R. Polet, J. Squifflet, M. Nisolle, M. Smets and J. Donnez

Introduction

According to the data available, approximately 20% of women of reproductive age suffer from menorrhagia. From the 600,000 hysterectomies performed each year in the USA, about 20% involve uteri that demonstrate no anatomic abnormality upon histological examination. Although curative, hysterectomy is not a trivial undertaking. Mortality ranges from 6 to 11 per 10,000 cases performed for non-obstetric, benign indications.

Though the precise level of bleeding that determines menorrhagia is difficult to pinpoint, its manifestations are tangible. Anaemia, fatigue, irritability, depression and discomfort result in a general deterioration in the quality of life of the menorrhagic patient. In some cases, blood loss may be severe enough to warrant blood transfusions and periods of hospitalisation. Excessive menstrual bleeding can be related to the presence of submucous myomas and frequently, the diagnosis of dysfunctional uterine bleeding, which is a diagnosis of exclusion, is made. In this chapter we describe the endometrial laser intra-uterine thermal therapy (ELITT) procedure pioneered by Donnez et al.

Description, specifications and safety features

The ELITT procedure employs a laser light to destroy the endometrium by thermal therapy increasing the temperature of the endometrium to induce coagulation. Unlike other global ablation modalities, ELITT does not require direct contact with the endometrium in order to induce coagulation. The laser light is diffused inside the uterine cavity in all directions, reaching the entire uterine cavity, including inaccessible areas such as the cornua. The 830 nm wavelength laser light penetrates the uterine wall to a precise depth and is absorbed by the haemoglobin. The absorbed light is then transformed to heat, which warms the endometrium and causes controlled coagulation. The inherent light scattering inside the endometrium contributes positively to the uniformity of the light distribution and resultant coagulation. The GyneLase® system used in the ELITT procedure is manufactured by ESC-Sharplan (Needham, MA, USA) and is composed of a compact tabletop 20 W, 83 0 rim diode laser and a disposable handset.

The system emits laser beams simultaneously through three separate parallel channels. Each channel delivers

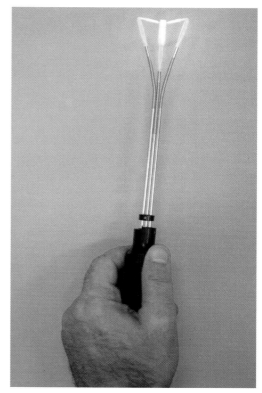

Figure 18.1 — The GyneLase® includes three optical light diffusers, which can be manipulated to conform to the shape as the uterine cavity.

equal laser power at any time, covering the laser beam to the target through an optical fibre. The idea of the handset (Fig. 18.1) was conceived by Donnez and preliminary results were published in 1995 and 1996. The handset includes three proprietary optical light diffusers, which are designed to transmit the laser in all directions to effect the destruction of the endometrial tissue in the fundus and cornua, away from the cervical opening. On each side of the handset, diffusers can be manipulated individually by the operator to conform to the shape of the uterine cavity.

The endocervical canal is dilated to 7 mm and the light diffuser hand piece is inserted into the uterus. The operator advances the distal end of the hand piece to the fundus and adjusts the side diffusers, forming a butterfly-wing contour, which conforms to the shape of the intra-uterine cavity. The laser is then activated for a 7 min pre-programmed cycle. The hand piece is then removed from the uterus.

From a technological standpoint, when compared with non-hysteroscopic endometrial ablation procedures, GyneLase® exhibits several specific features:

1. Maximum energy radiation occurs at the tip of the fibres with subsequent better cornual distribution of laser light.

2. The two-step opening of the device makes it fit in asymmetrical cavities.

3. No uncomfortable uterine distension is exerted before starting the procedure.

The device and the technique are safe. The fibres are solid and do not break. Breakage during laser emission should not be feared. Insertion is blind and allows dilatation of the cervix up to Hegar 7. In case of difficulty or doubt, the correct intra-uterine positioning and opening of the fibres can be checked by echography.

Taking all available data into account, the risk of perforation is very limited. The insertion of contraceptive intra-uterine devices, for example, is associated with a perforation risk of 8.7%. So far, no perforation has been observed. Also, practically, it would be impossible to open the device if it was in a wrong path inside the uterus. Conversely, a full perforation would be detected by the absence of resistance to the opening of the fibres.

In consideration of safety elements, it should be stressed that in contrast to traditional endometrial ablation with the Nd:YAG laser, the ELITT procedure does not require either intensive training or hysteroscopic control and it is inherently far less dangerous since the power used per unit area is 1000 times lower.

Practical aspects of treatment

1. Endometrial preparation
The use of gonadotrophin-releasing hormone (GnRH) before ablation has been shown to be beneficial, both by its well-known effects on the uterus and the clinical data obtained from the techniques of endometrial resection and laser ablation. Data regarding the transhysteroscopic destruction of the endometrium have clearly demonstrated that long-term results are poorer with bigger cavities. GnRH agonists shrink the cavity and allow a tighter fit of the device; they thin the endometrium and reduce the arterial blood perfusion, thereby lowering the heat sink effect of the uterus.

Endometrial laser destruction is proposed for uteri whose sounding ranges from 6 to 10 cm. Under 8 cm, the endometrium can be pre-treated by low dose contraceptive for 1 month, or is simply a direct post-menstrual phase. In bigger cavities, the use of GnRH increases the reduction in the menstrual score and the percentage of amenorrhoea.

2. Inclusion criteria
Dysfunctional uterine bleeding, with uterine sound between 6 and 10 cm, diagnosed by hysteroscopy and endometrial biopsy.

3. Exclusion criteria

- Fertility preservation
- Type I submucous myoma
- Endometrial polyp
- Endometrial atypical hyperplasia, endometrial carcinoma
- Synechiae
- Congenital uterine abnormalities
- Uterine cavity <6 cm or >10 cm

4. Anaesthesia
Approximately in one case out of three, the procedure is performed under local modality, using a paracervical block technique and intravenous sedation in patients who required it and who have shown a good tolerance to hysteroscopy. Otherwise, the choice is given to opt either for a general or local, regional anaesthesia.

Experimental studies

Thermal damage to viscera with incorrectly inserted device is not possible. The mathematical model on which this assumption is based demonstrates that the temperature on the serosa cannot rise significantly due to the heat sink effect of the uterus. *In vivo*, temperatures were measured on the serosa during laser emission and no significant variation was observed. Indeed, microelectrodes positioned 2–3 mm below the serosa failed to demonstrate any elevation of temperature, which remained constant during the entire procedure.

Results from histology tests have demonstrated that the ELITT procedure destroys the entire endometrium and an additional 1–3.5 mm of the adjacent myometrium. A minimum of 67% of the uterine wall remains intact leaving a sufficiently large safety buffer zone. Additionally, because of the design of the handset, the endocervical canal also remains untouched.

Results of treatment (Table 18.1)

Table 18.1 — Follow-up at 6 and 12 months: percentage of amenorrhoea rate

Bleeding status (*n* = 100)	6 months (%)	12 months (%)
Amenorrhoea	69	71
Spotting (<lp/day)	21	20
Hypomenorrhoea	5	5
Eumenorrhoea	4	2
Menorrhagia	1	2

From *Fertility and Sterility*, in press with permission.

Complications and adverse effects

Out of 99 patients, two did suffer dysmenorrhoea caused by cornual haematomata (<1 cm diameter) after exhibiting amenorrhoea for more than 6 months. They underwent laparoscopic subtotal hysterectomies, one at 9 months and the other at 14 months after the procedure. One patient had a cervical stenosis with subsequent haematomata and she was relieved by simple drainage of the uterine cavity. Another patient had a profuse cervical leucorrhoea for 3 weeks, probably as a consequence of an endocervical burn, similar to what is observed in cryotherapy of the cervix. Endometritis was reported in two cases, mainly when no pre-operative use of antibiotics had been set. The patient is now systematically given 2 g cefacidal pre-operatively. In case of mucopurulent cervicitis, the patient should be treated several days before the operation so that the cervix is sterilized at the time of the procedure. Several cases of severe cramping pain have been observed in the immediate post-operative phase requiring use of NSAID parenteral or in rare instances, dipidolor. We have added to the pre-operative preparation of the patient the systematic administration of NSAID intravenously or per rectum at the time of the antibiotic dose.

Conclusions

The endometrial ablation by the diode laser using the GyneLase® system has replaced, in our department, all the hysteroscopic surgery performed for dysfunctional uterine bleeding with anatomically (sub)normal cavity, with far better results in terms of amenorrhoea rate and general patient satisfaction. The ability to perform in a clinic set-up, speeds up the management of the menorrhagic patients and reduces the surgical suite occupation. The extreme simplification of the laser endometrial ablation achieved by the GyneLase® contrasts with its extreme effectiveness.

Myomatous uteri are not contraindication for the procedure. True amenorrhoea is simply not achieved so often and the patient should be informed about it.

Advantages	Inconvenients
Simple	Cost of the furniture
Inherently safe	Controlled randomised clinical trials not achieved yet
Effective (amenorrhoea rate)	
Multifunctionality of the laser source★	
Light and transportable	

★Indications other than endometrial ablation: condylomas, limited foci of epithelial dysplasia, cervical mucorrhoea, coagulation of cervix, and small endometrial polyps with 5 mm hysteroscope.

Bibliography

1. Hallberg L, Hogdahl A, Nilsson L. Menstrual blood loss — a population study. *Acta Obstet Gynecol Scand* 1966; 45: 320–351.

2. Decherney AH, Polan ML. Hysteroscopic management of intrauterine lesions and intractable uterine bleeding. *Obstet Gynecol* 1983; 61: 392–397.

3. Goldrath MH, Fuller FA, Segal S. Laser photovaporization of endometrium for the treatment of menorrhagia. *Am J Obstet Gynecol* 1981; 140: 14–19.

4. Basterday CL, Grimes DA, Riggs JA. Hysterectomy in the United States. *Obstet Gynecol* 1983; 62: 203–212.

5. Carlson KJ, Nichols DH, Schiff I. Indications for hysterectomy. *N Engl J Med* 1993; 83: 792–796.

6. Meyer WR, Walsh BA, Grainger DA, Peacock LM, Loffer FD, Steege JF. Thermal balloon and rollerball ablation to treat menorrhagia: a multicenter comparison. *Obstet Gynecol* 1998; 92: 98–103.

7. Amso NA, Stabinsky SA, McFaul P, Blanc B, Pendley L, Neuwirth R. Uterine thermal balloon therapy for the treatment of menorrhagia: the first 300 patients from a multi-centre study. *Br J Ob/Gynaecol* 1998; 105: 517–523.

8. Dequesne J, Galliant A, Garza-Leal JG. Thermoregulated radiofrequency endometrial ablation. *Int J Fertil* 1997; 42: 311–318.

9. Friberg B, Joergensen C, Ahlgren M. Endometrial thermal coagulation — degree of uterine fibrosis predicts treatment outcome. *Gynecol Obstet Invest* 1998; 45: 54–57.

10. Donnez J, Polet R, Mathieu PE, Konwitz E, Nisolle M, Casanas-Roux F. Nd:YAG laser ITT multifibre device (the Donnez device): endometrial ablation by interstitial hyperthermia. In: J Donnez, M Nisolle (Eds) *Atlas of Laser Operative Laparoscopy and Hysteroscopy*, pp 353–359, 1995. Parthenon Publishing.

11. Donnez J, Polet R, Mathieu PE, Konwitz E, Nisolle M, Casanas-Roux F. Endometrial laser interstitial hyperthermy: a potential modality for endometrial ablation. *Obstet Gynecol* 1996; 87: 459–464.

12. Higham JM, O'Brien PMS, Shaw RW. Assessment of menstrual blood using a pictorial chart. *Br J Obstet Gynaecol* 1990; 97: 734–739.

13. Donnez J, Vilos G, Gannon M, Stampe-Sorensen S, Klinte I, Miller R. Goserelin acetate (Zoladex) plus endometrial ablation for dysfunctional uterine bleeding: a large-randomised, double-blind study. *Fertil Steril* 1997; 68: 29–36.

14. Hawe JA, Chien FF, Martin D, Phillips AG, Garry R. The validity of continuous automated fluid monitoring during endometrial surgery: luxury or necessity? *Br J Obstet Gynaecol* 1998; 105: 797–801.

15. Overton C, Hargreaves J, Maresh. A national survey of the complications of endometrial destruction for menstrual disorders: the mistletoe study. *Br J Obstet Gynaecol* 1997; 104: 1351–1359.

16. Neuwirth RS. Endometrial ablation using a thermal balloon system. *Contemp Obstet Gynecol* 1995; 15: 35–39.

17. Singer A, Almanza R, Gutierrez A, Haber G, Boldue LR, Neuwirth R. Preliminary clinical experience with a thermal balloon endometrial ablation method to treat menorrhagia. *Obstet Gynecol* 1994; 732–734.

18. Vilos GA, Vilos EC, Pendley L. Endometrial ablation with a thermal balloon for the treatment of menorrhagia. *J Am Assoc Gynecol Laparosc* 1996; 3: 383–387.

19. Phipps JH, Lewis BV, Prior MV, Roberts T. Experimental and clinical studies with radio frequency induced thermal endometrial ablation for functional menorrhagia. *Obstet Gynecol* 1990; 76: 876–881.

20. Lewis BV. Radio frequency-induced endometrial ablation. *Baillier Clin Obstet Gynecol* 1995; 9: 347–355.

21. Donnez J, Polet R, Squiffiet J, Rabinovitz R, Levy U, Ak M, Nisolle M. Endometrial laser intrauterine thermotherapy (ELITT™): a revolutionary new approach to the elimination of menorrhagia. *Curr Opin Obstet Gynaecol* 1999; 11: 363–370.

22. Donnez J, Gillerot S, Bougonjon D, Clerckx F, Nisolle M. ND-YAG laser hysteroscopy in large submucous fibroids. *Fertil Steril* 1990; 54: 999–1003.

23. Donnez J, Nisolle M, Gillerot S, Smets M. Endometrial ablation in dysfunctional bleeding: size of the uterine cavity. In: J Donnez, M Nisolle (Eds) *Atlas of Laser Operative Laparoscopy and Hysteroscopy*, pp 312–322, 1995. Parthenon Publishing.

19

Hydrothermablation (BEI)

Milton Goldrath

Introduction

Efforts to find a safe, effective and easy to perform therapy for relief of menorrhagia can be documented back to the last century, with the introduction of superheated steam into the uterine cavity.[1] Other early methods included electrocoagulation of the endometrium as early as the 1930s and 1940s when a large round electrode was blindly introduced into the uterus.[2] Additional blind methods included the introduction of destructive materials, including radium[3] and various chemical agents.[4] Cryosurgical probes were blindly placed within the uterus in an attempt to produce the same effect as cervical ablation.[5] Recently, balloon devices containing heated fluid have been introduced.[6,7] All of these methods, while representing ingenious approaches to the destruction of endometrial tissue, suffer limitations that include the risks associated with blind introduction and blind application of destructive effect, as well as the inability to provide homogeneous delivery of energy throughout uterine cavities of varying sizes and shapes.

In 1981, an efficacious and cost-effective method of transcervical endometrial ablation utilising the neodymium:yttrium–aluminum–garnet (Nd:YAG) laser was first reported.[8] Subsequently, hysteroscopic methods utilising electrosurgical currents for destruction of the endometrium were developed.[9] While both of these treatment methods represent excellent treatment alternatives, outcomes are dependent on the experience and skill of the user. Absorption of significant amounts of the fluid used to distend the uterus can cause serious complications.[10]

The pursuit has continued for a new method of endometrial ablation that would be easy to learn, would provide clinical results less dependent on the experience and skill of the clinician would allow the procedure to be moved to an outpatient setting, and would reduce or eliminate the significant risks associated with existing methods of hysteroscopic endometrial ablation. Additionally, such a method should include hysteroscopic visualisation, be suitable for use with uterine cavities of varying sizes and shapes, provide the ability to effectively treat the cornual areas and eliminate the risk of fluid overload.

This pursuit led to the development of the Hydro ThermAblator® (HTA®) (BEI Medical Systems, Teterboro, New Jersey, USA) which allows the controlled circulation of heated saline within the uterine cavity under direct visualisation at pressures below the minimum required for Fallopian tube opening. Initial investigations of the HTA® concept focused on documenting that the external temperature of the uterus is not increased by the circulation of 90°C saline within the uterine cavity during the treatment cycle and that heated fluid does not escape from the Fallopian tubes due to the gravity limited, low pressure within the uterus.

The Hydro ThermAblator® (HTA®) system

The HTA® consists of a mobile, microprocessor controlled, main control unit (HTA®) with IV Pole, reusable Heater Canister (Fig. 19.1) and sterile HTA Procedure Kit (Fig. 19.3).

The HTA® main control unit consists of the following elements:

- front display panel,
- cassette plate and pump,
- HTA® IV Pole,
- support software and firmware.

The HTA® is intended to allow thermal ablation of endometrial tissue through heat transfer from re-circulating heated fluid. The HTA uses 0.9% NaCl solution ('normal saline') heated to 90°C, which is circulated into the uterine cavity through the inflow channel of a single patient use insulated hysteroscopic sheath. A reusable Heater Canister (Fig. 19.1) heats the saline solution externally to the patient. The saline solution is delivered to the patient's uterine cavity using pressure *only* sufficient to achieve the distention of the uterus and circulation of the heated saline solution. Distention of the uterus is achieved by raising the

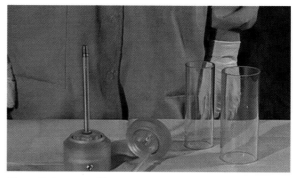

Figure 19.1 — Reusable Heater Canister.

IV Pole to position the mid-point of the fluid level reservoir (Fig. 19.4) at a height of 115 cm above the level of the patient's uterus. This height produces a net hydrostatic pressure of the circulating fluid of approximately 50–55 mmHg within the uterine cavity. This net hydrostatic pressure within the uterine cavity during fluid circulation is less than the static pressure created by a 115 cm column of normal saline that would actually be closer to 78 mmHg. This is due to the evacuation of fluid from the uterine cavity by the peristaltic circulation pump. Fluid flow to and from the patient's uterine cavity is controlled by valves which are only open during the stages of HTA® operation when the circulation pump is also in operation.

A necessary component of the HTA® system is the reusable Heater Canister (Fig. 19.1), which incorporates the fluid heating rod and temperature sensors.

Temperature measurement is achieved by use of two redundant temperature sensors (thermistors — Fig. 19.2) positioned inside the reusable Heater Canister. Accurate and precise temperature control is achieved by use of a programmable temperature controller. The HTA® system continuously monitors and displays temperature on the front display panel of the control unit. If the redundant temperature measurements do not comply with the preset temperature, an alarm will sound and a self-diagnostic message will be displayed informing the operator of the fault condition.

The sterile HTA® Procedure Kit (Fig. 19.3) consists of the following elements:

• sterile patient sheath assembly ('Sheath'),
• sterile cassette ('Cassette'),
• fluid level measurement reservoir ('Reservoir'),
• fluid collection bag.

The peristaltic re-circulation pump is used to remove saline solution from the uterine cavity and return the saline solution to the Reservoir at a flow rate of approximately 300 ml/min. This is accomplished with the use of the Cassette and Reservoir tubing sets. Saline solution from the Reservoir flows into the inlet port and exits from the outlet port of the reusable HTA® Heater Canister. As the saline solution passes through the Heater Canister, it is heated to 90°C. When the Sheath tubing set is connected to the output tubing of the Cassette, saline solution is delivered to the patient and is then returned from the patient to the Reservoir by the pump to complete a closed loop fluid path.

Five solenoid valves located on the Cassette mounting plate at the side of the main control unit are used to control the flow of saline solution during various stages of the HTA® operation (Fig. 19.4). The fill valve (source valve) allows saline solution from the saline source bag to enter the system during the filling, priming and cooling stages. The drain valve allows the system to remove saline solution during the flushing and draining stages. A bypass valve (re-circulation valve) is used so that the Heater Canister, Reservoir and Cassette tubing can be filled with saline solution prior to the Sheath being connected to the system. This allows self-diagnostic checks to be performed on the heating and temperature measurement systems of the unit and to the fluid loss detection system, prior to the insertion of the hysteroscopic sheath into the patient. The patient safety inlet valve allows saline solution to be delivered to the patient and the patient safety outlet valve allows saline solution to be returned from the patient to the Reservoir. The patient safety valves are open when the patient connection indicator on the front panel is illuminated. A sixth solenoid is used as a latch to secure the Cassette to the Cassette plate. A manual latch on the Cassette plate assembly is provided for additional security.

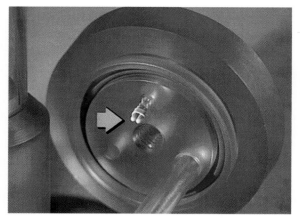

Figure 19.2 — Dual temperature sensors.

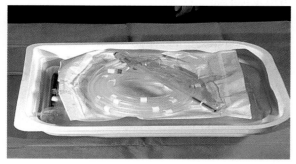

Figure 19.3 — Sterile HTA® procedure kit.

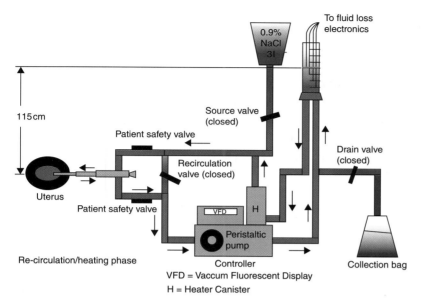

Figure 19.4 — Schematic diagram of the re-circulating and heating system. Note that gravity controls fluid flow through the Heater Canister and to the patient. The pump will withdraw fluid from the patient and return the fluid to the Reservoir. The Reservoir contains fluid from the pump that enters into the Heater Canister via gravity for re-heating.

The HTA® utilises a fluid measurement system located on the IV Pole, which monitors the saline solution level in the Reservoir during the procedure. If the system loses >10 ml of saline solution, either cumulatively or at one time, the flow of saline solution to the patient is stopped. An alarm will sound and an error message will warn the user that there has been a fluid loss. User action is required to continue the procedure. Likewise, if the saline solution level in the Reservoir rises >20 ml, saline solution flow to the patient will be interrupted. An alarm will sound to warn the user that fluid has reached an excessive level. The excess saline solution will automatically be drained to the Fluid Collection Bag. Normal operation can then be resumed. The '80' level on the Reservoir is considered the normal operating fluid level.

The HTA® uses a vacuum fluorescent display (VFD) (Fig. 19.5) located on the control unit to provide step-by-step message prompts to guide the user through the procedure. This display also presents warnings, self-diagnostic error messages and corrective action messages. In addition, front panel indicator lights are used to show the status of the Pump, heater, patient connection and Cassette. A blinking heater light indicates that the fluid has been heated, and a steady heater light indicates that there is power to the heater rod and the fluid is being heated. The Cassette light will blink and indicate when the Cassette can be installed or removed. The Cassette may be installed or removed by pressing the Cassette release button. Once installed and secured, the Cassette cannot be removed until the end

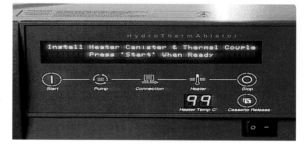

Figure 19.5 — Message display.

of the procedure due to the Cassette latch that engages and locks the Cassette in place. The HTA® is controlled by pressing the start and stop membrane buttons located on the front.

The Sheath is designed to accept many commercially available ≤3 mm hysteroscope telescopes by means of corresponding adapters. The Sheath is provided sterile and functions as the inflow and outflow channels for fluid circulation to the uterine cavity (Fig. 19.6). The Sheath is constructed of polycarbonate and incorporates air pockets within its outer wall that act as a thermal insulator to protect the cervix and endocervical areas from the temperature of the saline solution circulating within the Sheath.

The cervix is sufficiently dilated to allow introduction of the insulated Sheath (7.8 mm OD) which accommodates a 3 mm hysteroscope telescope. Over-dilation of the cervix should be avoided to assure a

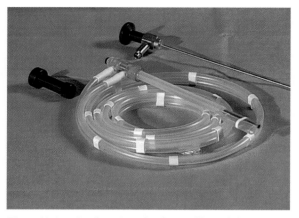

Figure 19.6 — Sterile patient sheath assembly with hysteroscope and adapter HTA® procedure.

snug fit around the Sheath. The HTA® sheath can be inserted under direct visual control, either by viewing directly through the eyepiece or attaching a video camera to the hysteroscope to allow observation on a video monitor. Initially, the uterine cavity is distended with unheated (room temperature) saline solution and the entire cavity is examined visually using the HTA® sheath as a diagnostic hysteroscope. This diagnostic hysteroscopy allows the uterine cavity to be examined for any unsuspected pathology and to confirm proper sheath placement in the lower uterine segment. If the cervix does not fit snugly around the Sheath, a cervical sealing tenaculum can be used to 'seal' the cervix as well as to stabilise the position of the Sheath. After satisfactory visualisation and inspection of the cavity with the unheated saline solution has been achieved, the fluid control system is switched to the re-circulating mode and the system fills to establish the nominal amount of fluid that will be re-circulated and monitored for loss throughout the remainder of the procedure. Since a fixed amount of fluid is re-circulated, any loss of fluid from the system will result in a measurable change in the level of fluid in the upper Reservoir. The fluid level monitoring system in the Reservoir is designed to detect a cumulative loss of 10 ml. In the event that such a loss is detected the system will interrupt fluid circulation and provide an alarm and appropriate self-diagnostic message.

Following the filling phase, the HTA® prompts the user to confirm their desire to proceed with heating of the fluid and treatment. The heating system is designed to gradually raise the saline temperature to therapeutic levels in approximately 3 min. During much of this time only mildly warmed fluid will be circulated and

circulating fluid volume is continuously monitored. This provides additional protection in the event that fluid loss is detected since the system will shut down before the operative temperature of the fluid is reached.

When the temperature of the circulating saline reaches 80°C, fluid circulation is momentarily interrupted and the level of the fluid in the Reservoir is re-confirmed. The unit then begins its 10 min treatment countdown as the temperature continues to rise to 90°C. Re-circulation of the heated saline at 300 ml/min and continuous monitoring of fluid level are maintained throughout the treatment cycle. Extensive testing has demonstrated that a temperature drop of only 2–3°C occurs between the heater and the output port of the hysteroscopic sheath due to the high re-circulation rate, Thus, no thermocouples need to be placed within the uterus. After completion of the treatment cycle, the system is flushed with room temperature saline which rapidly cools the Sheath and its tubing as well as the fluid in the uterus and the hysteroscope provides visual confirmation of the changes in the appearance of the uterine cavity. At the completion of the 1 min cooling cycle, the user is prompted that it is safe to remove the Sheath from the patient.

Inclusion/exclusion criteria

Patients who are in good general health and who do not desire future pregnancies are good candidates for treatment with the HTA®. The uterine cavity should measure ≤12 cm. Patients who present with intramural fibroids can be treated provided that the fibroids do not obscure visualisation of both cornua or distort the cavity to the extent that it would effect fluid flow.

Patients should be excluded from treatments with the HTA® if they have an abnormal cervical or endometrial pathology or large submucous fibroids and polyps. Patients who have had previous uterine surgeries where thinning of the uterine wall musculature could occur should be fully evaluated before treating with the HTA®. Any patient with a full septate or bicornuate uterus should be excluded for treatment, however, patients with partial septa can be included for HTA® treatment.

Phase I study

Studies by Ralph Richart et al, on uteri extirpated post-HTA® treatment were conducted to determine

Table 19.1 — Phase I time and temperature results

Patients	Treatment time (min)	Treatment temperature (°C)	Depth of necrosis (mm)	Uniformity	Cornual necrosis (mm)
1–2	3	85	0–1.5	Poor	0–1
3–11	5	85–88	1–3	Poor	1–2
12–14	7–8	85–87	1–3	Poor	1–2
15–20	10	85–87	2–3	Adequate	2
21–32	10	90	3–4	Good	2–3

the depth of destruction of tissue.[11] A total of 32 patients were included in the Phase I study, 10 of whom had patent Fallopian tubes. All patients received GnRH analogue before undergoing HTA treatment. The patients were treated at varying times and temperatures to establish optimal treatment parameters (Table 19.1).

The specimens were cut fresh within 30 min of their surgical removal and snap frozen in liquid nitrogen. They were cut on a microtome as a frozen section, stained histochemically for the presence of oxidative enzyme activity using standard methodology and examined microscopically. Cells that contained active oxidative enzymes could be identified by the presence of a black reaction product. Those with inactivated enzymes due to their denaturation by the HTA procedure did not contain the black reaction product (Figs 19.7 and 19.8).

The slides were also stained with a light counterstain, allowing the myometrium, endometrial and endocervical glands, blood vessels and other tissue components to be identified. The distribution of intact and inactive enzyme was noted and the depth of inactivation was measured under the microscope using a millimetre ruler. The results were tabulated and correlated with the time and temperature of the HTA treatment.

Based on this study conducted on patients treated for 10 min with heated 0.9% NaCl solution (USP Injection Grade) at 90°C, the depth of tissue destruction was 3–4 mm with no observable destruction in the cervical tissue.

Endometrial preparation

Optimal ablation with the HTA® occurs when the procedure is performed in a uterine cavity with a thin endometrium. Therefore, endometrial thinning must take place prior to the HTA® treatment in order to aid visualisation and to achieve the optimum heat penetration through the endometrium into the myometrium. Ideally, the endometrium should measure <4 mm at the time of treatment.

The following regimens have been tested using the HTA® procedure:

Option 1 One dose Lupron® Depot 3.75 mg IM or Zoladex® 3.6 mg IM given on day 1–5 of the patient's menstrual period. The treatment is performed between days 24 and 30 from the date of the injection.

Option 2 One dose of Lupron® Depot 7.5 mg IM or Zoladex® 7.2 mg IM is given on day 19–23 of the patient's menstrual period. The treatment is performed between days 19 and 28 from the date of the injection, provided a menstrual flow has occurred. If the patient does not have a menstrual period, an ultrasound must be performed to measure endometrial thickness and a pregnancy test must be performed to ensure that the patient has not become pregnant (GnRH agonists are not contraceptive drugs).

Option 3 Two doses Lupron® Depot 3.75 mg IM or Zoladex® 3.6 mg IM. The first injection may be given any time during the patient's menstrual period with the second injection occurring 4 weeks from the date of the first injection. The treatment is performed between 2 and 4 weeks after the date of the second injection.

Patients should be instructed to discontinue use of any other hormonal medications while receiving the described hormonal agents. Patients can become pregnant during administration of the pre-treatment hormonal medications and must be instructed to use barrier device methods for contraception.

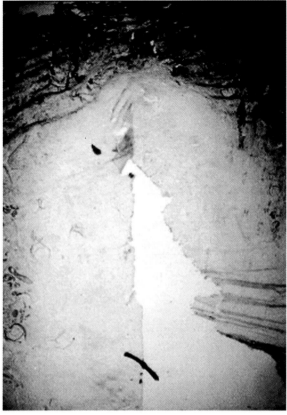

Figure 19.7 — Cornual pathology section with oxidative enzyme stain.

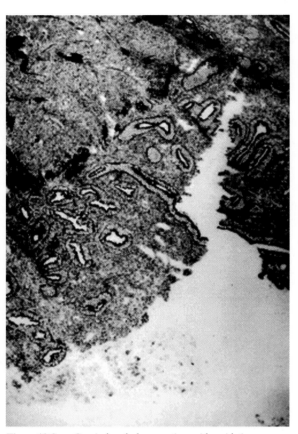

Figure 19.8 — Cervical pathology section with oxidative enzyme stain.

Adverse events/ complications

The HTA® should only be used by physicians who have been properly trained. There have been no serious adverse events reported to the company in over 850 cases performed. Some of the adverse events relating to the procedure are uterine cramping, ranging from mild to severe and lasting up to 4 h after completion of the procedure. Cases of haematometra have been reported (<1% of cases performed), however, the majority were resolved by sounding the uterus in the office.

Other potential complications do exist when using the HTA®, especially the risk of cervical leakage. The physician must not excessively dilate the cervix when inserting the Sheath. The cervix should form a tight seal around the Sheath to prevent retrograde flow back into the vagina. Physicians must position the distal tip of the hysteroscopic Sheath just inside the internal cervical os during treatment and resist the urge to manipulate the Sheath once the heater is activated. A cervical sealing tenaculum may be placed on the cervix to help stabilise the Sheath during therapy. The potential also exists for external burns as a result of the Sheath tubing resting on the patient during treatment. The incidence was <0.5% during clinical trials. The tubing assembly is being modified to prevent this type of occurrence.

Advantages and disadvantages of HTA® therapy

Advantages	Disadvantages
Integrated hysteroscope allows the physician to perform diagnostic hysteroscopy immediately	Endometrial suppression should be given before treatment using GnRH agonists or Danazol,

before treatment, properly position the Sheath for treatment and to observe treatment effect on tissue.

resulting is a delay before HTA treatment.

Per procedure cost is estimated to be below US $400.

Heated saline fully conforms to the endometrial lining for complete treatment of the endometrium, including the cornua.

Treatment outcomes are less dependent on the skill or experience level of the physician.

Treatments may be performed in the outpatient or office setting under local anaesthesia (paracervical block) only.

Results of HTA treatment

The FDA Phase II study was performed on menorrhagia patients who were not candidates for, or who did not desire, hysterectomy. Only patients with documented pictorial blood-loss assessment chart[12] (PBAC) diary scores of ≥150 were included in the study. The outcome measurement was the cessation or reduction of the amount of menstrual bleeding, documented by PBAC diary scores which directly affects the patient's quality of life. Performance of the HTA® also provided a demonstration of the safety of the equipment. Patients received two doses of GnRH analogue approximately 4 weeks apart, with the treatment occurring between

2 and 4 weeks after the second injection. All patients were treated at 90°C for 10 min. Results are listed in Table 19.2. All patients experienced mild to severe uterine cramping for up to 4 h after the treatment which was treated with non-steroidal anti-inflammatory drugs. No other adverse events occurred.

Prospective studies of HTA® efficacy have been conducted at various international sites, with the patients followed for at least 12 months after HTA treatment. The 12-month results of these studies are summarised in Table 19.3.

Patient treatments under the FDA Phase III multi-centre randomised clinical study to evaluate the safety and effectiveness of thermal endometrial ablation using the HTA®, when compared with existing ablation therapy using rollerball treatment to reduce excessive menstrual bleeding or menorrhagia, were completed in August 1999. The study is prospective and randomised 2:1 with a 2-week, 3-month, 6-month and 12-month clinical follow-up with 276 patients enrolled:

- 181 patients receiving treatment with the HTA®,
- 88 receiving treatment with rollerball,
- 7 patients not treated due to varying circumstances.

Six-month patient follow-up clinical data has been submitted to the FDA and it is anticipated that 12-month follow-up data will be submitted in September 2000.

Table 19.2 — Phase II efficacy results

Number of patients	20
Age	43.2 ± 5.01
Pre-operative PBAC diary scores	580 ± 392.82
6 months post-operative PBAC scores	58.33 ± 26.89
12 months post-operative PBAC scores	15 ± 21.21

Table 19.3 — International 12-month efficacy results

Authors	Number of patients	Amenorrhoea rate (%)	Success rate (%)
Romer and Muller[13]	18	50	94.4
Dores et al[14]	17	47	94.1
Jimenez et al[15]	59	44.1	93.2
Weisberg[16]	19	57.9	94.7
Romer et al[17]	60	45	95

Conclusion

Hydrothermablation under direct hysteroscopic visualisation is a safe method of ablating the entire endometrium in patients with menorrhagia. The safeguards built into the HTA system protect the patient from injury. The efficacy of the procedure is not dependent on the skill or experience of the surgeon and requires only basic diagnostic hysteroscopy skills.

The results of the HTA® treatment are favourable when compared to reported results using resectoscopic and rollerball techniques and does not require the degree of skill and experience necessary for those procedures. The free circulation of heated saline at low pressures allows uterine cavities of varying sizes and shapes to be effectively treated, without a need to exclude minor anatomical anomalies such as partial septa or small myomas.

The ability to use the HTA® to perform endometrial ablation under local anaesthesia with or without accompanying sedation enables the gynaecologist to perform the procedure in a clinic or office setting, making it a convenient and cost-effective alternative when compared to traditional methods of endometrial ablation.

References

1. Pinkus. *Apparat zur Atmokausis*. Euro-Med-Clinic, Fürth (textbook).

2. Bardenheuer FH. Electrokoagulation der Uterusschleimhaut zur Berhandlung Klimakterischer Blutugen. *Zentralbl Gynäcol* 1937; 4: 209–211.

3. Rogny AJ. Radium therapy in benign uterine bleeding. *J Mt Sinai Hosp* 1947; 14: 569.

4. Schenker JG, Polishuk WZ. Regeneration of rabbit endometrium following intrauterine instillation of chemical agents. *Gynecol Invest* 1973; 4: 1.

5. Droegemueller W, Greer BE, Makowski EL. Cryosurgery in patients with dysfunctional uterine bleeding. *Obstet Gynecol* 1971; 38: 256–259.

6. Singer A, Almanza R, Gutierrez A, Haber C, Bolduc CR, Neuwirth R. Preliminary clinical experience with a thermal balloon endometrial ablation method to treat menorrhagia. *Obstet Gynecol* 1994: 84: 732–734.

7. Friberg B, Persson BR, Willen R, Ahlgren M. Endometrial destruction by hypothermia — a possible treatment of menorrhagia. *Acta Obstet Gynecol Scand* 1996; 75: 330–335.

8. Goldrath MH, Fuller TA, Segal S. Laser photovaporization of endometrium for the treatment of menorrhagia. *Am J Obstet Gynecol* 1981; 140: 14–19.

9. De Cherney A, Desmond MC, Lavy G et al. Endometrial ablation for intractable uterine bleeding: hysteroscopic resection. *Obstet Gynecol* 1987; 78: 688–670.

10. Arieff AI, Ayres JC. Endometrial ablation complicated by fatal hyponatremic encephalopathy. *JAMA* 1993; 270: 1230–1232.

11. Richart RM, Dores GB, Nicolau SM, Focchi GR, Cordeiro VC. Histologic studies of the effects of circulating hot saline on the uterus before hysterectomy. *J Am Assoc Gynecol Laparosc* 1999; 6: 269–273.

12. Janssen CAH, Scholten PC, Heintz APM. A simple visual assessment technique to discriminate between menorrhagia and normal menstrual blood loss. *Obstet Gynecol* 1995; 85: 997–982.

13. Romer T, Muller J. A simple method of coagulating endometrium in patients with therapy-resistant, recurring hypermenorrhea. *J Am Assoc Gynecol Laparosc* 1999; 6: 265–268.

14. Dores GB, Richart RM, Nicolau SM, Focchi GR, Cordeiro VC. Evaluation of Hydro ThermAblator for endometrial destruction in patients with menorrhagia. *J Am Assoc Gynecol Laparosc* 1999; 6: 275–278.

15. Jimenez JS, Martin I, de la Fuente L, Munoz JL, Vaquero G, Ramirez M, Perez C, de la Fuente P. Severe menorrhagia due to glanzmann thrombasthenia treated with hydrothermal ablation. *J Am Assoc Gynecol Laparosc* 2000; 7: 265–267.

16. Weisberg M. Endometrial ablation using the Hydro ThermAblator®. Presented at the *ESGE Meeting*, September 1999, Stockholm, Sweden.

17. Romer T et al. Treatment of recurrent menorrhagia using the Hydro ThermAblfsator® — results of the prospective German multicenter study. Presented at the *ESGE Meeting*, September 1999, Stockholm, Sweden vol. 95; 312–322.

20

The EnAbl™ hydrothermal system for endometrial ablation

Rafael F. Valle and Michael S. Baggish

Introduction

Almost 20 years after a feasible, effective and practical method of endometrial ablation by laser photo vaporisation was introduced, multiple new methods have been developed or are under study in an attempt to simplify the original laser ablation procedure.[1,2] These new variations have included electro-surgery, radiofrequency, cryosurgery, microwaves and improved delivery of laser energy with or without tissue sensitisation.[3–8] These modern methods of endometrial destruction are certainly a far cry from the original attempts of using chemicals, cytotoxic agents and other more dangerous agents such as ionising radiation, that have shown to carry significant morbidity and poor efficacy. While laser energy and electro-surgery have proven efficient and relatively safe in accomplishing endometrial ablation and are considered today the standard methods to obtain endometrial destruction with an overall success rate of 85%, their performance and application requires considerable experience. The problems associated with excessive fluid absorption as well as less than desirable or excessive tissue destruction with possible uterine perforation are still a concen.[9–11] Additionally, a uterine cavity with variable distortions in its symmetry may not be reached adequately in its entirety and the endometrium may not be uniformly destroyed. Other significant factors are the subjective variables involved to accomplish uniform endometrial destruction, particularly with electro-surgery, be it by resection or by coagulation.[12–14] In order to address these concerns, new methods with built-in computerised systems are being introduced to reduce the inherent drawbacks involved in endometrial destruction using previous methods of endometrial ablation.[15] It is undeniable that such a method should remove what may be a significant factor in the outcome besides proper patient selection and preparation, i.e. individual subjectivity of assessing complete endometrial destruction. Heated fluids that can be delivered in the uterine cavity easily and safely with a computerised mechanism that involves its circulation, accurate control of the intra-uterine pressure and temperature are appealing due to their simplicity, removal of additional endoscopic methods with its ancillary equipment and applicable to an office setting. The only technical aspect of the method required will be the introduction of the device in the uterus, similar to the introduction of an intra-uterine device.

Description of the EnAbl™ device

The InnerDyne endometrial ablation catheter or EnAbl™ system is a small, single-use 5 mm diameter, 24 cm long thermal ablation device. It consists of an electrical resistance heater mounted in a semi-flexible shaft (12 French — 4 mm diameter). The fluid defuser is located within a cage-like structure which is collapsible to facilitate placement, expands within the uterus to support the organ walls and prevent the fluid defuser from making direct tissue contact. The temperature sensors are mounted on the ribs of the wall expander to monitor the fluid temperature adjacent to the organ wall. The catheter shaft incorporates a central lumen to permit infusion and aspiration of fluid and to provide for the cycling mixing action. An extension set, bonded to the catheter shaft and connected to a 3 mm syringe, is inserted in the micro-jet isothermal mixer. Power and sensor connections are located on the proximal shaft of the catheter (Figs 20.1 and 20.2).

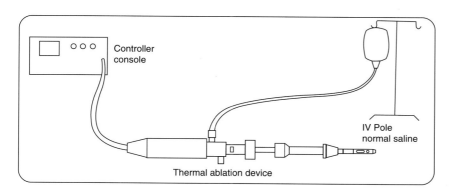

Figure 20.1 — Schematic representation of the EnAbl™ system.

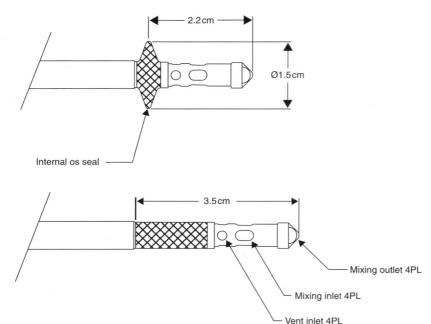

Internal os seal

Mixing outlet 4PL

Mixing inlet 4PL

Vent inlet 4PL

Figure 20.2 — Close up view of the thermal ablation device tip with an activated (top) and collapsed cervical stop (bottom) (Scale 2:1).

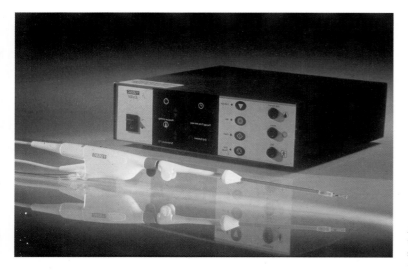

Figure 20.3 — The EnAbl™ cannula and control unit for monitoring of intra-uterine pressure and temperature.

A trans-cervical uterine access device consists of a 6.7 mm insulated shaft containing a 4.5 mm lumen through which the ablation catheter is placed. A side port with a stopcock is provided in the access device for fluid filling, evacuation of excess fluid or air and pressure monitoring (Fig. 20.3).

A treatment software version 4.26 and computer system is required for data acquisition. Thermal ablation power and connecting cables are also designed to meet UL544 requirements. The power unit supplies direct current to the thermal ablation catheter at a maximum of 26 V and 3.0 A (78 W). It is connected to the computer by a ribbon cable, which allows for monitoring and proportional, integral differentiation control feedback. It is also connected to the thermal ablation catheter by cables and carries the electrical power to the heater coil and the temperature monitoring signal to the system (Fig. 20.4).

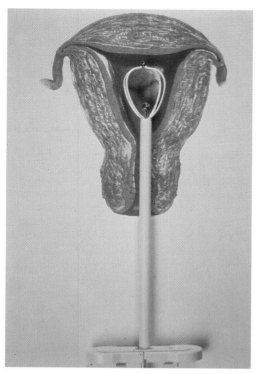

Figure 20.4 — EnAbl™ system in the uterine cavity with thermocouples in place.

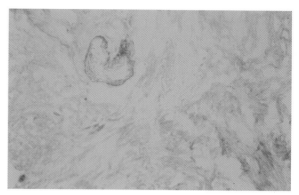

Figure 20.5 — Photomicrograph of treated endometrium with hot circulating saline. Negative NADH — diaphorase tissue staining confirms loss of tissue viability.

Micro-jet isothermal mixer

The micro-jet isothermal mixer is a pneumatically driven syringe pump. The mixer system is designed to achieve and maintain uniform temperature distribution within the uterus during thermal treatment and to optimise heat transfer from the ablation catheter. The micro-jet mixer uses a pneumatic logic control to provide the frequency of 30 cycles per minute and a stroke length of 2.5 cm (2.5 ml volume) (Fig. 20.5).

Pressure monitoring system

The pressure monitoring system consists of a Datascope 2002, a Cobe CDX 111 transducer and interconnect cable. The transducer is connected to the side port of the access device. Before thermal treatment, fluid filling of the intra-uterine cavity is provided through the annular space within the access device and out through the side port, stopcock and transducer. The inter-connect cable is attached to the electronic pigtail of the transducer at one end and to the Datascope 2002 at the other end. The Datascope 2002 provides continuous pressure monitoring. A possible perforation of the uterus will be signalled by loss of pressure.

In vitro and *in vivo* assessment of the EnAbl™ hydrothermal system

Baggish et al[16] evaluated this computer-controlled, continuous circulating, hot irrigating system for endometrial ablation in an *in vivo* sheep study as well as an *in vitro* human uterus perfusion. As shown by NADH-diaphorase staining, treatments at 80°C resulted in complete loss of viability at the mucosa and submucosal levels of the sheep uteri with little or no viability of the adjacent myometrium. Uterine segments treated at 70°C were characterised by consistent necrosis of the mucosa and evidence of myodegeneration and oedema. Most of the submucosal glands were necrotic but some of the deeper glands were spared. At 60°C treatments, a loss of viability (by NADH–diaphorase) of the mucosal layer was demonstrated. The myometrium was normal nonetheless (Fig. 20.6).

In the *in vitro* human uterus perfusion studies, when temperatures were sustained at more than 80°C or

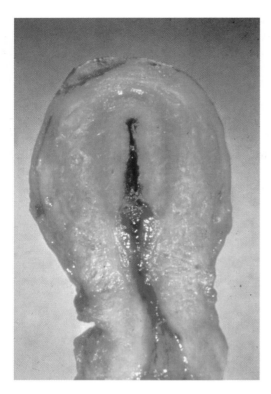

Figure 20.6 — Sagital view of divided uterus treated with hot circulating saline before hysterectomy. Note destruction of endometrial lining.

Assessment of intra-uterine instillation of heated saline safety in pre-hysterectomised patients

Bustos-Lopez et al[17] evaluated the safety of intra-uterine instillation of heated saline in women undergoing abdominal hysterectomy because of abnormal uterine bleeding. Before hysterectomy, the endometrial cavities were exposed to 15 min of re-circulatory normal saline heated to 70–85°C. The uteri were analysed for extent of thermal damage using standard histopathological techniques and tissue viability by histochemical staining. Intra-uterine pressures and serosal temperatures were continuously monitored by computer. In each treated specimen, histochemical staining demonstrated the depth of necrosis that extended throughout the entire endometrium and approximately 1–2 mm into the myometrium. No side effects or related complications were noted. In all 11 patients, serosal and subserosal temperatures were within safe limits (mean temperature 37°C). Four women with patent tubes did not show a spill of fluid during the procedure. The patients were pre-treated with a GnRH analogue, leuprolide acetate, 3.75 mg IM, to thin the endometrium uniformly in order to make a better assessment of the tissue penetration of the circulating heated saline. In this study, consistently low serosal and subserosal temperatures (less than 37°C) were detected. Thermal damage to the endometrium was homogenous along the uterine cavity, including the cornual regions. This is especially relevant given the diversity of uterine cavity configuration in humans. An average depth of 4.3 mm of destruction was obtained which is adequate to destroy the functional layers of the endometrium Tables 20.1–20.3 (Figs 20.7–20.9).

more for 15 min, the evaluation of the endometrium at gross examination showed complete destruction. Microscopically, the endometrial glands were disrupted and the stroma collagenised. Alternatively, the endometrium was converted into a structureless, coagulated amorphous mass (hematoxilin eosin stain). NADH-diaphorase stain evaluation of the tissues showed complete destruction of the endometrium. Additionally, no evidence of viability was found in the superficial myometrium (1–3 mm) next to the basalis. Importantly, a substantial margin (50–70%) of viable was demonstrated through the uterus, including the cornual regions. Peak serosal surfaces ranged from 35°C to 49°C. No uterine perforations were noted. Intra-uterine pressures were continuously monitored and ranged between 20 and 40 mmHg with a mean pressure of 26 mmHg. No leakage of fluid from the oviducts was observed. No retrograde leakage through the cervix (i.e. around the access device) was observed as well. The volume of saline solution required to fill the uterus ranged from 5 ml to 15 ml.

Clinical application of the EnAbl™ system

Patients' selection, preparation and technique for use

The appropriate selection (dysfunctional uterine bleeding) and preparation (thin endometrium) of patients for endometrial ablation remains one of the most important variables involved in achieving success of treating

Table 20.1 — Histology results

Number of patients	°C (time in min)	Thermal gross	Treatment H & E	Depth (mm) NADH
1	Control	0.0	0.0	0.0
2	70 (17)	4.8	4.9	4.9
3	70 (17)	4.8	5.1	5.1
4	80 (15)	3.5	3.7	3.7
5	80 (15)	4.0	4.0	4.0
6	80 (15)	2.0	2.3	2.4
7	80 (15)	4.1	4.1	4.2
8	85 (15)	4.0	4.0	4.1
9	85 (15)	5.3	4.7	4.9
10	85 (15)	4.8	4.7	4.7
11	85 (15)	6.0	4.0	4.5

Adapted from Bustos-Lopez et al.[17]

Table 20.2 — Subserosal temperatures (thermo couples) results

Area	n	$\bar{X}$	SD	Max	Min
Cervix	219	37	2	42	30
Anterior body	198	37	3	42	28
Fundus	219	37	3	45	28
Posterior body	219	38	3	45	28
L fimbria	219	35	1	37	26
R fimbria	219	35	1	38	26
Control	211	35	2	41	28
Total	1504	36.28°C			
$\bar{X}$ = intra-uterine pressures		45.77 ± 8.67			

Adapted from Bustos-Lopez et al.[17]

Table 20.3 — Serosal temperatures (infra red) results

Area	n	$\bar{X}$	SD	Max	Min
Right Oviduct	153	34	1	38	31
Left Oviduct	156	35	1	38	31
Right Cornu	153	35	2	40	29
Left Cornu	153	35	2	40	29
Control	152	34	1	36	30
Total	767	34.6			

Adapted from Bustos-Lopez et al.[17]

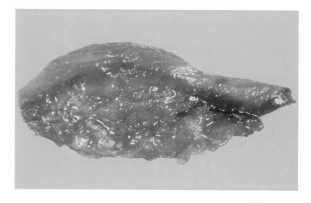

Figure 20.7 — Close up view of fundal area of uterus after ablation.

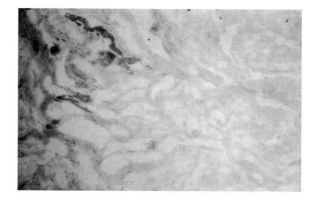

Figure 20.8 — Photomicrograph of endometrium after ablation. NADH — diaphorase staining demonstrates lack of stain uptake in devitalised tissue.

abnormal bleeding. Nonetheless, with the extended use of this method of treatment, they have frequently been ignored, deriving in variable results. Therefore, standardisation of these important variables is of utmost importance in the use of any method of endometrial ablation. Patients with organic uterine lesions causing the abnormal bleeding should be eliminated and the procedure done when the endometrium is thin, i.e. postmenstrual and mechanically or hormonally thinned.[18–20]

The technique of endometrial ablation with the EnAbl™ system is relatively simple. Once the patient has been selected and prepared for this procedure, the uterus is evaluated including an aspiration endometrial biopsy to rule out malignant and pre-malignant conditions. The uterus is then sounded to assess depth and the thermal catheter, adjusted for the appropriate length, is introduced. Because there is no need for routine cervical dilatation, analgesia or anaesthesia is optional. A mild sedation or analgesic, before the

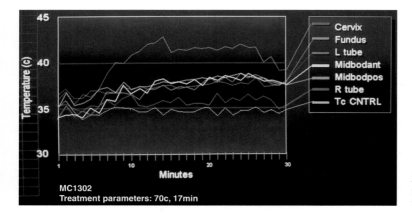

Figure 20.9 — Subserosal temperatures of uterus at different sites with measurement of temperature versus time of exposure.

procedure, may be helpful for some women to relieve apprehension. Alternatively, a local paracervical block, placed superficially at the base of each uterosacral ligament may be required should a need for uterine sounding or cervical dilatation arise. The system is checked for possible leakage and, if none, the unit activated for 15 min at 75–80°C temperature of the circulating saline. At the completion of the procedure, the patient is observed briefly and then discharged with instructions for care and follow-up.

Clinical trials and future improvements

The EnAbl™ system of computer-controlled, continuously circulating hot irrigating saline for endometrial ablation seems to be an efficient and safe method to accomplish uniform destruction of the endometrium in a simple and practical manner. An office-based self-contained catheter that can be placed within the uterine cavity without resorting to dilatation, that can circulate normal saline solution heated to temperatures high enough to obtain endometrial coagulation within a short time, seems attractive to patients, health care providers and insurance companies. Based on animal *in vivo* studies, as well as human *in vitro* and *in vivo* evaluations, this method of endometrial ablation seems to efficiently obtain uniform endometrial destruction with safety in controlling depth of penetration and fluid diffusion through patent fallopian tubes. Based on this evaluation with peak serosal temperatures under a safe range and with excellent endometrial destruction of all human uteri studied, including those with cavity deformities caused by submucous myomas, that were treated with about 80°C for 15 min showing

destruction of the endometrium and destruction below the endometrium into the myometrium extending 1–3 mm, efficacy is confirmed. Furthermore, the peak serosal temperature between 15°C and 49°C and the mean intra-uterine pressure of 26 mmHg demonstrates safety in avoiding excessive tissue destruction or damage to surrounding organs.

However, in view of the limited number of subjects treated in these preliminary evaluations, some larger studies, that also measure intra-uterine pressures serially, are needed to confirm these preliminary findings and assure safety, particularly of spilling heated fluid into the peritoneal cavity. The system could be improved with added safety valves preventing the increase of pressure even above 30 mmHg.[21]

Although the EnAbl™ unit senses a decrease in intra-uterine pressure automatically and shuts the system down and immediately stops the heating and circulation of the saline, leakage of fluid through the oviducts could trigger similar events by decreasing the intra-uterine pressure. Nonetheless, similar safety valves should apply to increased intra-uterine pressure above 30 mmHg.

The EnAbl™ system for endometrial ablation remains appealing due to its relative simplicity, office base applicability and uniform endometrial destruction coupled with safety of heat penetration. Extended clinical trials are eagerly awaited.

Summary and conclusions

A conservative surgical method of controlling abnormal uterine bleeding in patients who do not respond to hormonal treatment is highly desirable, particularly in women at high risk of major surgical interventions. In view of the fact that the ideal patients to be treated by endometrial ablation are those with dysfunctional uterine bleeding, i.e. no organic aetiology causing the problem, a hysterectomy, which after all cures these patients, seems to be too aggressive and an invasive method to treat this problem. Endometrial ablation is an excellent alternative under these circumstances. The methods employed today have, by far, addressed the problem adequately despite that in the long term only about 85% of women could be cured and 15% may require additional treatment for recurrent abnormal uterine bleeding. The standard methods of ablation utilised today, such as laser and electro-surgery used by most gynaecologists for endometrial ablation, whilst used in a significant number of patients, require an operating suite, skilful endoscopists and expensive array of instrumentation. Additionally, the inherent problems of possible fluid overload, uterine perforation and the subjective appraisal of endometrial destruction by physicians, makes the technique somewhat cumbersome by some and not applicable in all settings and for all potentially eligible women. New methods that remove subjective variables, reduce the need for hospital facilities and ancillary instrumentations and depend more on computerised systems to achieve uniform endometrial destruction not requiring cervical dilatation, are eagerly awaited and welcome by patients and clinicians alike. The EnAbl™ system seems to provide most of these features, while at the same time eliminates many of the drawbacks inherent in our standard methods of endometrial ablation used today.

Should extended clinical trials of the EnAbl™ hydrothermal system confirm the preliminary encouraging findings in the *in vitro* and *in vivo* studies so far performed, this computerised system of circulating heated fluid used in the uterus to accomplish endometrial ablation, will have a significant role in the treatment of those women with abnormal uterine bleeding unresponsive to medical therapy.

References

1. Goldrath MA, Fuller T, Segal S. Laser photovaporisation of the endometrium for the treatment of menorrhagia. *Am J Obstet Gynecol* 1981; 140: 14–19.

2. Baggish MS, Valle RF, Barbot J. Endometrial ablation. In: MS Baggish, S Barbot, RF Valle (Eds) *Diagnostic and Operative Hysteroscopy. A Text and Atlas,* 2nd edn, pp 289–306, 1999. London: Mosby.

3. DeCherney AH, Diamond MP, Lavy G et al. Endometrial ablation for intractable uterine bleeding: hysteroscopic resection. *Obstet Gynecol* 1987; 70: 668–670.

4. Drogemueller W, Greer BE, Makowski E. Cryosurgery in patients with dysfunctional uterine bleeding. *Obstet Gynecol* 1971; 38: 256–258.

5. Pittrof R, Majid S, Murray A. Initial experience with transcervical cryoablation of the endometrium using saline as a uterine distension medium. *Minimal Invasiv Ther* 1993; 2: 69–73.

6. Phipps JH, Lewis BV, Roberts T et al. Treatment of functional menorrhagia by radio frequency induced thermal endometrial ablation. *Lancet* 1990; 335: 374–376.

7. Sharp NC, Cronin N, Feldberg T et al. Microwaves for menorrhagia: a new fast technique for endometrial ablation. *Lancet* 1995; 346: 1003–1004.

8. Donnez J, Polet R, Mathieu PE et al. Endometrial laser interstitial hyperthermy: a potential modality for endometrial ablation. *Obstet Gynecol* 1996; 87: 459–464.

9. Garry R. Good practice with endometrial ablation. *Obstet Gynecol* 1995; 86: 144–151.

10. Phillips G, Chien PFW, Garry R. Risk of hysterectomy after 1000 consecutive endometrial laser ablations. *Br J Obstet Gynecol* 1998; 105: 897–903.

11. O'Connor H, Magos AL. Endometrial resection for the treatment of menorrhagia. *N Engl J Med* 1996; 335: 151–156.

12. Valle RF. Rollerball endometrial ablation. In: AG Gordon (Ed) *Endometrial Ablation,* vol 9, pp 299–316, 1995. London: Bailliére Tindall.

13. Onbargi LC, Hayden R, Valle RF et al. Effects of power and electrical current density variations in an *in-vitro* endometrial ablation model. *Obstet Gynecol* 1993; 82: 912–918.

14. Overton C, Hargraves J, Maresh M. A national survey of the complications of endometrial destruction for menstrual disorders: the MISTLETOE study. *Br J Obstet Gynaecol* 1997; 104: 1351–1359.

15. Baggish MS. Minimally invasive non-hysteroscopic methods for endometrial ablation. In: MS Baggish, J Barbot, RF Valle (Eds) *Diagnostic and Operative Hysteroscopy. A Text and Atlas,* 2nd edn, pp 325–332, 1999. London: Mosby.

16. Baggish MS, Paraiso M, Brezneck EM, Giffrey S. A computer-controlled, continuously circulating, heated irrigating system for endometrial ablation. *Am J Obstet Gynecol* 1995; 173: 1842–1848.

17. Bustos-Lopez HH, Baggish MS, Valle RF et al. Assessment of the safety of intrauterine instillation of heated saline for endometrial ablation. *Fertil Steril* 1998; 69: 155–160.

18. Valle RF. Should hysteroscopic ND-YAG endometrial ablation be used only for women in whom hysterectomy

will be contraindicated? *J Gynecol Surg* 1990; 6: 289–290.

19. Valle RF. Endometrial ablation for dysfunctional uterine bleeding: role of GNRH agonists. *Int J Gynecol Obstet* 1993; 41: 3–15.

20. Valle RF, Baggish MS. Endometrial carcinoma following endometrial ablation: high-risk factors predicting its occurrence. *Am J Obstet Gynecol* 1998; 179: 569–572.

21. Baker VL, Adamson GD. Threshold intra-uterine perfusion pressures for intra-peritoneal spill during hydrotubation and correlation with tubal adhesive disease. *Fertil Steril* 1995; 64: 1066–1069.

21

Photodynamic therapy

Michael J. Gannon, Mark R. Stringer and Stanley B. Brown

Introduction

Herodotus, the ancient Greek historian described the use of sunlight for treating skin lesions.[1] Phototherapy was developed as a science and popularised by Faroe Islands physician Niels Finsen who won the Nobel Prize in 1903. He showed that light from a carbon arc with a heat filter could be used to treat tuberculosis of the skin.[2] Administration of a sensitiser in addition to light has long been known to have a beneficial effect. Ancient Egyptians ingested plants containing light-activated psoralens and satin strong sunlight to treat vitiligo. Four thousand years later psoralen activated by ultraviolet A radiation (pUV A) is used in the treatment of psoriasis.[1] The process is known as photo chemotherapy.

Origin of photodynamic therapy

One hundred years ago, Oscar Raab, who was testing the effect of acridine against the malaria protozoan *in vitro,* performed two similar experiments with widely varying results in the rates of *Paramecia* destruction.[3] A thunderstorm which obscured daylight during the second experiment was the only difference in conditions. Raab, then a medical student, went onto demonstrate that light was required for acridine-induced destruction of *Paramecia.* Over the next few years it was recognised that oxygen was the essential component required for the destructive effect. The term 'photodynamische Wirkung' was coined to distinguish this oxygen-dependent phenomenon from the phototherapy described by the ancient physicians.

Photodynamic therapy (PDT) is now recognised as a medical treatment that uses a combination of visible light and a sensitising drug to destroy selected cells. In PDT, a drug without dark toxicity is introduced into the body and accumulates preferentially in rapidly dividing cells. When the drug, known as a photosensitiser, reaches an optimal concentration in target tissue a measured light dose of appropriate wavelength is shone onto the area. Light activates the drug and elicits the toxic reaction in the presence of oxygen.

Studies with haematoporphyrins

The porphyrins are the most widely studied of the many drugs with photosensitising properties. German scientist

Friedrich Meyer-Betz gave a compelling demonstration of the photodynamic properties of porphyrins in a celebrated experiment in 1913. He injected himself with 200 mg of haematoporphyrin and suffered photosensitivity associated with oedema and hyperpigmentation for 2 months.[4]

Haematoporphyrin derivative (HpD), which gave better fluorescence with a lower dose and shorter administration time than crude haematoporphyrin, was introduced in the early 1960s.[5,6] Richard Lipson used light from a direct current carbon arc lamp passed through a copper sulphate solution to remove the red component. This produced an intense blue beam between wavelengths 400 and 407 nm, suitable for diagnostic studies. Following systemic administration of HpD, the suspect area was viewed through a filter to block … activating light. Carcinoma of the cervix showed the typical salmon pink tumour fluorescence[7] and a good correlation between fluorescence and biopsy-proven malignancy was shown in several studies.[8,9] During tumour detection studies of breast cancer, Lipson realised that the porphyrins, which induced tissue fluorescence, at the same time would allow destruction of the fluorescent tissue by light at an appropriate wavelength.[10]

Modern development of PDT

Two American groups commenced research into PDT in 1972. Diamond and colleagues reported that the administration of haematoporphyrin followed by visible light therapy proved lethal to glioma cells in culture and produced massive destruction of porphyrin-containing gliomas which had been transplanted subcutaneously in rats.[11] This paper brought the term 'photodynamic therapy' into general use.[2] Dougherty demonstrated eradication of a transplanted mouse mammary tumour using HpD activated by red light from a filtered xenon arc lamp[12] and treated various malignant tumours with intravenous HpD and laser light.[13] The longer wavelength red light (650 nm) was chosen for treatment as it had better tissue penetration properties than shorter wavelength blue or green light.

Results from pre-clinical and clinical studies, conducted worldwide over the past 30 years, have established PDT as a useful treatment approach for some cancers. The clinical applications of PDT as a treatment modality have been directed to advanced or recurrent cancers unsuitable for curative surgery. PDT may provide an alternative or an adjunctive treatment for gynaecological cancers where other modalities fail.[14] Since 1993, regulatory approval for PDT using a purified preparation of HpD in patients with early and advanced stage cancer of the lung, digestive tract and genitourinary tract has been obtained in Canada, the Netherlands, France, Germany, Japan and the US.[15] Photofrin received UK approval in January 1999.

Mechanism of photodynamic therapy

Photosensitisers, in general, tend to accumulate in neoplastic tissues. The ratio of photosensitiser concentration between tumour and surrounding normal tissue varies with the photosensitiser and the tissue and forms the basis for successful PDT. Selective photosensitiser uptake in vascular, proliferative tissues is used to target certain non-neoplastic tissues, as well as tumours, for destruction. As a rule it can be stated that practically all photosensitisers that have been studied have a pronounced affinity for non-neoplastic tissues which are high in reticulo-endothelial components.[16]

Photodynamic action

A photosensitiser in tissue remains stable until excited by light of an appropriate wavelength and sufficient energy.[16] This rapidly causes a transformation from the ground singlet state to a photoactive, excited triplet state. The next step is crucially dependent on the presence of oxygen. Interaction of the metastable triplet state and molecular oxygen forms the electronically excited singlet oxygen. The process, known as photodynamic action, is responsible for cellular damage in PDT. Photosensitiser in the target tissue localises the toxicity of chemical reactions resulting from electrical excitation. Singlet oxygen, accompanied by other highly reactive intermediates such as free radicals,[17] is responsible for the irreversible oxidisation of essential cellular components.[18] The destruction of crucial cell membranes, organelles and vasculature leads to cell necrosis. Targets of PDT also include microvasculature both of the tumour and normal tissue as well as the inflammatory and immune host system. The photodynamic effect is dependent on an adequate supply of molecular oxygen for conversion to the highly toxic-activated species singlet oxygen.[17]

Light wavelength and penetration

Visible light is used in PDT. It is convenient to generate a fixed dose with a laser and deliver this to the target area via a fibre. The wavelength chosen for treatment depends on a number of considerations. Porphyrins generally absorb well in the low wavelength, blue range of the visible spectrum.[19] The porphyrin photosensitisers are thus most efficiently activated by blue light. Unfortunately, endogenous tissue chromophobes including haemoglobin also absorb well in the blue. The ubiquitous nature of haemoglobin means that blue light has a very limited capacity for penetration in living tissue. The haemoglobin absorption spectrum falls off rapidly above a wavelength of 600 nm in the red. Longer wavelengths are therefore chosen for PDT even though most photosensitisers absorb less well at these levels. The increased penetration depth of longer wavelength light is a major incentive for the development of new photosensitisers absorbing at such wavelengths.

About 30% of incident light between wavelengths 600 and 800 nm reflects off the surface layer.[20] This leaves about 70% of photons free to propagate into the tissue. These photons are subject to multiple scattering before they are absorbed. Scattering is caused by variations in refractive index which alter the direction of travel of individual photons. The initial forward direction is altered after about 1–2 mm to a nearly isotropic light distribution in most tissues. The path travelled by a photon is much longer than the linear distance covered. Scattering thus leads to increased absorption even though the process itself occurs without loss.

Optical dose

The fluence rate measures the quantity of photons per second passing through a defined area $(mW\,cm^{-2})$.[20] Light fluence in tissue decreases exponentially with distance due to absorption and scattering. The effective penetration depth of light is the distance (in mm) corresponding to a decrease in the fluence rate by a factor of $1 \cdot e^{-1}$ equivalent to 0.37 (where $e = 2.718$). Since it is determined by absorption and scattering and as both of these parameters differ between tissues, there is a characteristic optical penetration depth for each tissue. The average light penetration depth is about 1–3 mm at 630 nm and 2–6 mm at 700–850 nm of light.

Optical dose is a product of the incident fluence rate and the exposure time.[20] The amount of light delivered to a tissue is also influenced by propagation properties and geometry of the particular tissue. Back-scattered light enhances the fluence rate near the surface increasing light delivered to a superficial tissue. The suitability of PDT for the treatment of surface lesions has been exploited in recent studies of PDT for superficial lesions which are extensive or prove difficult to eradicate, such as pre-malignant conditions[21] and endometriosis.[22] Furthermore, in a hollow organ such as the uterus, the surface fluence rate may be increased by a factor of 5–6 due to the reflection of light from surrounding walls. The accessibility of the endometrium and the buffer provided by the myometrium make the prospect of safe endometrial destruction by PDT appealing.

Photodiagnosis

Photosensitisers produce fluorescence which may be used to identify photosensitisation. Earlier sensitisers such as HpD being mixtures of compounds with diverse photosensitisation and fluorescence properties were not well suited to quantitative detection. In contrast, the newer photosensitisers, which are based on a defined molecular structure, have the potential to give quantitative fluorescence detection. The best fluorescence differential is usually produced by relatively low doses of photosensitiser.

The photophysical properties required in a sensitiser for diagnosis are different from those required for treatment. Diagnosis by fluorescence is favoured by a high quantum yield of fluorescence whereas treatment requires high triplet yields. According to the law of photochemical equivalence (Stark-Einstein) the total of quantum and triplet yields cannot exceed unity. It is probable that distinct photosensitisers will therefore be developed for diagnosis and therapy.[2] Blue light, which is absorbed weakly, is used for fluorescence activation in the technique of photodiagnosis (PD). Developmental work is based on studies carried out for the detection of superficial bladder cancer.[23] Gynaecological, indications for PD include lower genital tract intraepithelial neoplasia, peritoneal or endometrial cancer and endometriosis.

Dysfunctional uterine bleeding

Current methods of endometrial ablation generally require anaesthesia and despite meticulous technique about one in five women subsequently need hysterectomy.[24] PDT is simple to perform and may give better results because of endometrial targeting.

Early studies on photodynamic endometrial ablation

The first attempt at photodynamic endometrial ablation was carried out on ovariectomised rats. Dihematoporphyrin ether (DHE) was taken up by the endometrial layer of the oestrogen-primed rat uterus. Photoradiation of the uterine surface, 72 h after DHE administration, caused selective coagulation necrosis in the entire endometrium and the inner part of the muscularis.[25] PDT endometrial ablation was also studied in rabbits which, like rats, have a double uterus providing a convenient treatment and control uterine horn in each animal. Bhatta[26] showed that Photofrin was retained preferentially by the endometrium, with, the greatest concentration observed in the stroma. Laser light was delivered using an optical fibre with a diffusing tip inserted in the rabbit uterus. When the uterus was examined after treatment, endometrial necrosis was confirmed and related to the dose of Photofrin. Despite the rabbit's relatively thin myometrium there was no full thickness uterine destruction.

Development of porphyrin photosensitisers

Many early studies were carried out using HpD which is a complex mixture of porphyrins including esters and ethers. A more efficient photosensitiser was obtained by removal of the monomers, which do not localise in tumour tissue to yield the proprietary preparation, Photofrin. This has specificity for malignant tissue, although it also accumulates in liver, spleen, kidneys and skin.

The latter may lead to photosensitisation lasting up to 6 weeks thus restricting the wider use of Photofrin.[27] Tumour selectivity over surrounding normal tissues is not always optimal. Moreover, Photofrin absorbs only weakly above 600 nm where light exhibits the deepest penetration of tissues.

The ideal tumour photosensitiser should be a pure, single substance, selective for tumour tissue over surrounding normal tissue, which achieves efficient photosensitisation, is non-toxic in the dark and rapidly excreted from the body. It is desirable that the sensitiser has a high triplet quantum yield and efficient transfer of excitation energy to produce singlet oxygen.[2] For optimum effect it should absorb well in the red part of the visible spectrum. Red light has less absorption and scattering, and penetrates tissue more deeply than shorter wavelength blue or green light.[28]

Chlorins, purpurins and phthalocyanines

Several strategies have been employed to increase porphyrin absorption in the red. The search for new photosensitisers is concentrated on preparations with relatively intense bands in the longer wavelength 650–800 nm region.[19] Chlorins and bacteriochlorins are formed by progressive reduction of porphyrins. The chlorin absorption spectrum shows a strong band in the red (650 nm) giving the substance a green colour. As its natural parent compound, chlorophyll is sensitive to autoxidation, studies have been performed on the PDT activity of less fragile derivatives such as mono-aspartyl chlorin e_6 (MACE-Nippon Petrochemical/Meiji Seika, Tokyo, Japan). A powerful photosensitiser causing better tumour necrosis than Photofrin *in vivo* tests is the synthetic chlorin meso-Tetra(m-hydroxyphenyl) chlorin (m-THPC) or temoporfin. It is undergoing clinical studies in PDT for various cancers and is available commercially as Foscan (Scotia Pharmaceuticals Ltd., Guildford, UK). Benzoporphyrin derivative (BPD), a chlorin in spite of its name, is also being developed commercially as BPD-monoacid ring A (BPD-MA, QLT PhotoTherapeutics Inc., Vancouver, Canada). The drug–light interval is short and generalised photosensitisation is low. BPD-MA has an interesting application in macular degeneration, a common cause of blindness. Neovascularisation near the macula is treated by PDT through an ophthalmoscope using a diode laser. Treatment produces selective closure of the leaky vessels without damage to overlying retina.

Chlorin substitution gives a puce coloured series of compounds called purpurins. The most active is the hydrophobic tin complex of etiopurpurin (SnEt2-Miravant Inc., formerly PDT Inc., Santa Barbara, California, USA). Further reduction produces the bacteriochlorins with an intensified absorption band which is shifted further to the red at around 735 nm. More extensive changes to the porphyrin structure produce the azaporphyrin derivatives phthalocyanine (pc) and the closely related naphthalocyanine (Nc). Sulphonation of the metal complex renders these extremely hydrophobic compounds water soluble. Various complexes of Pc with non-transition elements such as zinc (Zn phthalocyanine, Cuba Geiger, Basel, Switzerland), aluminium and silicon show photobiological activity against tumours. Absorption maxima are red shifted to around 670 nm for Pc and 750 nm for Nc. Although there is also a greater magnitude of light absorption than shown by Photofrin the evidence for its translation into photodynamic effect *in vivo* is limited.[29]

5-Aminolaevulinic acid

An alternative approach uses 5-aminolaevulinic acid (ALA) to produce protoporphyrin IX (PpIX), a precursor of haem in most body cells.[30] Administration of excess ALA leads to accumulation of PpIX which acts as an endogenous photosensitiser. Like the other porphyrins, PpIX accumulates preferentially in tumour tissue. As ALA is a natural body compound which is completely metabolised within 24 h, the problem of prolonged skin sensitivity is avoided by its use. ALA is commercially available as Levulan (DUSA Pharmaceuticals Inc., Valhala, New York, USA). Kennedy and Pottie[27] studied the distribution of ALA-induced PpIX in normal tissues and found that fluorescence occurred primarily in surface and glandular epithelium of the skin and the lining of hollow organs. Systemic ALA administration has been shown to induce a five-fold greater PpIX fluorescence in rabbit endometrium than in myometrium or stroma.[31]

Intrauterine photosensitisation

Topical administration has been investigated as a means of minimising photosensitiser-induced skin sensitivity.[32] Rats were randomised to receive intravenous, intraperitoneal or intrauterine Photofrin and the uterine porphyrin levels were determined. Intrauterine administration provided the best uptake and distribution within the uterus, at lower drug doses. The powerful photosensitiser BPD when instilled into the uterine cavity of rabbits was shown to accumulate in higher concentration in the endometrium compared to myometrium.[33] After PDT substantial, persistent endometrial destruction was generally observed, although there were regional variations in re-epithelialisation.

Intrauterine administration of ALA in rats enabled selective PDT endometrial ablation.[34] There was preservation of some glandular elements after treatment, yet no regeneration of endometrium was evident at 10 days.

The functional effect was confirmed by comparing pregnancy implantation in treated and untreated uterine horns. Those treated by means of ALA PDT showed a profoundly decreased rate of implantation as well as the absence of functioning endometrium.[35] This study suggests that, although complete endometrial destruction was not immediate, photoablation of the endometrium was achieved by direct tissue destruction combined with the effect of local toxicity from photoablated tissue.

Pharmacokinetics and safety of ALA

A study of ALA PDT in rats and rabbits explored the pharmacokinetics and effective distribution of intrauterine ALA.[36] Peak endometrial fluorescencing hence PpIX conversion, was observed at 3 h in both animal models. No significant dose-dependent fluctuations were observed in glandular, stromal and myometrial fluorescence when the ALA concentration was increased from 100 to 400 mg/ml. However, glandular uptake was significantly higher than that of the other structures regardless of drug concentration. Although the solution of ALA was highly acidic and potentially toxic, buffering to pH 5.5 did not affect the fluorescence levels. Histological appearances of the uteri were similar at 3 and 7 days, showing destruction of glandular epithelium with moderate stromal scarring.

Endometrial PpIX fluorescence was measured in monkeys after ALA was administered either via a needle into the uterine fundus, transcervically or by intravenous injection.[37] Hysterectomy specimens after 3 h showed selective accumulation of PpIX in endometrium and not in myometrium. Peak fluorescence occurred 4–5 h after injection and decreased gradually to less than 20% at 8 h. Monkeys were shown to tolerate large doses of ALA without ill effect.[37] The safety of a large dose of ALA was shown in a study of the pathogenesis of acute porphyrins in man.[38]

First human studies

The authors investigated the use of ALA PDT of the endometrium in model systems and in a series of patients.[39] In all of this work, the ALA was administered directly into the uterine cavity to reduce any possibility of systemic photosensitisation. In a series of experiments in perfused *ex vivo* uteri, ALA was introduced into the cavity and protoporphyrin formation was measured in the endometrium, the underlying myometrium and the perfusate. ALA transfer into the perfusate was also measured. This work demonstrated that protoporphyrin formation in the endometrium was approximately tenfold that in the underlying myometrium and that systemic photosensitisation would be unlikely to result from transfer of administered ALA from the uterus into the circulation. Similar results were found in studies carried out *in vivo*, where ALA was administered to patients scheduled for hysterectomy.

The optical parameters required for clinical treatment were estimated from previous experience of PDT of the oesophagus and the bladder, both of which can be treated as hollow organs. The authors carried out studies on a post-hysterectomy uterus to characterise the distribution of light and to predict an adequate treatment time.[40] A light delivery system was constructed using a balloon catheter, later developed into a shaped latex balloon. The catheter was introduced through the cervix and the balloon inflated inside the uterine cavity. Intralipid in solution was injected into the balloon to scatter light. Other workers designed a balloon made of elastomer loaded with highly scattering particles for intrauterine PDT.[41] Reflecting and scattering of light inside the balloon achieved an even fluence rate over the balloon surface.

Light delivery methods

Clinical activation of the photosensitiser was generally achieved by visible light derived from a laser and directed to the site by optical fibre.[40] In the authors' studies, a fibre modification was designed to emit light over a cylindrical terminal section 2 cm in length. When the tip was activated in the intralipid filled balloon a homogenous light delivery was ensured.[42] Tromberg derived a mathematical model to describe homogenous light distribution in the uterus without balloon distention.[43] It proved possible to apply sufficient light to the entire endometrium with three separate cylindrical diffusers placed horizontally in the uterine cavity in a manner similar to the introduction of an intrauterine device.[44] Two lateral fibres with 2 cm diffusing tips fed into the cornua and a 4 cm central diffusing tip extended from the central fibre. The intrauterine light probe's ability to deliver the required light dose for PDT was demonstrated on three surgically removed human uteri.

Until recently large, complex laser systems were needed to deliver sufficient power (up to about 1 W) for effective treatment. A primary pumping laser such as an argon-ion or a opper-vapour laser was coupled to a separate, tunable, dye laser.[45] The high capital and maintenance costs associated with these laser systems was a limiting factor in the widespread application of PDT. Simpler, more compact and less expensive sources such as diode lasers[46] and filtered arc lamps[47] are now becoming available for use in PDT.

Conclusion

Successful PDT depends on the critical interaction of several complex, inter-related factors. These include tissue thickness which determines penetration of both drugs and light. Pre-operative manipulation of endometrial depth is common to many endometrial ablation techniques. It may be that hormonal suppression of endometrium impairs oxygenation for PDT. Furthermore, oestrogen activation has been shown to be of benefit in some experiments. The choice of photosensitiser, vehicle and route of administration must be made. There has been a trend towards topical photosensitiser administration for accessible lesions. Light delivery will be facilitated by the various purpose-made devices which are becoming available for the treatment of the uterine cavity. Perhaps the biggest recent advance, which will allow more widespread use of PDT, is the development of a new generation of compact diode lasers capable of producing light at more than 600 nm on a narrow wavelength. This will allow the more widespread use of this very promising technique and, perhaps, the development of the ideal outpatient method of endometrial ablation.

References

1. Gannon MJ, Brown SB. Photodynamic therapy and its applications in gynaecology. *Br J Obstet Gynaecol* 1999; 106: 1246–1254.

2. Bonnett R. Photodynamic therapy in historical perspective. *Rev Contemp Pharmacother* 1999; 10: 1–17.

3. von Tappeiner H, Jesionek A. Therapeutische versuche mit fluoreszierenden Stoffen. *Muenchener Medizinische Wochenschrift* 1903; 47: 2042–2044.

4. Meyer-Betz F. Investigations on the biological (photodynamic) action of haematoporphyrin and other derivatives of blood and bile pigments. *Deutsch Arch Klin Med* 1913; 112: 476–503.

5. Lipson RL, Baldes EJ, Olsen AM. The use of derivative of haematoporphyrin in tumour detection. *J Natl Cancer Inst* 1961; 26: 1–1J.

6. Lipson RL, Baldes EJ. The photodynamic properties of a particular haematoporphyrin derivative. *Arch Dermatol* 1960; 82: 508–516.

7. Lipson RL, Pratt JH, Baldes EJ, Dockerty MB. Hematoporphyrin derivative for detection of cervical cancer. *Obstet Gynecol* 1964; 24: 78–84.

8. Gray MJ, Lipson RL, Van S Maeck I, Parker L, Romeyn D. Use of hematoporphyrin derivative in detection and management of cervical cancer. A preliminary report. *Am J Obstet Gynecol* 1967; 99: 766–771.

9. Kyriazis GA, Balin H, Lipson RL. Haematoporphyrin-derivative fluorescence test colposcopy and colpophotography in the diagnosis of atypical metaplasia, dysplasiamg carcinoma *in situ* of the cervix: uteri. *Am J Obstet Gynecol* 1973; 117: 375–380.

10. Lipson RL, Gray MJ, Baldes EL. Haematoporphyria derivative for detection and management of cancer. *Proceedings of the 9th International Cancer Congress* 1966; p 393.

11. Diamond I, McDonagh AF, Wilson CB, Granelli SG, Nielsen S, Jaenicke R. Photodynamic therapy of malignant tumours. *Lancet* 1972; ii: 1175–1177.

12. Dougherty TJ. Activated dyes as anti-tumour agents. *J Natl Cancer Inst* 1974; 51: 1333–1336.

13. Dougherty TJ, Kaufman lE, Goldfarb A, Weishaupt KR, Boyle D, Mittleman A. Photoradiation therapy for the treatment of malignant tumours. *Cancer Res* 1978; 38: 2628–2635.

14. Wierrani F, Fiedler D, Grin W et al. Clinical effect of meso-tetrahydroxyphenylchlorine based photodynamic therapy in recurrent carcinoma of the ovary: preliminary results. *Br J Obstet Gynaecol* 1997; 104: 376–378.

15. Dougherty TJ, Gamer CJ, Henderson BW et al. Photodynamic therapy. *J Natl Cancer Inst* 1998; 90: 889–905.

16. Henderson BW, Dougherty TJ. How does photodynamic therapy work? *Photochem Photobiol* 1992; 55: 145–157.

17. Fuchs I, Thiele I. The role of oxygen in cutaneous photodynamic therapy. *Free Radic Biol Med* 1998; 24: 835–847.

18. Dougherty TJ. Photodynamic therapy (PDT) of malignant tumours. *Crit Rev Oncol Hematol* 1984; 2: 83–116.

19. Bonnett R. Photosensitizers of the porphyrin and phthalocyanine series for photodynamic therapy. *Chem Soc Rev* 1995; 24: 19–33.

20. Wyss P, Svaasand LO, Tadir Y et al. Photomedicine of the endometrium: experimental concepts. *Hum Reprod* 1995; 10: 221–226.

21. Martin-Hirsch PL, Whitehurst C, Buckley CH, Moore N, Kitchener HC. Photodynamic treatment for lower genital tract intraepithelial neoplasia. *Lancet* 1998; 351: 1403.

22. Yang JZ, Van Dijk-Smith JP, Van Vugt DA, Kennedy JC, Reid RL. Fluorescence and photosensitization of experimental endometriosis in the rat after systemic 5-aminolevulinic acid administration: a potential new approach to the diagnosis and treatment of endometriosis. *Am J Obstet Gynecol* 1996; 174: 154–160.

23. Kriegmair M, Baumgartner R, Knuchel R, Stepp H, Hofstadter F, Hofstetter A. Detection of early bladder cancer by 5-aminolevulinic acid induced porphyrin fluorescence. *J Urol* 1996; 155: 105–110.

24. Gannon MJ, Holt EM, Fairbank J et al. A randomised trial comparing endometrial resection and abdominal hysterectomy for the treatment of menorrhagia. *Br Med J* 1991; 303: 1362–1364.

25. Schneider DF, Schellhas HF, Wesseler TA, Moulton BC. Endometrial ablation by DHE photoradiation therapy in oestrogen-treated ovariectomized rats. *Colposc Gynecol Laser Surg* 1988; 4: 73–77.

26. Bhatta Nmg erson RR, Flotte T, Schiff I, Hasan T, Nishioka NS. Endometrial ablation by means of

photodynamic therapy with photofrin II. *Am J Obstet Gynecol* 1992; 167: 1856–1863.

27. Kennedy JG, Pottier RH. Endogenous protoporphyrin IX, a clinically useful photosensitizer for photodynamic therapy. *J Photochem Photobiol B: Biol* 1992; 14: 275–292.

28. Wan S, Parrish JA, Anderson RR, Madden M. Transmittance of non-ionising radiation in human tissues. *Photochem Photobiol* l981; 34: 679–681.

29. Schmidt S, Wagner U, Oehr P, Krebs D. Clinical application of photodynamic therapy in patients with gynaecologic tumours — antibody-targeted photodynamic laser therapy as a new oncological treatment modality. *Zentbl Gynakol* 1992; 114: 307–311.

30. Kennedy IC, Marcus SL, Pottier RH. Photodynamic therapy (PDT) and photodiagnosis (PD) using endogenous photosensitization induced by 5-aminolevulinic acid (ALA): mechanisms and clinical results. *J Clint Laser Med Surg* 1996; 14: 289–304.

31. Judd MD, Bedwell I, MacRobert AJ. Comparison of the distribution of phthalocyanine and ALA-induced porphyrin sensitisers within the rabbit uterus. *Lasers Med Sci* 1992; 7: 203–211.

32. Chapman IA, Tadir V, Tromberg BI et al. Effect of administration route and oestrogen manipulation on endometrial uptake of Photofrin porfimer sodium. *Am J Obstet Gynecol* 1993; 168: 685–692.

33. Wyss P, Tadir V, Tromberg BI et al. Benzoporphyrin derivative (BPD): a potent photosensitizer for photodynamic destruction of the rabbit endometrium. *Obstet Gynecol* l994; 84: 409–414.

34. Yang JZ, Van Vugt DA, Kennedy JC, Reid RL, Intrauterine 5-aminolevulinic acid induces selective fluorescence and photodynamic ablation of the rat endometrium. *Photochem Photobiol* 1993; 57: 803–807.

35. Yang JZ, Van Vugt DA, Kennedy JC, Reid RL. Evidence of lasting functional destruction of the rat endometrium after 5-aminolevulinic acid- induced photodynamic ablation: Prevention of implantation. *Am J Obstet Gynecol* 1993; 168: 995–1001.

36. Wyss P, Tromberg BJ, Wyss MT et al. Photodynamic destruction of endometrial tissue with topical 5-aminolevulinic acid in rats and rabbits. *Am J Obstet Gynecol* 1994; 171: 1176–1183.

37. Yang JZ, Van Vugt DA, Roy BN, Kennedy JC, Foster WG, Reid RL. Intrauterine 5-aminolaevulinic acid induces selective endometrial fluorescence in the rhesus and cynomolgus monkey. *J Soc Gynecol Invest* 1996; 3: 152–157.

38. Mustajoki P, Timonen K, Gorchein A, Seppalainen AM, Matikainen E, Tenhunen R. Sustained high plasma 5-aminolaevulinic acid concentration in a volunteer: no porphyric symptoms. *Eur J Clint Invest* 1992; 22: 407–411.

39. Gannon MI, Johnson N, Roberts DM et al. Photosensitization of the endometrium with topical 5-aminolevulinic acid. *Am J Obstet Gynecol* 1995; 173: 1826–1828.

40. Stringer MR, Hudson EJ, Dunkley CP, Boyce JC, Gannon MI, Smith MA. Light delivery schemes for uterine photodynamic therapy. In: G Jori, J Moan, WM Star (Eds) *Photodynamic Therapy of Cancer, Proc SPIE* 1994; 2078: 41–49.

41. Bays R, Woodtli A, Mosimann L et al. A light distributor for photodynamic endometrial ablation. In: P Wyss, Y Tadir, BJ Tromberg, U Haller (Eds) *Photomedicine in Gynaecology and Reproduction,* pp 243–245, 2000. Basel: Karger.

42. Gannon MI, Vernon DL, Holroyd JA, Stringer M, Johnson N, Brown SB. PDT of the endometrium using ALA. *Proc SPIE* 1997; 2972: 2–13.

43. Tromberg BJ, Svaasand LO, Fehr MK et al. A mathematical model for light dosimetry in photodynamic destruction of human endometrium. *Phys Med Biol* 1996; 41: 223–237.

44. Tadir Y, Hornung R, Pham TH, Tromberg BJ. Intrauterine light probe for photodynamic ablation therapy. *Obstet Gynecol* 1999; 93: 299–303.

45. Fehr MK, Madsen SJ, Svaasand LO et al. Intrauterine light delivery for photodynamic therapy of the human endometrium. *Hum Reprod* 1995; 10: 3067–3072.

46. Ripley PM. The physics of diode lasers. *Lasers Med Sci* 1996; II: 71–78.

47. De Jode ML, Mccilligan J, Dilkes MG, Cameron I, Hart PB, Grahn MF. A comparison of novel light sources for photodynamic therapy. *Lasers Med Sci* 1997; 12: 260–268.

22

Mirena intra-uterine system

Lynne Rogerson and Sean Duffy

Introduction

Patients presenting with menorrhagia whose symptoms are refractory to conventional medical therapy, traditionally, face the choice of either undergoing a hysterectomy or more recently some other alternative less invasive surgical treatment. Endometrial resection is the alternative to hysterectomy that has been formally assessed in clinical trials. In a number of randomised controlled trials,[1-4] endometrial resection was found to be as effective as hysterectomy in terms of patient satisfaction. It has also been found to be less costly as an alternative even if repeat procedures and failed cases are taken into consideration.[5] The benefits to the patient include shorter hospital stay, less post-operative morbidity, quicker return to work, and quicker overall recovery. However, there are complications associated with endometrial resection, such as

- the risks associated with general anaesthesia,
- fluid intravasation and dilutional hyponatraemia,
- the risk of uterine perforation and subsequent intra-abdominal trauma.

Intermediate complications, due to sepsis and haematoma can occur in up to 13% of patients at 3 months.[4] Such complications have driven research into the development of alternative treatments for the management of menorrhagia.

The Mirena intra-uterine system (IUS) was originally developed as a contraceptive which has been reported as being as effective as female sterilisation but was also found to reduce menstrual blood loss (MBL). In addition to its contraceptive action, the levonorgestrel (LNG) system has a protective effect on the incidence of ectopic pregnancy. The ectopic rate with Mirena is 0.06 per 100 woman-years compared to 1.2–1.6 in women not using contraception. The progesterone release has a contraceptive action that complements the mechanical effect of the device but also has a direct effect on the function of the adjacent endometrium. The endometrium is rendered inactive and resistant to the proliferative effects of oestrogen. The primary mechanism of action is the effect of LNG locally on the uterine cavity (i.e. thickening of the cervical mucus, inhibition of sperm motility and function and prevention of endometrium proliferation). Suppression of ovulation may occur in some women using the Mirena IUS and the device may also have a weak foreign body effect.

Description of Mirena intra-uterine system

The Mirena IUS (Schering) is an LNG-loaded IUS. It comprises a T-shaped polyethylene frame carrying a white hormone cylinder around the vertical arm. The cylinder contains a mixture of polydimethylsiloxane (50%) and LNG (50%) and is covered by a polydimethylsiloxane membrane which regulates the release of the LNG. The total amount of LNG in the system is 52 mg. After insertion into the uterus, LNG is released from the reservoir at an initial rate of $20\,\mu g/24\,h$ directly to the endometrium.

The total length of the system is 32 mm and the width of the horizontal arms is also 32 mm. The hormone cylinder length is 19 mm with an outer diameter of 2.8 mm (Fig. 22.1).

The T-shaped frame is impregnated with barium sulphate to make the system X-ray detectable. Dark monofilament polyethylene threads are attached to the lower end of the vertical arm. The Mirena has been licensed in the UK for contraceptive use and has recently obtained a licence for use in menorrhagia. In many other countries menorrhagia and endometrial protection for women on HRT are additional licensed indications for Mirena. The recommended duration of use is 5 years after which time it can be replaced with a further system if desired.

Practical aspects

Suitable patients for treatment with Mirena IUS are those who have dysfunctional uterine bleeding.

Exclusion criteria include:

- pregnancy,
- recent pelvic inflammatory disease,
- previous intra-uterine device (IUD) expulsion,
- acute liver disease,
- lower genital and uterine tract infection.

The Mirena IUS may be inserted into a fibroid uterus where there is no significant distortion of the cavity.

Endometrial preparation is not necessary prior to treatment with Mirena IUS but the system should ideally be inserted within the first 7 days of a woman's menstrual cycle or she should have abstained from sexual intercourse or used additional contraception for the previous 5 days to exclude an early pregnancy.

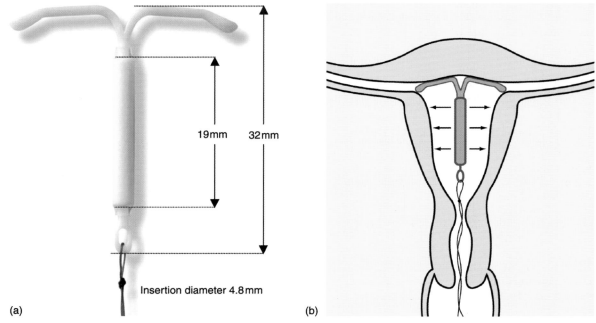

(a)   (b)

Figure 22.1 — Pictures of device (with scale) and hysteroscopic view.

Usually in an outpatient setting, the patient is placed in a modified lithotomy position and a pelvic examination is performed to clarify the size and position of the uterus. After visualisation of the cervix using a speculum, the vagina and cervix are cleansed with warm antiseptic solution. The anterior lip of the cervix can then be grasped using a tenaculum to facilitate gentle traction to reduce the angle between the cervical canal and the uterine cavity. This allows the introduction of a uterine sound which not only assesses the cavity length but also ensures that the cavity is unobstructed. Should the cervical canal be tight, cervical dilation may be necessary and anaesthesia such as 10 ml of local anaesthetic gel instilled into the cervical canal 5 min prior to insertion may therefore be required. In one study where Mirena was inserted into 50 women (nine of whom were nulliparous) for menorrhagia, only three required anaesthesia and all were parous.[5]

The Mirena IUS may then be inserted using an aseptic technique and the removal threads are trimmed so that 2 cm remain visible outside the cervix. These threads can also be used to check that the system is still *in situ* especially after a heavy period.

The whole procedure usually takes approximately 10–15 min and usually requires a doctor to insert the system and one assistant for psychological support for the patient. In a large contraceptive study in Finland[6] pain scores at insertion of the system were recorded — 17% felt no pain, 49% felt minimum pain, 28% moderate and 6% had severe pain.

Results of *ex vivo/in vitro* studies

The pharmacological properties of LNG and its toxicity profile after oral administration are well known, indicating that it is a safe drug. However, less is known about the effects in intra-uterine use. Since the shape and size of the LNG-IUS are unsuitable for the uteri of laboratory animals, LNG-releasing systems composed of similar components and materials have been tested. In spite of apparently high endometrial LNG concentration, no local intolerance or systemic toxic reactions have been observed. Compared to the oral administration of LNG, administration directly into the uterine cavity allows a very low systemic concentration in humans.

The inert carrier in the LNG-IUS, polydimethylsiloxane, is a biocompatible material that has shown no *in vitro*, local or systemic toxicity. Similar material has been widely used in implantable valves and prostheses. There is also extensive experience of the polyethylene frame, gained from studies with a copper IUD, Nova T which is used world-wide.

Very few pharmacokinetic studies have been performed with intra-uterine LNG system in animals but in a 1-year study in rhesus monkeys systemic LNG blood concentrations were measured. Toxicological studies showed limited systemic pharmacological effects of LNG. The local effects on the endometrium were a typical strong progestogenic effect including glandular atrophy, decidual changes and a foreign body reaction.[7–9] Safety evaluation of the silicone materials (membrane and core materials of the hormone reservoir) and polyethylene parts of the product (T body, removal threads and insertion tube) is based upon assessments of genetic toxicology in standard *in vitro* and *in vivo* test systems as well as assessments of biocompatibility in mice, guinea pigs, rabbits and *in vitro* test systems. In all biocompatibility tests the results showed acceptable biocompatibility.

Embryonic/fetal toxicity and teratogenic potential of an intra-uterine LNG system were studied in the rabbit. The treatment did not have any adverse effect on litter number, embryonic or fetal development.[10]

Endometrial, myometrial and fallopian tube concentrations of LNG have been studied after 4–6 weeks treatment with an LNG-IUS.[11] The endometrial tissue concentration of LNG was more than 100 times higher than that achieved with orally administered LNG at a daily dose of 250 μg. After insertion of the Mirena IUS, LNG can be detected in plasma in 15 min and the highest concentrations are reached within a few hours.[12]

The therapeutic effects of the Mirena IUS are based on local effects in the uterus. The proliferation of the endometrium has been shown to be prevented by the local administration of LNG which inhibits the function of oestradiol in the endometrium.[13] LNG thickens the cervical mucus thus also inhibiting sperm motility.[14] Ovulation is suppressed in some women and on average 75% of cycles have been shown to be ovulatory.[14,15] A weak foreign body reaction may also be present.[13]

Endometrial histology during the use of the Mirena IUS has been studied for up to 7 years after insertion in women of reproductive age. A few weeks after insertion endometrial glands became atrophic with a thin, inactive epithelium and the stroma undergoes an intense decidual reaction. The histology of the endometrium does not change during prolonged use. In a long-term contraceptive study endometrial histology was

evaluated at the removal of the Mirena from 100 women,[16] 92% showed endometrial suppression, with focal proliferative changes in 24%. The endometrium regenerated fully 2–6 months after removal.

In a study of Andersson et al[17] 79% of women wishing to conceive within 1 year did so and 87% within 2 years after removal of the Mirena. This shows that the function of the endometrium is restored even after prolonged suppression.

The efficacy of the LNG-IUS in the treatment of menorrhagia has been assessed in clinical studies of 183 women. A total of 107 took part in Leiras phase III studies comparing the LNG-IUS with oral norethisterone, tranexamic acid, endometrial resection and hysterectomy.[18–21]

In the study comparing the Mirena IUS with the most effective medical treatment for menorrhagia, tranexamic acid, the MBL decreased significantly during treatment in both groups.[18] However, at cycle 6 the MBL was 93.5% for Mirena and 62.1% for tranexamic acid. Mean ferritin levels increased significantly only in the Mirena group. The study of Lahteenmaki et al[22] suggests that Mirena may be a valuable alternative for hysterectomy in women with excessive bleeding as 60% of women with the Mirena cancelled their scheduled surgery whereas only 15% in the control did so.

Results of treatment

By rendering the endometrium inactive, Mirena has a potential role in the treatment of women with heavy and irregular menstrual bleeding. There are supportive studies that have investigated this potential. One of the first reports of the effect on locally released progesterone (norgestrel) on reducing MBL was by Nilsson in 1977.[23] Bergkveist and Rybo (1983) recorded a 65% reduction in MBL in women using the Progestasert device for contraception after 12 months of use.[24] Andersson and Rybo (1990) reported a 97% reduction in MBL volume after 12 months of use in those women who continued to use the device.[25] However, in this study 20% of the initial patients who had a device placed were withdrawn due to either spontaneous expulsion of the device or unwanted side effects (irregular bleeding or progestogenic symptoms, such as breast tenderness and bloating). The later study would therefore suggest a failure rate, after initial insertion, of 20%. In another study of patients taken off a waiting list for hysterectomy and offered the Mirena system 5, the failure rate was 24% including primary expulsions of

Table 22.1 — Results from trial by Crosignani et al[27]

	Mirena IUS n = 35	Endometrial resection n = 35
Failure rate (%)	11	8
Change in mean PBAC score★ (%)	79	89
Symptom improvement (%)	65	71
Satisfaction (%)	85	94

★ % Improvements on baseline mean values 12 months after treatment.

the device. This study did not have a control group. A more recent study[26] attempted to use a control group but the study was flawed as the control group consisted of women already on a waiting list for definitive surgery. Therefore, by definition, they were medical treatment failures and could not be classified as true controls.

There are two published randomised controlled trials of the Mirena system versus endometrial resection.[27,28] The first is that of Crosignani et al which assessed the effect of the Mirena system in terms of symptom chart score, patient satisfaction, effect on menstrual loss and failure rate. The period of follow-up was for 12 months but the total study number of 70 (35 to each arm) was relatively small. The study results are summarised in Table 22.1. The failure rate is defined by persistent menorrhagia and the unexpected loss of Mirena by expulsion from the uterus. Blood loss was assessed using the pictorial blood loss assessment chart[29,30] (PBAC). Symptomatic improvement is defined as amenorrhoea or oligomenorrhoea at 12 months. Satisfaction was assessed by simple questionnaire and responses of 'satisfied' or 'very satisfied' were recorded as successful outcomes. However, the study numbers would not be sufficient to demonstrate a clinically meaningful difference as statistically significant between the two groups.

The second study of endometrial resection versus Mirena by Kittleson[28] was again a relatively small study with only 60 patients in total. There were substantial numbers of patients who discontinued the Mirena prematurely (20%). In those who persisted with Mirena the mean (SD) blood loss score, as assessed by the PBAC, was reduced from 418 (349) at baseline to 42 (99.7) at 12 months. In the resection group, there were four failures (13%) and the mean PBAC score fell from 378 (463) to 6.6 (15.0). There was no data provided on patient satisfaction.

Endometrial resection has been compared to hysterectomy and has been found to be as effective and to have a cost advantage. The results of three randomised trials,[2–4] each with at least 100 patients randomised to endometrial resection and comprehensive follow-up, are shown in Table 22.2. Patient satisfaction rates in the two studies with 12-month follow-up[3,4] were 96% and 87% respectively. Symptomatic improvement rates were similarly high.

There has not been a randomised controlled trial comparing the LNG-IUS and hysterectomy but one study[5] recruited 50 patients with a history of failed medical treatment awaiting hysterectomy or transcervical resection of the endometrium. Following insertion of the Mirena system, 41 of the 50 patients recruited (82%) were taken off the waiting list for surgery because of a reduction in mean blood loss score, reduction of dysmenorrhoea (80%), and improvement in pre-menstrual syndrome (56%).

A larger randomised controlled trial comparing the LNG-IUS with hysteroscopic surgery for menorrhagia using quality of life assessments as its primary outcome measure is needed.

One such multi-centre study was commenced but had to be stopped due to poor patient recruitment as a result of patient preference for endometrial ablation. A study is now underway to find out more about the reasons for patient preference.

Complication

The incidence of complications during the insertion procedure are very small but include syncope usually due to dilation of the cervical os. This usually settles with a head down position but, rarely, atropine may have to be given. There is also a possibility of uterine perforation which again is usually when cervical dilation is used rather than on insertion of the actual Mirena IUS.

Table 22.2 — Results from the endometrial ablation arm of three important trials comparing endometrial ablation and hysterectomy and Crosignani et al's trial comparing Mirena and endometrial ablation

	n	Failure rate (%)	Symptom improvement (%)	Satisfaction* (%)
Mirena				
At 12 months				
Crosignani et al[27]	35	11	65	85
Endometrial ablation				
At 12 months				
Crosignani et al[27]	35	8	71	94
Pinion et al[3]	105	28	90	96
O'Connor et al[4]	116	25	–	87
At 4 months				
Dwyer et al[2]	100	15	89	85

*Percentage 'very satisfied' or 'satisfied' with treatment except O'Connor et al who presented only the percentage 'very satisfied'. Note these trials employed different 4 and 5 point satisfaction scales.

Other more long-term complications of the Mirena IUS are pelvic inflammatory disease as organisms can potentially be pushed up into the uterine cavity from the cervix and vagina. The Mirena IUS may also be spontaneously expelled especially in women who have high menstrual scores.

Side effects are most common during the first few months after the insertion and include irregular menstrual bleeding, intermenstrual spotting and hormonal side effects. The highest concentrations of LNG can be detected in the endometrium and the systemic levels are low.

Costs

The Mirena IUS costs approximately £100 (£89.25 + VAT) and covers a 5-year treatment period. The system may be replaced after this time period to continue the treatment. The other costs incurred are for a sterile pack to include a speculum, tenaculum, sponge forceps, cervical dilators, swabs and antiseptic solution.

Conclusions

Mirena appears to be an easy and effective method of treating menorrhagia and is being used regularly by many clinicians currently with a recently acquired licence for this indication. The potential advantage of the Mirena IUS is its ease of use and low complication rate. Its benefit will only be of interest if it is shown that it has a success rate in terms of patient satisfaction and symptomatic improvement comparable with the 'Gold Standard' of first-generation endometrial ablation. The treatment must also be of economic value. There is, therefore, a need to perform a large randomised controlled trial, to assess the efficacy of and tolerance to the Mirena IUS against the established and effective endometrial resection technique for controlling menorrhagia, before the method can be used confidently using evidence-based medicine.

Advantages	Disadvantages
Very economical	Syncope/bradycardia
Short treatment time	Perforation
Outpatient-based procedure	Expulsion
Avoids surgery	Spotting
Reversible	Lower abdominal pain
Not sterilising	Progestogenic side
Does not require good	effects:
hysteroscopic skills	Breast tenderness
	Acne
	Headaches
	Mood changes

References

1. Gannon MJ, Holt EM, Fairbank J, Fitzgerald M, Milne MA, Crystal AM et al. A randomised controlled trial comparing endometrial resection and abdominal hysterectomy for the treatment of menorrhagia. *Br Med J* 1991; 303: 1362–1364.

2. Dwyer N, Hutton J, Stirrat GM. Randomised controlled trial comparing endometrial resection with abdominal hysterectomy for the surgical treatment of menorrhagia. *Br J Obstet Gynaecol* 1993; 100: 237–243.

3. Pinion SB, Parkin DE, Abramovich DR, Naji A, Alexander DA, Russell IT et al. Randomised controlled trial of hysterectomy, endometrial laser ablation, and transcervical resection for dysfunctional uterine bleeding. *Br Med J* 1994; 309: 979–983.

4. O'Connor H, Broadbent JAM, Magos A, McPherson K. Medical Research Council randomised controlled trial of endometrial resection versus hysterectomy in management of menorrhagia. *Lancet* 1997; 349: 897–901.

5. Barrington JW, Bowen-Simpkins P. The levonorgestrel intrauterine system in the management of menorrhagia. *Br J Obstet Gynaecol* 1997; 104: 614–616.

6. Sommardahl C, Blom T. Five-year clinical performance of the new formulation of the levonorgestrel intrauterine system and serum levonorgestrel concentration with the new formulation compared to that with the original one. *Leiras Study Report* 102-89532-07, 1996.

7. Wadsworth PF, Heywood R, Allen DG, Sortwell RJ, Walton RM. Treatment of rhesus monkey with intrauterine devices loaded with levonorgestrel. *Contraception* 1979; 20: 177–184.

8. Sethi N, Agarwal K, Singh RK, Bajpai VK. Effect of 24 mm levonorgestrel IUD on uterine endometrium of female rhesus monkeys. *Contraception* 1988; 37: 99–108.

9. Schering. One year local and systemic tolerance study with a levonorgestrel-releasing intrauterine device in the rhesus monkey and determination of plasma concentration of levonorgestrel using a radioimmunoassay method. *Schering Study Report* 9725, 1992.

10. Argus Research Laboratories. Embryo/fetal toxicity and teratogenic potential study of levonorgestrel administered via a Silastic intrauterine device to pregnant New Zealand White rabbits, 1984.

11. Nilsson CG, Haukkamaa M, Vierola H, Luukkainen T. Tissue concentrations of levonorgestrel in women using a levonorgestrel-releasing IUD. *Clin Endocrinol* 1982; 17: 529–536.

12. Luukkainen T. Levonorgestrel-releasing intrauterine device. *Ann NY Acad Sci* 1991; 626: 43–49.

13. Silverberg SG, Haukkamaa M, Arko H, Nilsson CG, Luukkainen T. Endometrial morphology during long-term use of levonorgestrel-releasing intrauterine devices. *Int J Gynecol Pathol* 1986; 5: 235–241.

14. Barbosa I, Bakos O, Olsson SE, Odlind V, Johansson EDB. Ovarian function during use of a levonorgestrel-releasing IUD. *Contraception* 1990; 42: 51–66.

15. Nilsson CG, Lahteenmaki P, Luukkainen T. Ovarian function in amenorrhoeic and menstruating users of a levonorgestrel-releasing intrauterine device. *Fertil Steril* 1984; 41: 52–55.

16. Lahteenmaki P. Evaluation of endometrial biopsies at the time of and after the removal of LNG-IUS. *Leiras Study Report* 1204 ©, 1991.

17. Andersson K, Batar I, Rybo G. Return to fertility after removal of a levonorgestrel releasing intrauterine device and Nova T. *Contraception* 1992; 46: 575–584.

18. Pankalainen T, Blom T. Randomised comparative study of the efficacy of the levonorgestrel IUS and oral tranexamic acid for the treatment of idiopathic menorrhagia. Interim report of 6 cycle data. *Leiras Study Report* AV99, 1998(a).

19. Korpela I, Heikkila A. Efficacy and safety of the levonorgestrel intrauterine system compared with oral norethisterone in the treatment of idiopathic menorrhagia. *Leiras Clinical Study Report* 102-92549-01, 1996(a).

20. Korpela I, Blom T, Trauramo I. Conservative treatment of excessive uterine bleeding and dysmenorrhoea with levonorgestrel IUS as an alternative to hysterectomy. *Leiras Study Report* 102-90528-01, 1996(b).

21. Pankalainen T, Blom T. Randomised controlled study comparing the efficacy of LEVONOVA with surgical treatment of menorrhagia by transcervical endometrial resection. *Leiras Study Report* 102-93503-01, 1998(b).

22. Lahteenmaki P, Haukkamaa M, Puolakka J, Riikonen U, Sainio S, Suvisaari J, Nilsson CG. Open randomised study of use of levonorgestrel releasing intrauterine system as alternative to hysterectomy. *Br Med J* 1998; 7138: 1122–1126.

23. Nilsson CG. Comparative quantification of menstrual blood loss with a d-norgestrel releasing IUCD. *Contraception* 1977; 15: 295–306.

24. Bergqveist A, Rybo G. Treatment of menorrhagia with intrauterine release of progesterone. *Br J Obstet Gynaecol* 1983; 90: 255–258.

25. Andersson JK, Rybo G. Levonorgestrel releasing intrauterine device in the treatment of menorrhagia. *Br J Obstet Gynaecol* 1990; 97: 690–694.

26. Puolakka J, Nilsson C, Haukkamaa M et al. Conservative treatment of excessive uterine bleeding and dysmenorrhoea with levonorgestrel intrauterine system as an alternative to hysterectomy. *Acta Obstet Gynecol Scand* 1996; 75: 82.

27. Crosignani PG, Vercellini P, Mosconi P, Oldani S, Cortesi I, De Giorgi O. Levonorgestrel releasing intrauterine device versus hysteroscopic endometrial resection in the treatment of dysfunctional uterine bleeding. *Obstet Gynecol* 1997; 90: 257–263.

28. Kittleson N, Istre O. A randomised study comparing levonorgestrel intrauterine system and transcervical resection of the endometrium in the treatment of menorrhagia: preliminary results. *Gynaecol Endosc* 1998; 7: 61–67.

29. Higham JM, O'Brien PMS, Shaw RW. Assessment of menstrual blood loss using a pictorial chart. *Br J Obstet Gynaecol* 1990; 97: 734–739.

30. Janssen CAA et al. A simple visual assessment technique to discriminate between menorrhagia and normal menstrual blood loss. *Obstet Gynecol* 1995; 85: 977–82.

23

Bilateral uterine artery embolisation

W. Walker

History of arterial embolisation

Arterial embolisation is not a new technique, it was developed during the late 60s and 70s and used particularly for the treatment of haemorrhagic conditions, malignancies and arterial venous malformations. Although arterial embolisation became rapidly established in general surgery, neuro-radiology and urology utilisation of the technique in obstetrics and gynaecology was comparatively delayed.[1–4] It was realised that in cases of severe obstetric and gynaecological haemorrhage, particularly obstetric haemorrhage, uterine artery embolisation could be life saving[4] because of the ability of radiologists to carry out distal embolisation of vessels, as opposed to the more proximal occlusions caused by surgical ligature. This prevented perfusion of the bleeding site by collaterals and rendered radiologically mediated occlusions more effective.[3,5,6] Despite fibroids being a logical target for embolisation because of their relative central hypovascularity, accounting for their propensity to spontaneously infarct, it was not until 1995 that Professor Ravina's Group in Paris published their first series in the Lancet.[7] Initially, they employed the technique to reduce bleeding prior to embolectomy and hysterectomy but found that in a number of cases, the fibroids infarcted and shrunk and surgery was unnecessary.[7]

At the Royal Surrey County Hospital in Guildford, we commenced fibroid embolisation in 1996 and have so far treated over 350 patients.

Protocol and technique of embolisation

There are some variations between centres. The technique and protocol carried out at the Royal Surrey County Hospital in Guildford will be described.

After a decision has been made by the gynaecologist to recommend fibroid embolisation, in all cases the patient is interviewed by the consultant radiologist (WJW). During the interview, the technique and trial results are explained to the patient but emphasis is placed, in particular, on the complications encountered in our trial and also those described in the world experience. It is particularly important not to give the patient any false expectations of the technique and to explain that the fibroids are killed and, in most cases, undergo shrinkage only. In a minority of cases, fibroids may be expelled. The efficacy of fibroid embolisation in patients desiring pregnancy has not yet been fully assessed. In the author's view, it is unlikely that in patients with very large complex fibroid masses the prospects of a successful pregnancy will be significantly improved (see later).

At the Royal Surrey, unlike most centres, the radiologist looks after the patient during her admission and also follows up the patient at regular intervals following the embolisation. This is in addition to follow-up by the gynaecologist. The radiologist places himself on 24 h call for all his patients which is particularly important when patients are referred to a radiologist from different parts of the country. The radiologist will have an accumulated experience of the complications of fibroid embolisation and is thus well placed to advise the patient on post-procedural anxieties and complications and to liase with the gynaecologist, where necessary. It is vital that any patient who received a fibroid embolisation has a named, easily contactable individual who will take clinical responsibility for follow-up.

Our patients enter an ethically approved observational trial which is important in view of the SERNIP C rating (safety and efficacy not proven should be the subject of a trial) which the procedure has received. Patients are followed-up at 6 weeks, 3, 6 months and 6 monthly thereafter and have ultrasound scans, blood tests and MRI scans (at 0 and 6 months) and are required to fill in questionnaires at each visit.

Technique of fibroid embolisation

Prior to the procedure, Diclofenac Sodium 100 mg and 1 mg of Granisteron are administered rectally and intravenously, respectively. The procedure is carried out under local anaesthesia and intravenous sedation consisting of a mixture of Fentanyl 100 μg, Midazolam 10 μg and Metoclopromide 10 mg in saline. A right groin approach is used in most cases and following a flush pelvic arteriogram to map the pelvic vasculature, a 4F Cobra 2 catheter is passed into the internal iliac artery and then just into the origin of the uterine artery. Co-axially through this catheter, a 3F micro-catheter (Tracker 325 Boston Scientific) is inserted into the uterine artery. The micro-catheter is advanced approximately half way along the uterine artery and particles of polyvinyl alcohol (PVA), 355–500 μm, injected until oscillation of contrast medium is observed indicating distal blockade. If arterial spasm develops, Glycerol

Trinitrate 300 µg is administered intra-arterially in bolus form. Particle embolisation is followed by coil occlusion using 2–5 mm platinum coils. It is essential to catheterise and embolise both uterine arteries for the procedure to be successful.[8] After the procedure, a PCA pump is set up containing Morphine 60 mg with Droperidol 6 mg and further anti-inflammatory and oral analgesics. Gentomycin 120 mg, Ampicillin 500 mg and Metronidazole 500 mg are administered intravenously at the time of the procedure.

Results of fibroid embolisation

Interim results of our series have been reported elsewhere.[9–11,16] The average reduction in volume achieved is

- 40% at 6 weeks,
- 54% at 3 months,
- 63% at 6 months,
- 73% at 1 year.

Thus shrinkage continues up to 1 year following the procedure. Questionnaire response rate was 94% and indicated an average improvement in symptoms of 78%. Periods improving in 80%, pressure symptoms in 84% and abdominal discomfort in 71%. Ninety four percent of patients stated that they were satisfied with the procedure. Similar results have been reported in other centres.[8,12,14]

Complications

Infections

In our series, two patients have had infections leading to hysterectomy (less than 1%). One of our patients developed a tubeovarian abscess requiring hysterectomy at 3 weeks. At histology, PVA particles were found in the ovarian vessels. This demonstrated, conclusively, that injected particles can pass into ovarian vessels at uterine artery embolisation. However, in this particular patient, particles 150–200 µm in size as well as 355–500 µm had been used and it may be that use of the smaller particles pre-disposes to ovarian artery embolisation. Subsequently, we have only used 355–500 µm particles. The second patient developed chronic recurrent infection over a 3-month period due to a straightforward infection in the infarcted fibroid. In both patients, the organism causing the infection was *E. coli*. Similar infective complications have been reported by other authors.[12,13]

One of our patients, a 33-year old Afro-Caribbean, developed a chronic actinomycotic infection of her endometrial cavity 18 months following embolisation. This patient had a very large mass, the size of a 30-week pregnancy. A further patient with fibroids and adenomyosis haemorrhaged at 6 weeks requiring a blood transfusion.

Ovarian failure

This was studied in 153 patients under 45 years of age. Of these only one ceased having periods permanently. This patient had been embolised with small particles (150–200 µm in size) and it is possible that embolisation with these small particles caused passage into the ovarian arteries. A number of our patients developed transient ovarian failure which resolved over time.

Failures

Four of our patients elected to have hysterectomies because of inadequate response to the embolisation. In three patients embolisation failed because of difficult anatomy and two patients with adenomyosis and fibroids did not respond to embolisation.

Passage of fibroids

In most cases fibroids shrink following embolisation, but in some cases fibroids are passed intact per vaginum and this occurred in seven of our patients, the largest of these fibroids being 12 cm in diameter.[17] Many passed fibroids in fragments.

Pregnancies

Five of our patients have become pregnant. One of these has delivered following a caesarean section. A second patient elected to have an abortion early in the pregnancy as this was unplanned and the other three are on-going.

Radiation exposure

Dose data was collected on 250 patients. Average dose area product was 84 Gy cm^3 equivalent to an effective dose of approximately 14 msv, equivalent to approximately twice the typical dose for a barium enema examination.

Discussion

At the time of writing this chapter there have been at least 7000 embolisations carried out in the UK, France and the United States. Results of fibroids embolisation are similar in all reported series so far.[12,14,15] The technique of fibroid embolisation varies little from group to group but there is some difference in the type of catheter used to cannulate the uterine artery. In some cases, a 4F or 5F catheter is passed directly into the uterine artery and particles injected with very little flow in the vessel, thus particles are forced into the distal vessels in a situation of relative stasis. In the case of the author, micro-catheters are used and particles only injected when there is free flow around the catheter. If particles are injected without good vascular flow, it may be possible to force them into the ovarian arteries and this may account for a higher incidence of ovarian failure reported by the Ravina group, for example.[12] It needs to be remembered that premature menopause occurs in more than 3.3% of women under the age of 45[19] and that most women who have suffered ovarian failure following embolisation have not expressed any dissatisfaction with the result of the procedure. There are variations in the degree of shrinkage reported by various series.[12,14,15] Our group and the French group have reported higher shrinkages than the US group. This may be because the American groups used 500–700 μm particles whereas we and the French used smaller 150–200 μm and 355–500 μm particles. Smaller particles may cause a more complete distal block resulting in a greater amount of infarction.

Where possible MRI scanning should be included in the pre-embolisation assessment of patients. MRI of the pelvis is an extremely powerful diagnostic tool providing that state-of-the-art equipment is used. It is very accurate in the diagnosis of adenomyosis and can readily detect all but Stage I carcinoma of the endometrium. Ovaries are easily visualised. This can be a problem when ultrasound is used in patients with very large fibroids where the ovaries may be obscured. MRI can also pick up non-gynaecological pathology such as bowel tumours. We believe that the diagnosis of adenomyosis is particularly important in patients as this may be a contraindication to embolisation. In both our patients with adenomyosis embolisation failed. This may be due to the fact that in adenomyosis there is a diffuse hypervascularity throughout the adenomyotic area. In contrast to the situation with fibroids where there is peripheral hypervascularity and relative central hypovascularity. Essentially fibroids are an infarction waiting to happen but this may not be the case with adenomyosis.

It is likely that infection will continue to be the main serious complication of fibroid embolisation. Prophylactic antibiotics are unlikely to be effective due to the inability of the substance to permeate the necrotic fibroid and in both our infective cases leading to hysterectomy, prophylactic antibiotics had been administered for five days after the procedure. In the world experience, there has been a death from infection following embolisation reported in the Lancet.[20] So far this is the only death that has been reported from fibroid embolisation and a recent survey by the Society of Cardiovascular & Interventional Radiology on 4500 patients undergoing fibroid embolisation in the United States, did not indicate any mortality. It should be remembered that the mortality rate for hysterectomy for benign disease, excluding pregnancy, is 1:1600.[21] A recent survey of 923 patients undergoing hysterectomy specifically for fibroids found a serious complication rate of 6% and one death.[22]

How can we avoid serious complications resulting from infection following fibroid embolisation? The author feels that it is important to monitor patients carefully. They should be told that if they have a sudden temperature spike above 100°F, particularly if associated with increasing pain, they should contact the doctor. In such situation, the safest course of action is to admit the patient and monitor her. In most cases no treatment, not even antibiotics, will be required and the patient will improve. Embolisation of fibroid material itself causes a pyrexia and the sudden breakdown of fibroids following embolisation may be delayed. Should a patient be admitted for assessment, it is important to obtain an MRI scan as this may indicate the presence of pus in the uterine cavity and the need for surgical intervention. It is better to risk an unnecessary hysterectomy than to delay and risk the life of the patient.

Inadvertent embolisation of a uterine sarcoma is a significant cause of concern. These tumours are not detectable either by ultrasound or MRI as there are no specific features differentiating them from necrotic fibroids. However, uterine sarcomas are extremely rare and are often missed clinically, the sarcoma only being diagnosed following surgical resection and often in the UK preceded by a long wait for operation. It should be borne in mind that the mortality 1:1600 for hysterectomy for benign disease, excluding pregnancy, is greater than the incidence of uterine sarcoma.

Unfortunately, there is inadequate data on the efficacy of fibroid embolisation in pregnancy. However, undoubtedly, patients who were previously infertile before fibroid embolisation have been rendered fertile and have had successful pregnancies and deliveries. We have had a case in which there was a large conglomerate fibroid mass on MRI with no normal myometrium and no discernible endometrial cavity. Following embolisation, the fibroids were all eliminated resulting in a normal uterus and a successful pregnancy with delivery following elective caesarean section. Where a surgical myomectomy is feasible with a good chance of success it is probably the procedure of choice but in patients who have had previous myomectomies, or in whom the only treatment on offer is hysterectomy, there is a clear indication for embolisation in patients who wish to conceive. It is also an obvious option in patients in whom surgery is contraindicated for medical reasons or, for example, in Jehovah's Witnesses.

So far the results of fibroid embolisation are very encouraging. It would appear to be effective with a high patient satisfaction rate and a complication rate of morbidity and mortality less than surgery. The short hospital stay (usually two nights) and short convalescent period (2–3 weeks) is significantly less than with hysterectomy or myomectomy.

References

1. Walker WJ, Goldin AR, Shaff MI, Allibone GW. Per catheter control of haemorrhage from the superior and inferior mesenteric arteries. *Clin Radiol* 1980; 31: 71–80.

2. Wells I. Internal iliac artery bleeding in the management of pelvic bleeding. *Clin Radiol* 1996; 825–827.

3. Vedantham S, Goodwin SC, McLucas B, Mohr G. Uterine artery embolisation: an underused method of controlling pelvic haemorrhage. *Am J Obstet Gynaecol* 1997; 176: 938–948.

4. Walker WJ. Successful internal iliac artery embolisation with glue in a case of massive obstetric haemorrhage. *Clin Radiol* 1996; 51: 442–444.

5. Clark SL, Phelan JP, Yeh SY, Bruce SR, Paul RH. Hypogastric artery ligation for obstetric haemorrhage. *Obstet Gynecol* 1985; 66: 353–356.

6. O'Leary JA. Uterine artery ligation in the control of post-Caesarean hemorrhage. *J Repro Med* 1995; 40: 189–193.

7. Ravina JH, Herbreteau C, Ciraru-Vigneron N. Arterial embolisation to treat uterine myomata. *Lancet* 1995; 346: 671–672.

8. Worthington-Kirsch RL, Popky GL, Hutchins FL. Uterine arterial embolization for the management of leiomyomas: quality-of-life assessment and clinical response. *Radiol September* 1998; 208: 625–629.

9. Walker WJ. Bilateral uterine artery embolization for fibroids. In: S Scheth, C Sutton (Eds) *Menorrhagia*, pp 185–194, 1999. Oxford: Isis Medical Media.

10. Goodwin SC, Walker WJ. Uterine artery embolization for the treatment of uterine fibroids. *Curr Opin Obstet Gynaecol* 1998; 10: 315–320.

11. Walker W. Arterial embolization in obstetrics and gynaecology with particular reference to uterine fibroids. *Adv Gynaecol Obstet* 1999; 16: 2–8.

12. Ravina JH et al. Particulate arterial embolization: a new treatment for uterine leiomyomata-related hemorrhage. *La Press Medicale* 1998; 27(7): 299–303.

13. Goodwin SC, Vedantham S, McLucas B et al. Preliminary experience with uterine artery embolisation for uterine fibroids. *J Vascu Interven Radiol* 1997; 8: 517–526.

14. Goodwin SC, McLucas B, Lee M, Chen G, Perrella R, Vedantham S et al. Uterine artery embolisation for the treatment of uterine leiomyomata midterm results. *J Vascu Interven Radiol* 1999; 10: 1159–1165.

15. Hutchins FL, Worthington-Kirsch RL, Berkowitz RP. Selective uterine artery embolization as primary treatment for symptomatic leiomyomata uteri. *J Am Assoc of Gynecol Laparosc* 1999; 6(3): 279–284.

16. Walker W, Green A, Sutton C. Bilateral uterine artery embolisation for myomata-results, complications and failures. *J Minimal Invasiv Ther* 1999; 8(6): 449–454.

17. Jones K, Walker WJ, Sutton C. Sequestration and extrusion of intramural fibroids following uterine artery embolisation. *Gynaecol Endosc* (in press).

18. Ravina JH, Bouret JM, Ciraru-Vigneron N et al. Recourse to particular arterial embolisation in the treatment of some leiomyoma. *Bull Acad Med* 1997; 181(2): 223–243.

19. Cassou B, Derriennic F, Monfort C et al. Risk factors of early menopause in two generations of gainfully employed French women. *Maturitas* 1997; 26(3): 165–174.

20. Vashisht A, Studd J, Carey A et al. Fatal septicaemia after fibroid embolisation. *The Lancet* 1999; 354(July 24): 307–308.

21. Wingo PA, Huezo CM, Rubin GL et al. The mortality risk associated with hysterectomy. *Am J Obstet Gynecol* 1986; 152(7, Pt 1): 803–808.

22. Takamizawa S, Minakami H, Usui R et al. Risk of complications and uterine malignancies in women undergoing hysterectomy for presume benign leiomyomas. *Gynecol Obstet Invest* 1999; 48(3): 193–196.

24

Laparoscopic myomectomy

Kailash Nakade and Adrian Lower

Introduction

Uterine fibroids are benign smooth muscle tumours that are found in 20% of all women of reproductive age group. They are often detected incidentally during a routine pelvic examination following cervical smear. Asymptomatic fibroids may be present in 40–50% of women older than 40 years of age[1] and have been reported in up to 50% of women at post-mortem examination.

The symptoms caused are related to the site of the fibroids and include pelvic pain, dyspareunia, abnormal uterine bleeding, pelvic pressure, urinary frequency (pressure on bladder) and/or constipation (pressure on colon). Submucous and intramural fibroids may also be associated with infertility or recurrent pregnancy loss. However, most of the fibroids are asymptomatic and only 25% of cases are thought to cause significant symptoms.[2]

Not all fibroids need to be treated. Asymptomatic leiomyomas discovered incidentally can be monitored by observation only. Treatment is recommended when symptoms become significant and can be directly attributed to the uterine fibroids. There is an argument for treating asymptomatic fibroids that are growing rapidly whilst they are still relatively small since surgery is less complicated and the risk of hysterectomy is reduced. With appropriate training, smaller intramural and subserosal fibroids can be dealt with laparoscopically avoiding laparotomy. Rarely, fibroids undergo rapid growth due to sarcomatous change so that a tissue diagnosis in such cases can be helpful.

Abdominal myomectomy has been the standard surgical treatment for women desiring to maintain their reproductive potential. Hysterectomy, either by vaginal or abdominal route, is the most common surgical procedure for women not wishing further pregnancies and indeed uterine fibroids are the most common cause of abdominal hysterectomy in premenopausal women. With the development and improvement of endoscopic equipment, surgical techniques and skill, laparoscopic myomectomy has now become feasible and offers an alternative to the major abdominal surgery. This novel technique has been reported by a few centres and the results are encouraging.[3–6]

Preoperative evaluation and patient selection

A thorough preoperative evaluation of patients with uterine fibroids is required to determine whether surgery is necessary and if so, what procedure is to be recommended. The decision is based on the size, site and number of fibroids, the woman's desire for further pregnancies and the extent of symptoms she is experiencing.

The primary investigation for any pelvic mass is ultrasonography. Transvaginal ultrasonography allows higher frequency sound waves to be used which give better resolution but lack penetration. Abdominal ultrasonography is required for masses of greater than 10 cm in diameter. The use of saline within the endometrial cavity (saline sonography) can provide further information about the extent to which the cavity is distorted by the fibroids and whether they are predominantly intramural or submucous type 1 or 2 (Fig. 24.1). Type 1 submucous fibroids are relatively superficial and have the greater part of the fibroid within the endometrial cavity. Type 2 submucous fibroids lie with the greater part of their diameter within the myometrium. Magnetic resonance imaging (MRI) can provide much more accurate information about the location and number of fibroids than conventional ultrasound and the hard copy films are much easier to interpret. More importantly, MRI can better differentiate between focal adenomyosis and fibroids. Adenomyosis is much more difficult to remove and no clear plane of cleavage can be identified. Often, more damage is created by trying to remove areas of adenomyosis than by managing conservatively with gonadotrophin-releasing hormone agonists (GnRH-a). Hysterosalpingography (HSG) can be extremely useful in preoperative assessment of patients with submucous myoma as it outlines the intrauterine portion of the myoma and defines its relationship with the fallopian tubes.

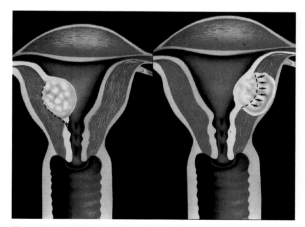

Figure 24.1 — Type 1 and type 2 fibroids.

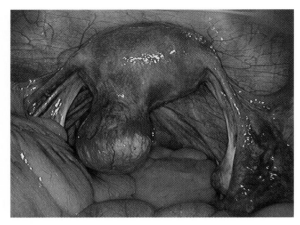

Figure 24.2 — Pedunculated fibroid.

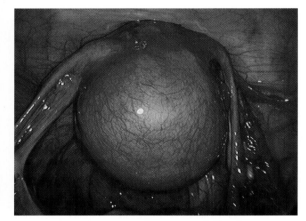

Figure 24.3 — 5-cm Intramural posterior wall fibroid.

Type 1 and type 2 submucous fibroids are best removed hysteroscopically. Subserous and intramural fibroids can be removed laparoscopically. Pedunculated fibroids (Fig. 24.2) are relatively straightforward, and, depending on the site, fibroids of up to 12 cm in diameter can be managed laparoscopically. Less superficial subserous and intramural fibroids (Fig. 24.3) are more difficult and a maximum diameter of 10 cm is recommended for fundal and posterior wall fibroids. Anterior, cervical or broad ligament fibroids present greater difficulty in removal and smaller fibroids should be tackled in these locations where access is restricted. The patient's habitus may also make access difficult and obesity or short stature may restrict further the maximum size of fibroid which can be safely removed laparoscopically. Where multiple fibroids are present the maximum individual diameter should be less than 8 cm and total diameter of

fibroids less than 15 cm. Careful selection of patients can decrease the likelihood of inappropriate performance of laparoscopic myomectomy and avoid the need to convert to laparotomy.[7] Using multiple preoperative criteria for selection of patients, conversion to laparotomy could be avoided in 90% of patients.[8]

Preoperative preparation

Laparoscopic myomectomy is a difficult endoscopic procedure and should be performed only by those with extensive experience in operative laparoscopy. Several operative principles need to be observed to minimise the morbidity associated with this procedure such as massive blood loss, infection, and uterine rupture during pregnancy, postoperative adhesions and damage to surrounding structures.

Preoperative treatment with GnRH analogues for 2–4 months prior to surgery has been shown to reduce the intraoperative blood loss in myomectomy.[9] The advantages of preoperative GnRH-a administration may include a reduction in uterine bleeding and an improvement of haemoglobin, reduction in uterine volume and size of fibroids. There is also a reduction in uterine blood flow and myometrial vascularity with preoperative GnRH-a therapy. The disadvantage of GnRH-a therapy is that it may cause some fibrosis around the fibroid, which can make it difficult to find the correct plane of cleavage. For this reason the author generally restricts the use of GnRH-a to fibroids of around 10 cm or more in diameter where access is likely to be difficult in an attempt to reduce the risk of reversion to open surgery.

The surgeon, patient and theatre staff should be prepared for an abdominal myomectomy as laparotomy may be necessary in the event of bleeding or technical difficulties. As with open myomectomy, the patient should be informed that emergency hysterectomy may need to be performed in the event of uncontrollable bleeding or if attempts at uterine repair are unsuccessful. This should be extremely rare with fibroids of a size where a laparoscopic approach is contemplated.

The patient should have her blood cross-matched for a possible blood transfusion. The patient may require postoperative admission for close observation of bleeding, infection, or other complications. Prophylactic antibiotics should be administered with laparoscopic myomectomy. Thromboprophylaxis should be given using TED stockings and clexane. A Foley catheter is usually placed to drain the urinary bladder if operating time is prolonged (more than $1\frac{1}{2}$ h) or if the fibroid is low on the anterior wall. A uterine cannula or manipulator is necessary to inject methylene blue dye and allow uterine manipulation.

Operative procedure

Instrumentation

Laparoscopic instruments necessary for myomectomy are similar to those required for other extensive laparoscopic procedures. A good telescope, video monitor, continuous CO_2 insufflator and electrosurgical unit are essential. Four trocar placements (three suprapubic and one intraumbilical) are generally necessary. A laparoscopic needle and syringe are required if the myometrium is to be injected with pitressin.

A 5-mm monopolar scissors or hook is used for coagulation and making a serosal incision. A grasper with teeth is used to grasp the fibroid and provide traction. Sharp scissors are necessary for dissection of the fibroid from the psuedocapsule. A good suction and irrigation system is mandatory. Laparoscopic suturing equipment should be readily available. An adhesion barrier is an added advantage. Instruments for laparotomy or colpotomy should be readily available, should this become necessary.

Anaesthesia and patient's position

Laparoscopic myomectomy is performed under general anaesthesia. The patient is placed in low lithotomy stirrups, a Foley catheter may be inserted in the bladder. Some surgeons may wish to stain the endometrium with methylene blue dye both as an aid to identification of the endometrial cavity and to test tubal patency for fertility patients. A good quality uterine manipulator such as a Valchev or Pelosi manipulator is essential to allow adequate anteversion or retroversion of the uterus to improve access.

Position of trocars

The laparoscope is introduced through a 10 mm intraumbilical incision. Two 5 mm lateral ports are sited lateral to the inferior epigastric arteries and a further midline suprapubic trocar is sited suprapubically 1–2 cm above the symphysis pubis (higher for larger fibroids) just above the fundus of the uterus. A 10–12 mm trocar is used in the midline with a reducer to allow the passage of needles. Some surgeons prefer to use two 5 mm trocars on the same side as they stand. This can allow a more relaxed and ergonomic position but makes the angle of interaction of the instruments less efficient.

General principles

It is important to accurately determine the anatomical relationship of the fibroid to the round ligaments and fallopian tubes. Ureters should be identified if the fibroid is located in the broad ligament. Since myomectomy is usually performed in a woman who wishes to conserve fertility, it is important to bear in mind the principles of infertility surgery. Care should be taken to prevent excessive bleeding. Meticulous haemostasis and impeccable closure of the myometrium will help prevent adhesions and postoperative complications. Excessive use of diathermy for myometrial haemostasis should be avoided as this may weaken the uterine scar by delaying healing. An adhesion prevention barrier should be used at the end of the procedure.

Removal of pedunculated subserous fibroid

An incision is made across the pedicle close to the fibroid. The fibroid is placed on stretch and using diathermy armed scissors or needle-point the pedicle is divided close to the base of the fibroid. An 'onion skinning' technique is used. There should be little haemorrhage provided that the plane stays close to the fibroid. Occasionally bipolar diathermy is required for persistent bleeding or a figure-of-eight suture may be placed. The serosa can be closed over the defect and sutured in place to decrease adhesion formation. Occasionally very small fibroids with very narrow pedicles can be removed using bipolar diathermy to the pedicle. The pedicle can also be ligated using a pre-tied loop of absorbable material (e.g. Endoloop) to secure the base.

Removal of sessile subserous or intramural fibroids

The location of fibroids at these sites presents more of a challenge to the laparoscopic surgeon than does resection of pedunculated subserous fibroids. The operative principles should be same as those used in open myomectomy. The most important factor is the citing of the uterine incision. This should be parallel to the line of the needle holder in the dominant hand. A longitudinal midline incision is used for posterior wall

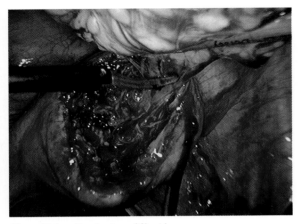

Figure 24.4 — Enucleation of fibroid

fibroids and an oblique tranverse incision is used for anterior wall fibroids. This allows a curved needle to be driven through the edge of the wound by simple pronation and supination of the dominant hand. Trauma to the surrounding myometrium should be kept to a minimum. Pitressin may be used to minimise blood loss. A solution of 20 units pitressin in 20 ml saline is favoured by the author and 10 ml is injected at the insertion of each round ligament. This leads to a rapid blanching of the whole of the uterus.

An incision is then made over the fibroid using a fine tip monopolar cautery, diathermy-armed scissors or harmonic scalpel. The incision is carried into the body of the myoma so that the pseudocapsule can be identified and stripped away from the myometrium. This is usually easily achieved using either a myoma screw or 10 mm claw grasping forceps and is surprisingly bloodless providing the correct plane is chosen (Fig. 24.4).

After the myoma is enucleated, it is placed in posterior cul-de-sac. If additional myomas are found, they should be removed through the initial incision if possible. Haemostasis is confirmed using bipolar diathermy where required. The operative field should be kept irrigated using heparinised Hartmanns solution or a proprietary adhesion prevention product such as icodextrin (Adept, Shire Pharmaceuticals).

The myometrial defect is repaired in two layers using 2-0 vicryl to the deep myometrial layer and 3-0 monocyl to the serosa.[10] Interrupted intracorporally tied sutures are usually employed. Opening of the endometrial cavity happens rarely. If the cavity is breached it should be repaired as a separate layer using 3-0 vicryl. Adhesions are expected after laparoscopic myomectomy[11] and some sort of adhesion preventive barrier is advisable. A barrier such as Interceed (Johnson & Johnson) can be used to mask the suture line and prevent adhesions at the site of repair. Adept will also protect the suture line but also prevent adhesion formation remote from the site of surgery.

Removal of the myoma from pelvic cavity

Fibroids should always be removed to avoid peritoneal reimplantation, and allow histological examination. A fibroid of less than 1 cm in diameter can be pulled directly through the 10-mm trocar with grasping forceps or a myoma screw. Larger myomas can be removed by enlarging the suprapubic trocar site. The trocar is removed and the resected myoma is brought to the port site where it is held with a grasper or myoma screw. The myoma is then pressed against the peritoneum to prevent the loss of pneumoperitoneum and then fragmented using a small blade passed through the incision. This procedure is time consuming and difficult especially with large myomas and overweight women. It is also dangerous if there is a sudden loss of pneumoperitoneum. The skin of the posterior vagina is more elastic than the anterior abdominal wall and larger fibroids can be removed by a posterior colpotomy.

The authors' preferred method of fibroid removal is using an electrosurgical morcellator. These have concentric cylinders of 10–15 mm in diameter with a knife blade on the inner, rotating cylinder. The instrument is introduced through the suprapubic incision after removal of the trocar and the fibroid is rapidly cut into long cylinders which are removed through the morcellator using grasping forceps. This is an extremely dangerous instrument and should only be used by the most experienced laparoscopic surgeons as it is all too easy to lose orientation and damage bowel or blood vessels with catastrophic results (Figs 24.5 and 24.6).[12]

Need for laparotomy

Laparotomy may be necessary in case of a difficulty or complications. It should not be considered the procedure of last resort. Indications for laparotomy include significant bleeding that cannot be controlled, long or deep myometrial incisions that cannot be repaired laparoscopically, if multiple myomas are unexpectedly identified or myomas are too large or too deep in the myometrium to be removed safely. Laparotomy is also

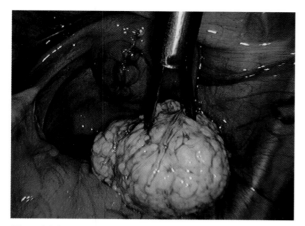

Figure 24.5 — Morcellation and suture line.

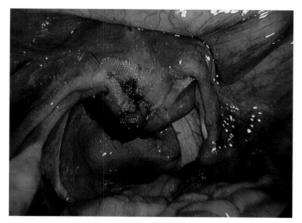

Figure 24.6 — Suture line masked with interceed.

indicated if the uterine cavity is entered during the procedure and the endometrium cannot be sufficiently repaired laparoscopically. Laparotomy should not be perceived as defeat, but rather as a prudent step to ensure the safety and well-being of the patient in case of a difficult procedure or significant complications.

Postoperative and complications

Same day discharge can be expected after removal of pedunculated subserous fibroids, however in case of intramural laparoscopic myomectomy, the patient should be hospitalised for 24 h. Serial haemoglobin levels should be obtained and vital signs monitored every 4 h.

Bleeding may occur from intra-abdominal operative sites making the patient haemodynamically unstable. This may be confirmed and treated with laparoscopy. However if it cannot be dealt with by laparoscopy, then laparotomy may be required.

Postoperative pyrexia is common with abdominal myomectomy and can also occur with laparoscopic myomectomy. It should be evaluated and managed as in the case of open myomectomy. However, unsuspected bowel injury should be kept in mind. A laparotomy is warranted if there is suspicion or evidence of bowel injury, or temperature does not respond to aggressive antibiotic therapy.

Extensive adhesion formation and bowel obstruction may occur after laparoscopic myomectomy. Various adhesion preventive measures are now available and should be used with laparoscopic myomectomy. Early second look laparoscopy for adhesiolysis has also been mentioned.[13]

Uterine rupture following laparoscopic myomectomy is rare but has been reported.[14–16] The incidence of uterine rupture will be kept to a minimum by meticulous surgical technique and accurate closure of the uterine defect. Routine elective caesarean section is not mandatory after laparoscopic myomectomy unless complicated by infection or haematoma at the uterine incision site, uterine defect was deep or the endometrial cavity was entered. However, all patients should be informed about this complication before considering laparoscopic myomectomy.

Results

Published results of laparoscopic myomectomy are encouraging. Compared with abdominal myomectomy, laparoscopic myomectomy has lower morbidity, no increased hospital cost, minimal hospital stay and fewer complications.[17,22] Relief of pressure symptoms and pain following laparoscopic myomectomy is excellent.[5,18,19] The pregnancy rate and obstetric outcome after laparoscopic myomectomy is reported to be the same as open procedures[20,22–24] and depends on patients age, duration of infertility before myomectomy and the existence of any other infertility factors.[21] The Cumulative risk of recurrence after laparoscopic myomectomy has been reported as 10.6% after 1 year, 31.7% after 3 years and 51.4% after 5 years.[25] It is suggested that this may be higher than abdominal myomectomy, however another study reports it to be similar to abdominal myomectomy.[26]

One must remember that many surgical series are biased and go unreported if results are poor. Also, the number of patients in many series is small. Therefore, until larger studies are published, laparoscopic myomectomy should be offered to a carefully selected group of patients.

Summary

Advances in the laparoscopic instruments and endoscopic skills have made laparoscopic myomectomy a feasible operation. It is a difficult technique and requires an experienced endoscopic surgeon with considerable experience in endoscopic suturing skills. There are many advantages of laparoscopic myomectomy to the patient as well as health care providers. In a group of properly selected patients and in the hands of experienced endoscopic surgeons, this procedure appears safe. The results are encouraging, however larger studies are necessary to confirm all its advantages over conventional abdominal myomectomy.

References

1. Hillard PA. Benign diseases of the female reproductive tract: symptoms and signs. In: JS Berek, EY Adashi, PA Hillard (Eds) *Novak's Gynecology*, 12th edn, pp 331–397, 1996. Baltimore: Williams & Wilkins.

2. Buttram VC, Reiter RC. Uterine leiomyomata: etiology, symptomatology and management. *Fertil Steril* 1981; 36(4): 433–445.

3. Dubuisson JB, Lecuru F, Foulot H, Mandelbrot L, Aubriot FX, Mouly M. Myomectomy by laparoscopy — a preliminary report of 43 cases. *Fertil Steril* 1991; 1(56): 827.

4. Daniell JF, Gurley LD. Laparoscopic treatment of clinically significant symptomatic uterine fibroids. *J Gynecol Surg* 1991; 7: 37–40.

5. Hasson HM, Rotman C, Rana N, Sistos F, Dmowski WP. Laparoscopic myomectomy. *Obstet Gynecol* 1992; 80: 884–888.

6. Nezhat C, Nezhat F, Silfen SL, Schaffer N, Evans D. Laparoscopic myomectomy. *Int J Fertil* 1991; 36: 275–280.

7. Parker WH, Rodi IA. Patient selection for laparoscopic myomectomy. *J Am Assoc Gynecol Laparosc* 1994; 2(1): 23–26.

8. Dubuisson JB, Fauconnier A, Fourchotte V, Babaki-Fard K, Coste J, Chaperon C. Laparoscopic myomectomy: predicting the risk of conversion to an open procedure. *J Reprod Med* 2001; 16: 1726–1731.

9. Lethaby A, Vollenhoven B, Sowter M. Pre-operative GnRH analogue therapy before hysterectomy or myomectomy for uterine fibroids. *Cochrane Database of Systematic Reviews* 2002; Issue 1.

10. Dubuisson JB, Chapron C, Chavet X, Morice P, Aubriot FX. Laparoscopic myomectomy: where do we stand? *Gynaecol Endosc* 1995; 4: 83–86.

11. The Myomectomy Adhesion Multicentre Study Group. An expanded polytetrafluoroethylene barrier (Gore-Tex Surgical Membrane) reduces post-myomectomy adhesion formation. *Fertil Steril* 1995; 63: 491–493.

12. Steiner RA, Wight E, Tadir Y, Haller U. Electrical device for laparoscopic removal of tissue from the abdominal cavity. *Obstet Gynecol* 1993; 81: 471–474.

13. Ugur M, Turan C, Mungan T, Aydogdu T, Shani Y, Gokmen O. Laparoscopy for adhesion prevention following myomectomy. *Int J Gynaecol Obstet* 1996; 53: 145–149.

14. Seidman DS, Nezhat CH, Nezhat FR, Nezhat C. Spontaneous uterine rupture in pregnancy 8 years after laparoscopic myomectomy. *J Am Assoc Gynecol Laparosc* 2001; 8: 618–619.

15. Pelosi MA 3rd, Pelosi MA. Spontaneous uterine rupture at thirty-three weeks subsequent to previous superficial laparoscopic myomectomy. *Am J Obstet Gynecol* 1997; 177: 1547–1549.

16. Friedmann W, Maier RF, Luttkus A, Shafer AP, Dudenhausen JW. Uterine rupture after laparoscopic myomectomy. *Acta Obstet Gynecol Scand* 1196; 75: 683–684.

17. Stringer NH, Walker JC, Meyer PM. Comparison of 49 laparoscopic myomectomies with 49 open myomectomies. *J Am Assoc Gynecol Laparosc* 1997; 4: 457–464.

18. Nezhat C, Nezhat F, Bess O, Nezhat CH, Mashiach R. Laparoscopically assisted myomectomy: a report of a new technique in 57 cases. *Int J Menopause Stud* 1994; 39: 39–44.

19. Mettler L, Semm K. Pelviscopic uterine surgery. *Surg Endosc* 1992; 6: 23–31.

20. Rosseti A, Sizzi O, Soranna L, Mancuso S, Lanzone A. Fertility outcome: long-term results after laparoscopic myomectomy. *Gynecol Endocr* 2001; 15: 129–134.

21. Dessolle L, Soriano D, Poncelet C, Benifla JI, Madelenat P, Darai E. Determinants of pregnancy rate and obstetric outcome after laparoscopic myomectomy for infertility. *Fertil Steril* 2001; 76: 370–374.

22. Seraccchioli R, Rossi S, Govoni F, Rossi E, Venuroli S, Bulleti C, Flaming C. Fertility and obstetric outcome after laparoscopic myomectomy of large myomata: a randomized comparison with abdominal myomectomy. *Hum Reprod* 2000; 15: 2663–2668.

23. Seinera P, Farina C, Tordos T. Laparoscopic myomectomy and subsequent pregnancy: results in 54 patients. *Hum Reprod* 2000; 15: 1993–1996.

24. Ribeiro SC, Reich H, Rosenberg J, Guglieminetti E, Vidali A. Laparoscopic myomectomy and pregnancy outcome in infertile patients. *Fertil Steril* 1999; 71: 571–574.

25. Nezhat FR, Roemisch M, Nezhat CH, Seidman DS, Nezhat CR. Recurrence rate after laparoscopic myomectomy. *J Am Assoc Gynecol Laparosc* 1998; 5: 237–240.

26. Rosseti A, Sizzi O, Soranna L, Cucinelli F, Mancuso S, Lanzone A. Long-term results of laparoscopic myomectomy: recurrence rate in comparison with abdominal myomectomy. *Hum Reprod* 2001; 16: 770–774.

25

Avoiding complications in hysteroscopic surgery

Kailash Nakade, K. Johnson, T.C. Li,
P. McGurgan and P.J. O'Donovan

Introduction

There is little doubt that Minimal Access Surgery (MAS) presents many advantages over conventional surgery:

- smaller scars,
- reduced post-operative pain,
- shorter hospital stay,
- speedier recovery.

Complications may occur in any surgical procedure. These may be due to those associated with anaesthesia and risks specific to the procedure performed. Hysteroscopic procedures involve introduction of instruments into the uterus and distension of the uterine cavity with media in a fashion not used conventionally. Any surgery has a potentially increased risk of iatrogenic complications, particularly during the learning phase of the surgeon. It is vital that every effort is made to reduce the complication rate of hysteroscopic procedures. This review focuses on practical and technological advances whereby complications may be decreased during hysteroscopic surgery.

The scale of the problem

Complication rates for hysteroscopic surgery will vary with the complexity of the procedure and experience of the operator. The following tables represent an overview of complication rates. Table 25.1 gives the complication and emergency hysterectomy rate for the Minimally Invasive Surgical Techniques — Laser, Endothermal, or Endoresection (MISTLETOE) Study.[1]

Table 25.2 demonstrates the increase in laparoscopic and hysteroscopic complications noted by the American Association of Gynecological Laparoscopists.[2]

It can be seen that minimal access procedure related complications are relatively infrequent. However, there is no room for complacency as rare complications for an individual surgeon can still represent a major problem on an international scale. We should not be lulled into a false sense of security by having no personal experience of complications, whilst using a technique which, on a larger scale, may be suboptimal.

As seen in Table 25.2, minimal access surgical complications appear to be on the increase. In this study, whilst the overall complication rate was low, there was a steep increase in complications as more advanced operative procedures were performed. This change over time may reflect the attempt by less skilled surgeons to perform increasingly complex procedures, or less reticence by surgeons to report on their complications as hysteroscopic surgery has become more widely accepted in the surgical community. Alternatively, it may be due to

Table 25.1 — Complications associated with endometrial ablation or resection[1]

Technique	Complication rates (%)	Emergency hysterectomy
Resection alone	10.9	13/1000
Roller-ball alone	4.5	3/1000
Combined resection/roller	7.7	5/1000
Laser	5.5	2/1000

Table 25.2 — Comparison between complication rates between two AAGL★ surveys[2]

Complication rate★★ per 1000 cases

Hysteroscopic	1998 Survey	1999 Survey	Change since 1988	
Uterine perforation (not requiring transfusion)	13	11.1	↓	×0.9
Haemorrhage requiring transfusion	1.0	0.3	↓	×0.3
Laparotomy to manage haemorrhage	0.5	1.4	↑	×2.9
Laparotomy to manage visceral injury	0	0.3	↑	
H_2O intoxication/pulmonary oedema	3.4	1.4	↑	×1.4
Death	0	0.1	↑	

★American Association of Gynaecological Laparoscopists.
★★Results are from a confidential survey with a 15% response rate — this may not represent true incidences.

inclusion of cases where the morbidity was intrinsically higher due to the pre-existent pathology. The lack of a definitive answer underlines the need for continuous audit of these techniques and the appropriate emphasis on training and accreditation.

One of our main concerns is the fact that whilst tremendous advances in the ability to perform minimal access procedures have been made, there is a surprising lack of quality research on the optimum approaches to perform basic and safe hysteroscopic surgery. In the absence of established optimum techniques, we present an overview of different attempts to decrease the risk of complications in hysteroscopic surgery.

General principles of safe hysteroscopic surgery

- Appropriate case selection
- Pre-operative preparation
- Proper equipment
- Optimal view
- Knowledgeable use of electrical sources
- Awareness of the learning phase.

Case selection

Appropriate case selection is one of the most import-ant factors in reducing complication rates of any surgery. First, one must accept that not all cases are suitable for hysteroscopic surgery. What might be tech-nically possible may not be the safest option. For example, there are uncertainties as to whether hystero-scopic surgery for large (>5 cm) type II submucous fibroids (Table 25.3) is appropriate. Whilst there are claims by experienced surgeons that it is feasible to carry out these procedures by hysteroscopic means, it is important to appreciate that what may be achieved by a few gifted surgeons may not be readily achievable by the average general gynaecologist.

Table 25.3 — Classification of leiomyomas

Type	Location
0	Pedunculated
I	<50% intra-mural
II	>50% intra-mural

Appropriate case selection is of particular importance in the 'learning phase'. As a rule one should start with simple cases. For example, when performing hystero-scopic resection of fibroids, start with small Type 0 or Type I submucous fibroids (Table 25.3). Once experi-ence and confidence have been gained, more difficult cases may be undertaken.

Pre-operative preparation

Appropriate patient preparation will make the proced-ure easier and reduce complication rates.

Pre-operative counselling and accurate documentation

The most important factor in decreasing litigation is a fully informed patient, particularly if there are known risk factors for performing surgery. Patients may have unrealistic expectations about these new procedures. A leaflet explaining the procedure is a useful adjunct to a full discussion. A plan of 'worst case scenario' should be made; for instance the need for a laparotomy or hys-terectomy in the event of a uterine perforation. When complications do occur, this should be fully documented and remedial surgery instituted as soon as possible.[3]

Endometrial preparation in hysteroscopic surgery

The need for endometrial preparation prior to endo-metrial ablation is well recognised. However, there is no consensus on endometrial preparation for other hysteroscopic surgery such as removal of septae or sub-mucous fibroids, but this is generally advisable except for those who are very experienced. The method of preparation varies — being either mechanical (curet-tage)[4] or pharmacological[5] (gonadotrophin releasing hormone, GnRH analogues and danazol). GnRH ana-logues add to the overall cost of the procedure and may cause difficulties in cervical dilation.

Appropriate equipment

It is essential to be properly equipped before embark-ing on hysteroscopic surgery. The minimum require-ments should include a good quality camera system, light source and image recording facilities. Both the surgeon and theatre staff should be familiar with the equipment and how it works.

Use of electrical sources

Hysteroscopic electrosurgical techniques conventionally use a non-ionic distension medium for obvious reasons. Glycine 1.5% and sorbitol 3% are commonly used for operative hysteroscopy. As we know, considerable amounts of these non-iso-osmotic substances can be absorbed systemically, with resultant morbidity and mortality (Table 25.2). The introduction of a bipolar electrosurgical device (Versapoint, Ethicon, USA) which operates in an ionic saline medium represents a considerable feat of engineering. This is a valuable new instrument for hysteroscopic surgery. The instrument's small diameter means that operative procedures may be performed on conscious patients in an out patient setting. Our experience agrees with the very positive initial reports.[6] Care must still be taken to avoid fluid overload, although the osmotically induced fluid shifts, characteristics of other media are minimised.

Learning phase

It is a well-recognised fact that complication rates are higher for cases performed by surgeons during their learning phase, than experienced operators. The following recommendations may help to reduce complication rates:

1. There are different levels of complexity of hysteroscopic surgery.[7] One should begin with simple procedures (level I and II) and not undertake complex procedures (level III and IV) until enough experience has been acquired (Table 25.4).

Table 25.4 — Examples of Hysteroscopic procedures by levels of training[7]

Level		Hysteroscopic procedures
I	Diagnostic procedures	Hysteroscopy and target biopsy
		Removal of polyps/IUCD★
II	Minor operative procedures	Minor Asherman's syndrome
		Proximal tubal cannulation
III	More complex (additional training)	Endometrial resection/ablation
		Resection of submucous leiomyomas
		Resection of uterine septum

★Intra-uterine contraceptive device.

2. In some cases, hysteroscopic surgery may be safer with concurrent laparoscopic control, for example, resection of a Type II submucous fibroid, (especially if situated over the cornual region), removal of uterine septum or dense intra-uterine adhesions (Asherman's syndrome). An experienced assistant, with a second camera and light source, continuously monitors the amount of light transmitted across the uterine wall and keeps the bowel away from the uterus. The amount of light transmitted should be compared with that via the cornual region and should be no more than the latter. Combined synchronous laparoscopic control should be considered in all difficult hysteroscopic cases and during the learning curve of beginners.

3. The RCOG has published a list of more than 100 preceptors in MAS in various parts of the United Kingdom. Gynaecologists should contact preceptors in their region to discuss individual training and preceptorship. The initial cases should be proctored by an experienced colleague or supervised by a recognised trainer until competence has been achieved.

Complications of hysteroscopy

Operative hysteroscopy is a new and valuable technique in the management of non-malignant pathology of the uterine cavity. As with any surgical procedure, there are potential complications due to the mode of access and also the actual surgical procedure performed. In this section we confine ourselves to the general principles of hysteroscopic surgery with emphasis on specific complications and strategies to avoid them. Appropriate training in this new field is vital, with staged levels of procedures, progressing only after adequate experience is developed at each stage in training (Table 25.4).

The main complications of hysteroscopic procedures result from perforation of the uterus or fluid overload through the use of distension media.

Dilation and perforation

Dilatation of cervix forms an essential part of the operative hysteroscopy, however the patients for operative hysteroscopy will often have received GnRH analogues. Whilst these drugs are an important part of pre-operative endometrial preparation, they can have a significant stenotic effect on the cervix. In these instances options include traditional methods of cervical dilation such as laminaria stents (Lamicel, Cabot Medical, PA, USA) or the more commonly administered pharmacological methods, for example, prostaglandins such as PgE2 or PgF2α. GnRH analogues decrease the uterine size and this increases the risk of initial perforation during dilation and possible subsequent perforation by the instrument during operative hysteroscopy.

The management of perforation depends largely on the instrument being used. If a perforation occurs during uterine sounding a conservative approach can be followed by, stopping the procedure, treatment with antibiotics and overnight stay. After perforation with a large dilator or operative hysteroscope it is usually advisable to perform a laparoscopy to evaluate the extent of trauma. Occasionally it may be necessary to perform a laparotomy, particularly if a perforation by a 'hot' instrument has occurred, or even a hysterectomy if bleeding is heavy. The incidence of perforation during operative procedures is very experience dependent and is estimated at 1–2% of operations.[8]

Distension media

Gas or liquid distension media are needed as a prerequisite for hysteroscopic surgery, in order to keep the uterine walls separated and obtain a clear view. It is the use of these media which creates complications specific to hysteroscopy.

Rubin first described the use of carbon dioxide in 1925. Its advantages are that it is cheap, easily available in theatres, non-flammable and relatively soluble in blood. It has a similar refractive index to air and allows good quality images to be obtained. The disadvantages of CO_2 are that it causes bubbling in the presence of excess fluid or any bleeding this effectively limits its use to diagnostic hysteroscopy. If intravasation occurs, deaths have been reported due to CO_2 gas embolism — therefore flow rates of less than 100 ml/min are fixed (a flow rate of 30–40 ml/min is usually satisfactory).

Liquid distension media include high viscosity fluids such as dextran 70 (Hyskon) and low viscosity fluids, such as 5% dextrose, 1.5% glycine, 3% sorbitol and 0.9% saline. Different experts have their preferences. Hyskon is immiscible with blood and its high viscosity decreases the risk of intravasation to some extent. However, the high viscosity makes it difficult to work with and necessitates immediate washing of instruments in contact

with it. Although intravasation is uncommon, a volume of only 300 ml is sufficient to cause pulmonary oedema. This is because dextran 70 is hydrophilic and in the circulation it osmotically shifts 6 times its own volume of water into the intravascular compartment. It also has an effect on blood coagulation and may rarely cause a disseminated intravascular coagulation type consumptive coagulopathy and has been linked to adult respiratory distress syndrome.[9] At present there is a suspicion that these features are due to an allergic type reaction.

Low viscosity fluids are more commonly used in the UK, although they are miscible with blood, they are not associated with any coagulopathic, or allergic complications. Dextrose 5% is rarely used; it has no advantage over saline and has the side effect of being hypo-osmolar. The solutions mainly used for operative hysteroscopy are 1.5% glycine and 3% sorbitol. Both of these are non-ionic and therefore suitable for mono-polar electrosurgery. Glycine, used originally by the urologists, is hypo-osmolar and excess absorption results in a dilutional hyponataemia, which can be further complicated by a subsequent hyperammonaemia due to glycine's intrahepatic metabolism causing the 'TURP Syndrome'. As with all of these compounds, vigilance is mandatory and deaths have been reported.[2] Sorbitol is similar to glycine in being hypo-osmolar (approximately 170 m Osmol) and it may also have metabolic complications, causing a hyperglycaemia due to its breakdown. Mannitol[10] is a relatively new medium being used with the advantage that it is iso-osmolar (approximately 285 m Osmol) and a natural osmotic diuretic. Little experience exists in the literature, so far, of any complications. However, mannitol will cause a volume overload if large intravasation occurs.

Until recently operative hysteroscopic surgery was limited to requiring a non-ionic medium, as electrosurgery in an ionic environment could not be performed, as electric current would simply disperse throughout the medium. However, Versapoint (Ethicon, USA) can operate in an ionic saline medium (Fig. 25.1). This represents a considerable feat of engineering and we feel this will ultimately become a valuable instrument for hysteroscopic surgery. The instrument's small diameter (5 French) means that operative procedures may also be performed on conscious patients in an out patient setting. Our experience[6] agrees with the very positive initial reports, however, care must still be taken to avoid fluid overload, although the osmotically induced fluid shifts, characteristics of other media are minimised.

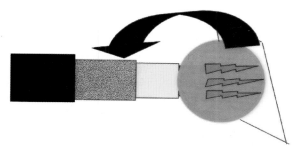

Figure 25.1 — Versapoint (Ethicon, USA) bipolar electrode. Path of current during vaporisation.

Table 25.5 — Management for iatrogenic hysteroscopic fluid overload

Deficit	Management
<0.5 L	Continue surgery
<1 L	Continue surgery
<1.5 L	Expedite procedure, check electrolytes, catheterise to monitor input:output
<2 L	Give frusemide 40 mg intravenously, terminate procedure if possible
>2 L	Terminate procedure, recheck haematocrit and electrolytes

It is essential that all theatres performing hysteroscopic surgery should have a system for monitoring fluid deficits during the procedure and a protocol for the management of excessive deficits (Table 25.5).[11]

Preventing fluid overload is important and there are many devices attempting to calculate the amount of fluid absorbed during the procedure. These range in sophistication from using syringes, calibrated fluid bags hung at a certain height over the level of the uterus (60–100 cm) with a collecting bucket or pouch in the subperineal drapes, to calibrated spring weight gauges. If any of these simpler devices are used the fluid balance must be checked every 5 min.

A biochemical method used for the assessment of absorbed fluid is the addition of a small (2%) amount of ethanol to the distension media, this measures the systemic fluid absorption by analysing the alcohol expired by the patient. There is very little literature on this area, being mostly small trials with poor design[12] and the potential complications of systemic alcohol in a post-operative patient are cause for concern.

There are a wide variety of pump systems, ranging from simple pumps where a constant rate of flow of fluid is produced at a given pump rate up to sophisticated pressure controlled pump systems. There are a variety of these devices available. Our experience is with the pressure limited rotary pump system (this avoids the catastrophic complications due to the gas driven variety); the Hamou Endomat (Karl Storz, Tuttlingen, Germany). Our experience agrees with Hamou's findings[13] of decreased fluid absorption and decreased morbidity. At present there is no consensus on hysteroscopic monitoring, however, in France, government legislation forbids hysteroscopic surgery unless a pump system is being used.

Conclusions

This review is an evaluation of the different methods that can be used to decrease the risk of complications in hysteroscopic surgery. We have focused on the prevention of those complications which are related to the basic principles of hysteroscopic surgery, rather than a discourse on specific operative complications.

Despite the tremendous advances in this area of gynaecological surgery and the appropriate emphasis on training, accreditation and critical appraisal of new techniques, there is a surprising lack of consensus on even the most basic techniques. Due to lack of quality research on what are the safest approaches, we have been unable to give any didactic opinions, instead, we offer a critical account of current practices and look forward to the time when we can give more definitive answers. MAS has now proved its superiority over conventional open surgery in a range of operations; it is now time to firmly establish what are the acceptable and safest methods for performing these operations.

Extensive international surveys have shown that hysteroscopic surgery is associated with very few complications but these surveys have noted a slight rise in complications. The reasons for this are not clear; it may reflect the advances in our surgical ability, where the morbidity will be intrinsically higher as a result of operating on cases with extensive pathology. Less reassuringly, it may indicate the attempt by less skilled surgeons to perform increasingly complex procedures or less reticence by surgeons to report on their complications as hysteroscopic surgery is more accepted in the wider surgical community. Our inability to explain this trend underlines the need for continuous audit of these techniques and the appropriate emphasis on training and accreditation.

We have attempted to give as comprehensive an overview of the equipment as possible. There have been remarkable and welcome developments in this area, notably in improving the safety aspects of these potentially lethal devices. Good quality trials to confirm, clinically, the theoretical advantages these instruments possess are awaited.

Key points for good clinical practice

General

- Appropriate case selection is vital
- Patient preparation both physically and psychologically are equally important
- Confidence in surgery depends on appropriate training and the use of quality equipment with which the surgeon and theatre staff are familiar.

Hysteroscopic surgery

- Beware of the difficult cervical dilation, in our experience, the degree of force is proportional to the complication rate
- Select the distension media to suit the procedure and the patient, always monitor flow rates and fluid balance
- If the uterine cavity collapses, this is uterine perforation until proven otherwise. Have a low threshold for investigating iatrogenic trauma if this occurs in operative procedures.

References

1. Overton C, Hargreaves J, Maresh M. A national survey of the complications of endometrial destruction techniques for menstrual disorders: the MISTLETOE study. Minimally Invasive Surgical Techniques — Laser, Endothermal or Endoresection. *Br J Obstet Gynaecol* 1997; 104(12): 1351–1359.

2. Hulka JF, Peterson HB et al. American Association of Gynecologic Laparoscopists' Survey 1972–1993. *J Am Assoc Gynecol Laparosc* 1972–1993.

3. Report of the Audit Committee's Working Group on Communication Standards Gynaecology: Surgical Procedures. Royal College of Obstetricians and Gynaecologists 1995R.

4. Lefler H, Sullivan G, Hulka J. Modified endometrial ablation: electrocoagulation with vasopressin and suction curettage preparation. *Obstet Gynecol* 77: 949–953.

5. Fraser I, Healy D, Torode H, Song J, Mamers P, Wilde F. Depot goserelin and danazol pre-treatment before rollerball endometrial for menorrhagia. *Obstet Gynecol* 87: 544–550.

6. O'Donovan P, Mc Gurgan P, Jones SE, Versapoint: a novel technique for operative hysteroscopy in a saline medium. *J Am Assoc Gynecol Laparosc.* Abstract: Atlanta 1998.

7. Report of the RCOG Working Party on Training in Gynaecological Endoscopic Surgery. Royal College of Obstetricians and Gynaecologists Press, 1994.

8. Hulka J, Peterson H, Phillips J, Surrey M, 1995 Operative hysteroscopy. AAGL 1993 Membership Survey 2: 133–136.

9. Manager D, Gerson JI et al. Pulmonary oedema and coagulopathy due to Hyskon. *Anesth Analg* 1989; 68: 686–687.

10. Kim AH, Keltz MD et al. Dilutional hyponatraemia during hysteroscopic myomectomy with sorbitol–mannitol distension media. *J Am Assoc Gynecol Laporosc* 1995; 2(2): 237–242.

11. O'Connor H. How to avoid complications at hysteroscopic surgery. In J Bonnar (Ed) *Recent Advances in Obstetrics and Gynaecology*, 20th edition. Churchill Livingstone.

12. Allweiner D et al. Addition of ethanol to the distension medium in surgical hysteroscopy as a screening test to prevent 'fluid overload'. *Geburtshilfe und Frauenheilkunde* 1996; 56(9): 462–469.

13. Hamou J, Fryman R, McLucas B, Garry R. A uterine distension system to prevent fluid intravasation during hysteroscopic surgery. *Gynecol Endoscopy* 1996; 5: 131–136.

26

Randomised controlled trials in second-generation endometrial ablation

Paul McGurgan, Peter J. O'Donovan and W. Prendiville

'Make the operation suit the patient, rather than the patient suit the operation'
Dr Charles Mayo

'Not wrung from speculations and subtleties but from common sense and observation'
T. Browne — 1663–1704

Introduction

The idea of destroying the endometrium and creating an iatrogenic 'Asherman's syndrome' as a treatment for dysfunctional bleeding is not new. Many attempts have been made in the past using a variety of chemical and physical agents — ethanol, formalin, copper sulphate, talc, quinacrine, fibroblast-impregnated sponges and even radiotherapy.[1] These methods were best characterised by their variable efficacy and high complication rates. It is only since the 1980s that endometrial destruction procedures have possessed adequate efficacy and sufficient safety to successfully compete with hysterectomy as a surgical treatment.

The so-called 'first-generation' techniques (resection,[2] laser[3] and rollerball[4]) have been extensively evaluated in national audits,[5,6] randomised controlled trials (RCTs)[7–10] and meta-analysis.[11] Indeed, endometrial ablation has been described as 'one of the most carefully evaluated surgical procedures'.[12] However, despite their efficacy, the first-generation methods have a number of drawbacks. They require a skilled hysteroscopic surgeon and despite having a significantly lower morbidity than conventional hysterectomy the national audits demonstrated incidences of uterine perforation ranging from 0.6% to 2.5% and fluid deficits >21 ranging from 1% to 5%.[5,6] Based on these findings, there was a need to develop alternative methods that could compare to the efficacy of the first-generation techniques but be safer and technically simpler to perform.

For a successful technique, the potential market is huge as menorrhagia is a significant health care problem in the developed world. In the UK alone, 5% of women of reproductive age will seek help for this symptom annually[13] and by the end of reproductive life the risk of hysterectomy (primarily for menstrual disorders) is 20%.[14] Menorrhagia is precisely defined as a menstrual loss of 80+ ml per month. Population studies have shown that this amount of loss is present in 10% of the population,[15] yet nearly a third of menstruating women consider their periods to be excessive.[16] This symptom thus creates a significant workload for health services.

The role of evidence-based practice

In clinical practice, the paradigm of evidence-based medicine currently holds away. Evidence-based medicine implies not only the application of effective treatments but their rational use within a comprehensive

Table 26.1 — Classification of evidence levels

Ia	Evidence obtained from meta-analysis of RCTs
Ib	Evidence obtained from at least one RCT
IIa	Evidence obtained from at least one well-designed controlled study without randomisation
IIb	Evidence obtained from at least one other type of well-designed quasi-experimental study
III	Evidence obtained from well-designed non-experimental descriptive studies, such as comparative studies, correlation studies and case studies
IV	Evidence obtained from expert committee reports or opinions and/or clinical experience of respected authorities

management framework. One of the paradoxes in the modern surgical management of excessive menstrual loss is that it was not until the surgical alternatives to hysterectomy were being evaluated that a proper critical reappraisal for our existing methods of treatment (both medical and surgical) occurred. Evidence is now classified (Table 26.1)[17] based on the scientific robustness of the source. A well-conducted RCT (or preferably a few, thereby increasing the generalisability) is the pinnacle of the evidence pyramid.

Increasingly, from this 'evidence', regulatory bodies such as the Royal College of Obstetricians and Gynaecologists (RCOG) and Scottish Intercollegiate Guidelines Network (SIGN), are formulating guidelines. Clinical guidelines are an increasingly familiar part of clinical practice and are systematically developed statements which assist clinicians and patients in making decisions about appropriate treatment for specific conditions. The principle aim is to improve the effectiveness and efficiency of clinical care through the identification of good clinical practice and desired clinical outcomes.[17] The RCOG has now published guidelines for the management of menorrhagia in primary and secondary care.[18,19]

Menorrhagia is a good example of the potential benefits to be gained through the introduction of guidelines. It is common, debilitating and despite having a variety of treatment options, it is frequently poorly managed. In the UK, more than a third of general practitioners prescribe norethisterone — arguably the least effective option — as first-line treatment, whereas only 1 in 20 prescribe tranexamic acid — probably the most effective first-line treatment.[20] The problem is not just confined to primary care or the

Table 26.2 — Grades of recommendations

A	Requires at least one RCT as part of a body of literature of overall good quality and consistency addressing the specific recommendation (evidence levels Ia, Ib)
B	Requires the availability of well-controlled clinical studies but no RCTs on the topic of recommendations (evidence levels IIa, IIb, III)
C	Requires evidence obtained from expert committee reports or opinions and/or clinical experiences of respected authorities. Indicates an absence of directly applicable clinical studies of good quality (evidence level IV)

Table 26.3 — SERNIP categories and definitions

SERNIP category	Definition
A	Safety and efficacy of the procedure established
B	Sufficiently close to an established procedure to give no reasonable grounds for questioning safety and efficacy; procedure may be used subject to continuing audit
C1	Safety and/or efficacy not yet established; procedure requires a fully controlled evaluation and may be used only as part of systematic research, consisting of an observational study in which all interventions and their outcomes are systematically recorded
C2	Safety and/or efficacy not yet established; procedure requires a fully controlled evaluation and may be used only as part of systematic research, consisting of an RCT and advise the Standing Group on Health Technology accordingly
D	Safety and/or efficacy shown to be unsatisfactory; procedure should not be used

UK. In New Zealand, where the use of tranexamic acid is restricted to secondary care, 50% of gynaecologists still use luteal phase progestogens and less than 10% use tranexamic acid.[21]

One of the strengths of these bodies recommendations is that they have had sufficient quality published data, in the form of RCTs, to provide mainly grade 'A' recommendations for practice in general.[18,19] This includes their recommendations on the use of endometrial ablation techniques. Based on the extensive cohort and randomised data for the first-generation techniques, the RCOG Guideline Development Group has stated, as a grade 'A' recommendation, that 'endometrial ablative procedures are effective in treating menorrhagia'.[19] Of course, this raises the issue of the generalisability of this statement concerning the newer second-generation methods (Table 26.2).

The current methods of second-generation endometrial ablation are:

1. cryotherapy: Cryogen™, Soprano™;
2. radiofrequency: Menostat™;
3. microwave: MEA™;
4. fluid balloon: Cavaterm™, ThermaChoice™, Menotreat™;
5. electrode: Mesh —Vesta™, Balloon — NovaSure™;
6. interstitial laser: ELITT™;
7. hydrothermal ablation: BEI™, Enabl™;
8. photodynamic therapy.

The Safety and Efficacy Registrar of New Interventional Procedures (SERNIP) of the Academy of Medical Royal Colleges is a 'quango' (quasi-autonomous non-governmental organisation) set up to evaluate new surgical procedures. SERNIP have five categories

defining the safety and efficacy of these procedures (Table 26.3). At present, only three of the second-generation endometrial ablation techniques have achieved category B status (ThermaChoice™, Vesta™ and MEA™). This is, in large part, due to the quality of scientific data available on the instruments.

Only Vesta™ and MEA™ have been rigorously compared to the acknowledged 'gold standards' — transcervical resection or laser ablation. Two other devices (ThermaChoice™ and Cavaterm™) have been compared to rollerball ablation — a technique which itself has never been directly compared in a RCT setting to hysterectomy. The remaining instruments' results are all based on case series and cohorts (Table 26.4) with the limitations that are inherent in these studies (see Appendix).

Randomised controlled trials — Thermachoice™

The first published RCT assessing a second-generation technique was Meyer et al's multicentre study

Table 26.4 — Published studies on second-generation endometrial ablation

Instrument	Type of study
Enabl™	Cohort
BEI™	Cohort
ThermaChoice™	Cohort, RCT
Cavaterm™	Cohort, RCT
Menotreat™	Cohort
MEA™	Cohort, RCT
NovaSure™	Cohort
Vesta™	Cohort, RCT
ELITT™	Cohort
Menostat™	Cohort
First Option™	Cohort
Cryogen™	Cohort
Photodynamic therapy	Case reports

Table 26.5 — Results of RCTs in endometrial ablation — ThermaChoice™

	ThermaChoice™ (*n* = 128)	Rollerball (*n* = 117)
Procedure time	<30 min in 71%	<30 min in 29%
GA used (%)	53	84
Peri-operative complications	0	4
Post-operative hysterectomy	2	3
Results (in %) at 1 year (n = 239)		
Mean menstrual diary scores decreased	85.5	91.7
Menstrual diary score <100	80.2	84.3
Amenorrhoea	15.2	27.2
Dysmenorrhoea decreased	70.4	75.4
Satisfaction	85.6	86.7

comparing ThermaChoice™ and rollerball endometrial ablation.[22]

Inclusion criteria were pre-menopausal women aged at least 30 years old, with completed families and prospectively documented menorrhagia as assessed by a pictorial menstrual diary scores (PBAC).[23] Women with PBAC scores of >150 (an estimated doubling of 'normal' menstrual loss) were entered into the study if the uterine cavity was anatomically normal (using hysterosalpingography, hysteroscopy or ultrasound) and between 4 and 10 cm in length. Exclusion criteria were women with abnormal Papanicolaou smears or endometrial biopsies within the previous 6 months, suspected genital tract infection or a previous endometrial ablation. Participating women were also questioned about the severity of their dysmenorrhea and pre-menstrual symptoms.

Two hundred and seventy-five women were initially randomised within their study centre to treatment with either ThermaChoice™ (*n* = 128) or rollerball (*n* = 117) ablation on a 1:1 basis using a random numbers table. This size of study could detect a 20% difference between the two methods, assuming that 85% of patients would have a beneficial response to the rollerball treatment (0.05 level of significance, 90% power).

Of the 275 women prospectively randomised, 255 were eventually treated as part of the study, 15 patients electively withdrew from the study prior to treatment, five other women were protocol violations, two had submucous fibroids, two had cavities larger than 30 ml

volume, one patient sustained a uterine perforation during the rollerball.

There were no significant differences in the two group's mean age (40.5) body mass index, PBAC scores or haemoglobin levels.

The only endometrial preparation used before either technique was a 3-min curettage using a 5 mm suction curette. The choice of anaesthesia was left to the individual surgeon — 84% of women undergoing rollerball compared to 53% of women undergoing ThermaChoice™ had a general anaesthetic (Table 26.5). There were no intra-operative complications noted amongst the thermal balloon-treated women, but in the rollerball group there were (3.2%). These complications were

• two cases of fluid overload,
• one uterine perforation,
• one cervical laceration.

There were no long-term sequelae.

Post-operatively, the balloon group reported one urinary tract infection and three cases of suspected endometritis — all resolved with oral antibiotics. In the rollerball group, there was one case of endometritis (treated with oral antibiotics), one case of haematometra (treated by dilatation and curettage, D&C) and a late presentation after 1 year with tubal sterilisation syndrome (treated by laparoscopic salpingectomy). Within 1 year of treatment, five women had undergone a hysterectomy — two in the balloon group (one for persistent menorrhagia, one for pain) and three in the rollerball group (one for persistent menorrhagia, one for pain and one for atypical hyperplasia in the curettage specimen). The outcomes for menstrual diary scores, amenorrhoea, dysmenorrhoea and patient satisfaction at 1-year post-treatment are listed in Table 26.5.

ThermaChoice™ was found to be significantly quicker to perform ($p < 0.05$) but had a lower rate of amenorrhoea ($p < 0.05$) at 1 year compared to rollerball. Despite this, there was no statistical difference in the decreased menstrual diary scores between the two groups; these decreased by 90% in 68.4% and 61.6% for the rollerball- and ThermaChoice™-treated women respectively. Similarly, both procedures had an equivalent impact on the incidence of anaemia — pre-existing anaemia decreased by approximately 60% after treatment in the two groups.

Myer's study was a landmark in the validation of the new second-generation endometrial ablation techniques and their results were generally re-assuring. However, the study had two fundamental weaknesses that limited its generalisability. The first potential flaw was their comparison with rollerball, a technique which in itself had never been validated in the form of a RCT (although observational series do suggest equivalent results to resection and laser[24-26]). The other issue was the *explanatory*, rather than *pragmatic* design of the trial, manifest by the strict study entry criteria. The authors do not mention how many women were deemed ineligible for trial entry because of their uterus being <4 or >10 cm in length or having an irregular endometrial cavity. A rough estimate for the incidence of women with these features may be more than 30% (based on Wilcox et al's study analysing the indications for women requiring hysterectomy, 29% and 61% of caucasian and black women respectively had fibroids[27]).

Nevertheless, Myer's study demonstrated that ThermaChoice™ was a safe, effective and satisfactory treatment in appropriately selected women requiring only pre-operative suction curettage giving equivalent results to rollerball endometrial ablation. Although the paper did not discuss methods used to provide analgesia to the 47% of women having ThermaChoice™ in an office setting, the numbers suggested its applicability in this environment.

Randomised controlled trials — Cavaterm™

Another fluid balloon device, the Cavaterm™ system, has also been compared in an RCT to rollerball endometrial ablation. Romer's study[28] assessed the outcomes of Cavaterm™ versus rollerball in 20 women (10 patients in each arm of the study). Again, women were excluded if they had any intrauterine abnormalities (submucous myomas, uterine septae, suspicion of uterine wall weakness or uterine cavity length <4 cm or >10 cm) or histological pathology. However, Romer pre-treated both groups with two injections of gonadotrophin-releasing hormone analogues (GnRHa). Follow-up at 15 months found almost identical results in the two treatment arms of the study with all 20 women expressing satisfaction with their treatment.

This study has gross methodological weaknesses — there is no power study to calculate the number of women needed to demonstrate if a statistically significant difference exists between the two treatments and it shares the limitations of Myer's work in using strict entry criteria and comparison with rollerball ablation.

Randomised controlled trials — Vesta™

The Vesta™ system for electrosurgical ablation consists of an inflatable balloon with 12 electrodes placed in contact with the endometrium. Interim data from a multicentre RCT comparing Vesta™ to a combined trans-cervical loop resection and rollerball (RR) technique, has been published by Corson et al.[29]

Inclusion criteria were pre-menopausal women aged between 30 and 49 years old, with completed families and had previously failed medical treatment for menorrhagia. Menorrhagia was assessed prospectively using pictorial menstrual diary scores (PBAC)[23] and women with scores >150 were entered into the trial. The patients uterine cavity was required to be anatomically normal (evaluated by hysteroscopy or ultrasound) and less than 9.75 cm in length. Exclusion criteria were women with abnormal Papanicolaou smears or endometrial biopsies within the previous 6 months, suspected genital tract infection, a previous endometrial ablation/myomectomy or the use of long acting hormonal therapy within 3 months of treatment.

Of 637 women initially screened with PBAC scores >150, 361 women were excluded (57%). The most common reason for exclusion was due to an unacceptable uterine cavity (138 women). This emphasises the limitations regarding the generalisability of these studies, due to their strict entry criteria. Two hundred and seventy-six women were then randomised on a 1:1 basis using sealed envelopes to treatment with either Vesta™ ($n = 150$) or RR ($n = 126$) ablation.

Of the 276 women prospectively randomised to treatment, nine were not treated (six in the Vesta™ group and three in the RR group):

- one woman refused pre-treatment;
- two had cancers: one endometrial, one breast;
- one responded to hormonal therapy;
- five withdrew for 'logistic' reasons;

Five were also lost to follow-up (one in the Vesta™ group and four in the RR group). There were no significant differences between the two groups' pre-operative PBAC scores.

Pre-operative endometrial preparation consisted of 2 weeks use of oral contraceptive pills. The procedure was performed immediately after withdrawal bleeding. The choice of anaesthesia was left to the individual surgeon. In those patients randomised to Vesta™ only 16.7% required a general or epidural anaesthetic compared to 80% of women in the RR group.

Minor muscular fasciculation occurred during the Vesta™ treatment in 18 patients (12%) but in only one case was it necessary to halt the procedure. The only other Vesta™ treatment protocol violation was a case where the balloon appeared to have entered a weak caesarean scar and the procedure performed was stopped but Corson did not describe the patient's outcome. The RR groups' complications were one fundal perforation (again no outcome was reported in the paper), two cervical lacerations, one haematometra, one myometritis and one fluid deficit of 1.3l.

There were 132 and 123 Vesta™- and RR-treated patients at 1-year follow-up respectively. Due to the paper's interim format, Corson only evaluated the bleeding patterns amongst the treated patients as an end-point. In comparison to the ThermaChoice™ study, Corson reported no significant difference in amenorrhoea rates between the Vesta™ and RR groups (31.8% and 39.6% respectively). The outcomes for menstrual diary scores and amenorrhoea at 1-year post-treatment are listed in Table 26.6.

Based on the interim data, Corson's study demonstrated that Vesta™ was a potentially safe and effective treatment in appropriately selected women, requiring

Table 26.6 — Results of RCTs in endometrial ablation — Vesta™

	Vesta ($n = 150$)	RR ($n = 126$)
Procedure time	Not noted	Not noted
GA used (%)	16.7	80
Peri-operative complications	2	6
Post-operative hysterectomy	Not noted	Not noted
Results (in %) at 1 year	$n = 132$	$n = 123$
Mean menstrual diary scores decreased	94	91
Menstrual diary score <76	87.9	82.9
Amenorrhoea	31.8	39.6
Dysmenorrhoea	Not noted	Not noted
Satisfaction	Not noted	Not noted

minimal pre-operative endometrial preparation and giving equivalent results to the accepted gold standard RR endometrial ablation. Although the paper did not detail the methods used to provide analgesia to the 83.3% of women undergoing Vesta™ in an office setting or the effect of the Vesta™-induced muscular fasciculation on patient acceptability, the numbers suggested its applicability in this environment.

Corson's, albeit limited, data on Vesta™ is generally re-assuring. The study had more generalisable results due to its comparison with the extensively validated RR method. However, it was still an explanatory rather than pragmatic design, manifest by the strict study entry criteria.

Two points of the trial were worth discussing in more detail. The first is the data on the numbers of potentially eligible women who were excluded, 361 women from a total of 637 screened women (57%). This emphasises the limitations regarding the use of these ablative methods in all menorrhagic women, a group who will often have an irregular or large endometrial cavity.

Corson's study is also the first to describe the incorrect placement of a second-generation endometrial ablation instrument in a RCT setting. Although the procedure was stopped, Corson does not describe the patient's outcome. The worry with any 'blind technique' is that the instrument will be incorrectly placed and activated, thereby ablating adjacent viscera and not endometrium. The data on all second-generation technologies for this complication is sparse. We have accurate data on first-generation techniques from the national audits which reported incidences of uterine perforation ranging from 0.6% to 2.5%. In fact, one of the pressures towards developing second-generation devices was an attempt to decrease this perforation rate. However, whilst perforation rates with the first-generation methods were relatively high, the advantage was that if a perforation did occur it was generally detected, thereby allowing reparative measures to be taken. With most second-generation methods, the cavity is not routinely visualised during the procedure (the exception being the Hydro ThermAblator™, BEI Medical Systems, NJ, USA) hence an unrecognised incorrect placement may not be detected. The clinical picture of damage of this nature to bowel, for example, would cause peritonism usually 24–48 h after the patient is discharged. Whilst abdominal signs may then be present, their significance might not be recognised. The resultant diagnostic and therapeutic delay can easily convert a 'sick' patient into a moribund patient.

There are no published cases reported on Medline/PubMed of any of the second-generation methods being incorrectly placed. However, the UK Medical Devices Agency have reports of serious complications occurring with most of these methods (R. Glover, personal communication). This area is intensely competitive for the 12 instruments currently in production. Any adverse publicity, however slight, could have a disastrous effect. Only one has to recall the fate of Menostat™ (a radiofrequency device) which was withdrawn due to the complications associated with its use.[30]

Randomised controlled trials — MEA™

Microwave endometrial ablation (MEA™) was pioneered in the UK by Sharp who published his first cohort results in 1995.[31] The method utilises the local heating effect of microwaves released from an 8 mm applicator. This gives a consistent, reproducible maximum depth of coagulation of 6 mm at 9.2 GHz frequency.[32] Cooper et al published their results from an RCT comparing MEA™ to RR in 1999.[33]

Two hundred and sixty-three women were initially randomised within their study centre to treatment with either MEA™ ($n = 129$) or RR ($n = 134$) ablation on a 1:1 basis using sequentially numbered opaque envelopes. The sequence was predetermined by using balanced blocks derived from computer-generated random number tables. This size of study had an 80% chance of detecting a minimum of 15% difference in satisfaction between the two methods, assuming that 78% of patients would be satisfied by the RR treatment (0.05 level of significance, 80% power).

The study was performed on a pragmatic basis to enable results to be as generalisable as possible. Therefore, trial exclusion criteria were minimal. Patients were deemed eligible for trial entry if they were premenopausal with no wish for fertility and had intolerable dysfunctional uterine bleeding (defined in this study as the complaint of menorrhagia in women with normal endometrial histopathology and a uterine size ≤10-week pregnancy). Pre-operative assessment using ultrasound or hysteroscopy was discouraged unless indicated by clinical examination or an endometrial biopsy could not be obtained. Notably, whilst the two lead surgeons were experienced hysteroscopic surgeons (had performed at least 50 endometrial resections) they had only performed five MEA™ procedures when the trial was started.

All of the 263 women prospectively randomised received 3.6 mg goserelin 5 weeks pre-operatively in order to promote endometrial thinning. A general anaesthetic was used for all procedures (MEA™ or RR). This was the practice of the surgeons at that time and, as one of the primary end-points of the study was patient satisfaction, it eliminated any potential bias from using different methods of analgesia.

Intra-operatively, submucous fibroids of greater than 2 cm were found in 32 women. In these cases the treatment proceeded as originally intended with the exception of one woman in the RR group who required a two-stage procedure and one woman in the MEA™ group who underwent an endometrial resection. Four other women originally randomised to MEA™ underwent RR as a result of the MEA™ equipment failing (this study used an earlier model to the device currently available, I. Feldberg, personal communication, Microsulis Plc.). In those women randomised to RR, one woman underwent MEA™.

Blunt perforation with an inactive hysteroscope or MEA™ probe occurred to one patient in each group, the MEA™ patient with perforation declined an attempt at a repeat procedure and later requested a hysterectomy. The perforation in the RR patient caused bleeding into the broad ligament which was managed intra-operatively by converting to a hysterectomy. A hysterectomy was also required in another of the RR-treated patients who presented 2 weeks after the original procedure with abdominal/pelvic pain.

Table 26.7 — Results of RCTs in endometrial ablation — MEA™

	MEA™ (*n* = 129)	RR (*n* = 134)
Procedure time	11.4 ± 10.5	15 ± 7.2
GA used (%)	100	100
Peri-operative complications	17	14
Post-operative hysterectomy	9	12
Results (in %) at 1 year	*n* = 116	*n* = 124
Mean menstrual diary scores	92	91
Menstrual diary score <100	Not noted	Not noted
Amenorrhoea	40	40
Dysmenorrhoea	80	82
Satisfaction	77	75

Primary haemorrhage occurred in five patients treated by RR which was managed by inserting a 14 gauge Foley catheter into the uterus for 6 h. There were no cases of primary haemorrhage in the MEA™ group. Re-admission after discharge occurred in six women treated by RR; three complained of pelvic pain, two required repeat procedures and one patient had chest pain. Four women treated by MEA™ were subsequently re-admitted; three with minor secondary haemorrhage treated by antibiotic therapy.

Rates of satisfaction and acceptability of treatment were high for both techniques (Table 26.7) at 12-month follow-up and the results were similar to previous trials of endometrial ablation. Of the eight health-related quality of life dimensions in the Short Form-36, all were improved after MEA™ (six significantly) and seven were improved after TCRE (all significantly). Although amenorrhoea was not used as an outcome to define success, this was achieved in 40% of treated patients for both techniques. Dysmenorrhoea and peri-menstrual symptoms also improved in most treated women. Only 4% and 8% of MEA™ and RR-treated women respectively complained of 'new' pelvic pain after treatment.

Cooper et al's study represents the most robust RCT in this area to date. As in Corson's study using Vesta™, the MEA™ had more generalisable results due to its comparison with the extensively validated RR method.

However, it was the pragmatic rather than explanatory design of the study that meant that the results obtained should be reproducible in other settings. The pragmatic approach was derived from the study's minimal exclusion criteria combined with the instrument's ability to treat relatively large (up to 10-week size) uterine cavities containing fibroids — factors that are often contraindications to other methods of endometrial ablation.

The MEA™ RCT (as in the Vesta™ study) also reported one case of uterine perforation when inserting the applicator. As previously discussed, this once again emphasises the need for prompt recognition of this complication by the operating surgeon in order to avoid iatrogenic injury. The MEA™ User Group, who independently audit all the results of MEA™ procedures, have had four reported blunt perforations (rate 2.6/1000), two of which have occurred during the initial dilatation (D. Parkin, personal communication). This represents approximately one-tenth of the perforation rate associated with first-generation techniques. There is no data available on the other second-generation techniques by which to compare the different methods.

Conclusions

The ideal technique for endometrial ablation would be

- safe,
- scientifically validated,
- simple,
- economical,
- outpatient based,
- provide contraception.

At present, there are 12 different instruments available for endometrial ablation. Concerning safety, some mechanisms are now discredited (Menostat™). Most techniques appear satisfactory and are easy to perform, based on the data available, providing in some cases that strict entry criteria are met. Disappointingly, only three instruments have had RCTs performed. No technique at present has been proven to be effectively contraceptive and all potential patients should be strongly advised to ensure they should continue to use contraception after the ablative procedure. There is little data on the economical implications of introducing these new second-generation endometrial ablation methods. They are likely to be equivalent in cost to the first-generation techniques but this area needs further study.

References

1. Punnonen R, Gronroos M. Cathetron and radium in the treatment of functional uterine bleeding. *Ann Chir Gynae Fenniae* 1972; 61: 215–219.

2. Neuwirth RS, Amin HK. Excision of submucus fibroids with hysteroscopic control. *Am J Obstet Gynecol* 1976; 126(1): 95–99.

3. Goldrath MH, Fuller TA, Segal S. Laser photovaporization of endometrium for the treatment of menorrhagia. *Am J Obstet Gynecol* 1981; 140(1): 14–19.

4. Vancaillie TG. Electrocoagulation of the endometrium with the ball-end resectoscope. *Obstet Gynecol* 1989; 74(3 Pt 1): 425–427.

5. Scottish Hysteroscopy Audit Group. A Scottish audit of hysteroscopic surgery for menorrhagia: complications and follow-up. *Br J Obstet Gynaecol* 1995; 102: 249–254.

6. Overton C, Hargreaves J, Maresh M. A national survey of complications of endometrial destruction for menstrual disorders: the MISTLETOE study. *Br J Obstet Gynaecol* 1997; 104: 1351–1359.

7. Gannon MJ, Holt EM, Fairbank J. A randomised trial comparing endometrial resection and abdominal hysterectomy for the management of menorrhagia. *Br Med J* 1991; 303: 1362–1364.

8. Dwyer N, Hutton J, Stirrat GM. Randomised controlled trial comparing endometrial resection with abdominal hysterectomy for the surgical treatment of menorrhagia. *Br J Obstet Gynaecol* 1993; 100: 237–243.

9. Pinion SB, Parkin DE, Abramovich DR et al. Randomised trial of hysterectomy, endometrial laser ablation and transcervical resection for dysfunctional uterine bleeding. *Br Med J* 1994; 309: 979–983.

10. O'Connor H, Broadbent JAM, Magos AL, McPherson K. Medical Research Council randomised trial of endometrial resection versus hysterectomy in the management of menorrhagia. *Lancet* 1997; 349: 897–901.

11. Lethaby A, Shepherd S, Cooke I, Farquhar C. Endometrial resection and ablation versus hysterectomy for heavy menstrual bleeding. *Cochrane Menstrual Disorders and Subfertility Group*, Update Software 1999.

12. Garry R. Endometrial ablation and resection: validation of a new surgical concept. *Br J Obstet Gynaecol* 1997; 104: 1329–1331.

13. Vessey MP, Villard-Mackintosh L, McPherson K, Coulter A, Yeates D. The epidemiology of hysterectomy: findings in a large cohort study. *Br J Obstet Gynaecol* 1992; 99: 402–407.

14. Coulter A, McPherson K, Vessey M. Do British women undergo too many or too few hysterectomies? *Soc Sci Med* 1988; 27: 987–994.

15. Hallberg L, Hogdahl A, Nilsson L, Rybo G. Menstrual blood loss — a population study: variation at different ages and attempts to define normality. *Acta Obstet Gynecol Scand* 1966; 45: 320–351.

16. MORI. *Women's Health in 1990*. Market Opinion and Research International, 1990 (Research study conducted on behalf of Parke-Davis Research Laboratories).

17. RCOG Press. *Guidance for the Development of RCOG Clinical Guidelines*, August 1999. http://www.rcog.org.uk/guidelines/gt_guidelines.html

18. RCOG Press. *Evidence-Based Clinical Guideline No. 1. The Initial Management of Menorrhagia*, 1998. http://www.rcog.org.uk/guidelines/menorrhagia.html

19. RCOG Press. *The Management of Menorrhagia in Secondary Care. Evidence-Based Clinical Guideline No. 5*, 1999. http://www.rcog.org.uk/guidelines/menorrhagiasc.html

20. Intercontinental Medical Statistics. UK and Ireland. Middlesex: IMS, 1994.

21. Farquhar CM, Kimble R. How do NZ gynaecologists treat menorrhagia? *Aust NZ J Obstet Gynaecol* 1996; 36(4): 1–4.

22. Meyer WR, Walsh BM, Grainger DA et al. Thermal balloon and rollerball ablation to treat menorrhagia: a multicentre comparison. *Obstet Gynecol* 1998; 92(1): 98–103.

23. Higham JM, O'Brien PMS, Shaw RW. Assessment of menstrual blood loss using a pictorial chart. *Br J Obstet Gynaecol* 1990; 9: 734–739.

24. Townsend DE, McCausland V, McCausland A, Fields G, Kauffman K. Post-ablation tubalization sterilisation syndrome. *Obstet Gynecol* 1993; 82: 422–424.

25. Chullapram T, Song JY, Fraser IS. Medium-term follow-up of women with menorrhagia treated by rollerball endometrial ablation. *Obstet Gynecol* 1996; 88(1): 71–76.

26. Fraser IS, Angsuwathana S, Mahmoud F, Yezerski S. Short and medium term outcomes after rollerball endometrial ablation for menorrhagia. *Med J Aust* 1993; 158(7): 454–457.

27. Wilcox LS, Koonin LM, Pokras R, Strauss LT, Xia Z, Peterson HB. Hysterectomy in the United States, 1988–1990. *Obstet Gynecol* 1994; 83(4): 549–555.

28. Romer T. Die therapie rezidivierender menorrhagien — Cavaterm-ballon koagulation versus roller-ball endometrium koagulation — eine prospektive randomiserte vergleichstudie. *Zentralblatt fur Gynakologie* 1998; 120(10): 511–514.

29. Corson SL, Brill AI, Brooks PG et al. Interim results of the American Vesta Trial of Endometrial Ablation. *J Am Assoc Gynecol Laparosc* 1999; 6(1): 45–49.

30. Thijssen RF. Radiofrequency induced endometrial ablation: an update. *Br J Obstet Gynaecol* 1997; 104(5): 608–613.

31. Sharp NC, Cronin N, Feldberg I, Evans M, Hodgson D, Ellis S. Microwaves for menorrhagia: a new fast technique

for endometrial ablation. *The Lancet* 1995; 346: 1003–1004.

32. Hodgson D, Feldberg IB, Sharp N, Cronin N, Evans M, Hirschowitz L. Microwave endometrial ablation: development, clinical trials and outcomes at three years. *Br J Obstet Gynaecol* 1999; 106: 684–694.

33. Cooper KG, Bain C, Parkin DE. Comparison of microwave endometrial ablation and trans-cervical resection of the endometrium for treatment of heavy menstrual loss: a randomised trial. *Lancet* 1999; 354: 1859–1863.

Appendix: Global endometrial ablation techniques — what the literature says

The ideal treatment

- Safe
- Satisfactory with minimal exclusion criteria
- Simple
- Economical
- Scientifically validated
- Outpatient based
- Effect on fertility

Current methods of second-generation endometrial ablation

- Cryotherapy: Cryogen™, Soprano™
- Radiofrequency: Menostat™
- Microwave: MEA™
- Fluid balloon: Cavaterm™, ThermaChoice™, Menotreat™
- Electrode: Mesh — Vesta™, Balloon — NovaSure™
- Interstitial laser: ELITT™
- Hydrothermablation: BEI™, Enabl™
- Photodynamic therapy

How do we grade evidence?

Evidence-based medicine:

- Grade A: Well-conducted RCTs
- Grade B: Collective data from cohort-based studies
- Grade C: Consensus opinion from expert bodies

Current published studies on second-generation endometrial ablation

- Cryotherapy: Cohort studies
- Radiofrequency: Cohort studies
- Interstitial laser: Cohort studies
- Hydrothermablation — BEI™ and Enabl™: Cohort studies
- Photodynamic therapy: Case reports
- Fluid balloon —
  Cavaterm™ and Menotreat™: Cohort studies
  ThermaChoice™: RCT
- Electrode
  NovaSure™: Cohort studies
  Vesta™: RCT
- Microwave
  MEA™: RCT

Cryotherapy: Cryogen™, Soprano

First reported in 1980 by Waldron, *Phys Med Biol* 1980; 25(2): 323–331

- *Ex vivo* studies using N_2O and liquid N_2
- $-20°C$ causes complete cell death
- Theoretically and experimentally effective

Pittrof et al, *Int J Gynecol Obstet* 1994; 47: 135–140

- 67 women; pre-operative GnRHa, progesterone or danazol
- 15 min duration, using a $-45°C$ saline ice ball
- No serious adverse complications, but device failure in 36%

Cryogen™

Dobak et al, *J Am Assoc Gynecol Laparosc* 1998; 5(1)

- *Ex vivo* studies; 10 uterii used

- 3–5 min duration, using a 170°C lubricant ice ball under US control
- Tissue necrosis 9–12 mm, no adverse complications

Rutherford et al, *J Am Assoc Gynecol Laparosc* 1998; 5(1)

- Cohort 15 patients; pre-operative D&C
- Seven OPD-based procedures
- 3–5 min treatment duration, using a 170°C lubricant ice ball under US control
- End-point amenorrhoea in 50% at 22 months, no adverse complications

Cryotherapy: conclusions

- Limited published data, cohort-based studies
- Cheap technology, uses US Guidance
- Can be OPD based
- Not limited to regular cavity
- Large zone of tissue necrosis

Radiofrequency: Menostat™

Phipps et al, *Lancet* 1990; 335

Thijssen, *Br J Obstet Gynaecol* 1997; 104

- Cohort 1280 women, pre-operative danazol or GnRHa; treatment time 20 min, 'satisfaction' in 78%, 20% require further treatment
- Complications:
  Alternate site burns in 11
  VVF in five
  Bowel burn in one
  Cervical burn in one

Radiofrequency: conclusions

- 20% require further treatment
- Not OPD based
- Unsatisfactory complication rate alternate site burns, bowel and cervix, VVF

Fluid balloon: Cavaterm™, ThermaChoice™, Menotreat™

Menotreat™

- Cohort-based studies, nil published in Medline cited journals

Cavaterm™

- Cohort-based studies published, RCTs ongoing

Friberg et al, Genolet et al, Hawe et al, *Br J Obstet Gynaecol* 1999; 106

Hawe et al, *Br J Obstet Gynaecol* 1999; 106

- 50 women, normal cavities, pre-operative GnRHa, danazol or D&C
- OPD based for 12 women
- 200 mmHg, 75°C for 15 min
- Amenorrhoea in 68%, further surgery in 7%

Cavaterm™: conclusions

- Cohort-based studies appear effective
- Can be OPD based
- Limited to regular uterine cavity

ThermaChoice™

Meyer et al, *Obstet Gynaecol* 1998; 92(1)

- 255 women randomised to treatment with either ThermaChoice™ ($n = 128$) or rollerball ($n = 117$)
- Age range 29–51 (mean 40.5) years old
- Inclusion criteria:
  Normal uterine cavity depth 4–10 cm
  +30 years, accept infertility, failed medical therapy
  Normal smear and endometrial biopsy
- Pre-treatment: curettage used

For results of RCTs in endometrial ablation: ThermaChoice™ see Table 26.5.

Electrode: Vesta™, NovaSure™

Novacept™

- Cohort-based studies, bi-polar mechanism
- Nil published on Medline cited journals

Vesta™

- Corson et al, *J Am Assoc Gynecol Laparosc* 1999; 6(1)
- 276 women were randomised to treatment with either Vesta™ ($n = 150$) or RR ($n = 126$)
- Of 361 patients, 158 were excluded due to myoma, polyps or abnormally sized cavities
- Age range 30–49 (mean 40.5) years old
- Inclusion criteria:
  Normal uterine cavity depth 4–10 cm
  +30 years, accept infertility, failed medical therapy
  Normal smear and endometrial biopsy
- Pre-treatment: OCP for 2/52 used

For results of RCTs in endometrial ablation: Vesta™ see Table 26.6.

Interstitial laser: ELITT™

Donnez et al, *Obstet Gynecol* 1996; 87(3)

- Diode laser 830 nm
- 8 *Ex vivo* uterii studied
- Cohort 10 patients; pre-operative GnRHa
- 7 min treatment time
- 7 patients follow-up to 6/12 - 100% amenorrhoea, two hysterectomies (one for cervical ca)
- No adverse complications

ELITT™: conclusions

- Cohort-based studies
- Can be OPD based, advise US guidance in original study
- Notable high amenorrhoea rate
- Limited to regular cavity

Hydrothermablation: BEI™, Enabl™

Enabl™

Baggish et al, *Am J Obstet Gynecol* 1995; 173(6)

- 32 *ex vivo* uterii studied; heated saline
- 80°C for 15 min; thermal necrosis up to 3 mm myometrium with no fluid leaks

Bustos-Lopez et al, *Fertil Steril* 1998; 69(1)

- 11 *ex vivo* uterii studied; pre-operative GnRHa; heated saline 70–85°C for 10–17 min thermal necrosis up to 6 mm depth with no fluid leaks

Enabl™: conclusions

- Ongoing (unpublished) cohort studies
- Treatment time 15 min
- Optimum *ex vivo* results with a regular cavity
- Variation in depth of destruction noted

BEI™: Hydro ThermAblator

Richart et al, *J Am Assoc Gynecol Laparosc* 1999; 6(3)

- 32 *ex vivo* uterii, pre-operative GnRHa
- Heated saline 90°C for 10 min; thermal necrosis 3–4 mm (2–3 mm in cornua)
- No leaks if pressure <70 mmHg (advise 50 mmHg pressure)

Romer et al, *J Am Assoc Gynecol Laparosc* 1999; 6(3)

- Cohort 18 women, pre-operative GnRHa
- Heated saline 90°C for 10 min; under continuous visualisation; no leaks (at 50 mmHg pressure)
- 50% amenorrhoea at 1 year; one hysterectomy — adenomyosis
- No adverse complications

das Dores et al, *J Am Assoc Gynecol Laparosc* 1999; 6(3)

- Cohort 26 women, pre-operative GnRHa
- Heated saline 90°C for 10 min; under continuous visualisation; no leaks (at 50 mmHg pressure)
- 47% amenorrhoea at 1 year; one hysterectomy — not noted why
- No adverse complications

BEI™: conclusions

- Small cohort-based studies
- Able to visualise cavity
- Does not require normal-shaped cavity but no results on potential effect of this
- Treatment time 10 min

Microwave endometrial ablation: MEA™

Cooper et al, *Lancet* 1999; 354

- 263 women were randomised to treatment with either MEA (*n* = 129) or
- RR (*n* = 134)
- Mean age 41 years old (SD = 6.7–8.4)
- Inclusion criteria:
    Uterine cavity depth up to 10/52 size
    Presence of submucous fibroids
    +30 years accept infertility, failed medical therapy
    Normal smear and endometrial biopsy
- Pre-treatment: GnRHa for 5/52 used

For results of RCTs in endometrial ablation: MEA™ see Table 26.7.

Photodynamic therapy

- No established companies — experimental technology

Bhatta et al, *Am J Obstet Gynecol* 1992; 167(6)

- Photofrin II — animal-based studies

Wyss et al, *Int J Obstet Gynecol* 1998; 60

- ALA — 3 patients OPD based, decreased bleeding, no complications

3 RCTs in endometrial ablation (Table 26.A1)

- ThermaChoice™: Meyer et al, *Obstet Gynecol* 1998; 92(1)
- Vesta: Corson et al, *J Am Assoc Gynecol Laparosc* 1999; 6(1)
- MEA: Cooper et al, *Lancet* 1999; 354

Table 26.A1 — Comparison of cohort and RCT studies for different methods of endometrial ablation

	ThermaChoice™	Vesta™	MEA™
Procedure time	<30 min in 71%	Not noted	11.4 ± 10.5
OPD based	37%	83%	Being evaluated
Cavity required	Normal	Normal	Myoma >2 cm in 11%
Peri-operative complications (%)	0	1	5
Post-operative hysterectomy (%)	2	Not noted	7
Results (in %) at 1 year			
Mean menstrual subjective scores (%)	85.5	94	92
Amenorrhoea	15.2	31.8	40
Dysmenorrhoea	70.4	Not noted	80
Satisfaction (%)	85.6	Not noted	77

The ideal technique

- Safe
- Satisfactory with minimal exclusion criteria
- Scientifically validated
- Simple
- Economical
- Outpatient based
- Effect on fertility

- Satisfactory with minimal exclusion criteria: RCTs so far validate this but exclusion criteria still a problem
- Outpatient based: majority are applicable
- Simple: all techniques are easy to operate
- Effect on fertility: no technique at present is proven effectively contraceptive
- Economic criteria: appear equivalent to first-generation techniques but needs further study

Conclusions

Eight mechanisms, 12 instruments for endometrial ablation.

- Safety: some mechanisms now being discredited

27

What is the best surgical method for the conservative management of menorrhagia: A personal view

David E. Parkin

235

I am usually asked to write a contribution based on evidence-based practice but for once I can give my own view of the merits, disadvantages and evidence that I base my practice upon. Before continuing, there is no doubt that the days of hysterectomy as the only surgical option are long gone and endometrial ablation especially by the hysteroscopic methods has an evidence based, proven, long track record which is now unarguable.

My background is in hysteroscopic surgery, with my team having performed over 3600 endometrial ablations in the past 11 years. These have been split approximately into 2400 transcervical resections of the endometrium (TCRE), 600 endometrial laser ablations (ELA) and 600 microwave endometrial ablations (MEA). My personal series is of over 1500 TCREs carried out rapidly, effectively and safely, and this may explain my final conclusions. In my team's hands, TCRE has an operating time of 15 min,[1] an amenorrhoea rate of 40% at 2 years[2] and 60% at 5 years,[3] a hysterectomy rate of 12% at 2 years[2] and 19% at 5 years[3] with 80% patient satisfaction at 5 years.[3,4] These results are from a total of over 1000 women reported in randomised trials with wide inclusion criteria and with about 30% having a fibroid uterus. During this time, we have had only one emergency hysterectomy, no bowel damage (though there was one case of bowel damage following ELA in a patient operated on by another consultant[5]). There was one death, however, from toxic shock syndrome following a TCRE.[6]

So what is the best method? It must be proven in well-designed randomised studies to be effective, safe, rapid, inexpensive, and adaptable to irregular uterine cavities, easy to learn and to be possible under local anaesthetic. TCRE fulfils all those criteria with the exception of being easy to learn and being possible under local anaesthetic. It does have the advantage over all other methods of giving tissue for histological examination. Over 11,000 hysteroscopic procedures were included in the two large prospective audits confirming their safety.[7,8] Three well-designed randomised trials have compared TCRE to hysterectomy, all showing satisfaction similar to hysterectomy, faster recovery and less complications than hysterectomy.[5,9,10]

TCRE and ELA have shown that they give similar results and safety in a randomised trial, though TCRE was faster, had less fluid absorption and is less expensive.[11] TCRE has been compared to medical treatment and been shown to be far superior with ultimately no increase in final surgery rates when offered as an initial treatment.[3,12] These trials have led to a review produced by the Cochrane group[13] and evidence-based guidelines from the Scottish Intercollegiate Guidelines Network (SIGN)[14] supporting the use of TCRE.

The major problem with TCRE is the fact that it is difficult to learn and teach. The learning curve for TCRE is long and results from myself and my series of trainees and research fellows have always been disappointing in the first 30–50 cases. Teaching TCRE is difficult even with well-designed courses. The Scottish video-hysteroscopic surgery course has had over 160 participants since it started but perhaps only 20 do TCRE as a routine. This is despite using potatoes as a plentiful, easily produced and very realistic model for trainees to practice on.[15] In Scotland, out of 160 Consultant Gynaecologists around only 20 carry out TCRE or ELA with any degree of regularity, and of these five are in Aberdeen. The result is that if only the hysteroscopic methods are to be used then most patients will not be able to access endometrial ablation. These resection or laser skills, if able to be learnt, are useful for other procedures such as resection of fibroids or uterine septae or full thickness endometrial/myometrial biopsies in women with abnormal bleeding on Tamoxifen therapy.

Where does that put the role of the second-generation methods? Having had the opportunity to read most of this book prior to writing this chapter one thing becomes obvious, there are too many claims made about second-generation methods with no reliable evidence to back them up. Many observational studies that are reported use outcome measures such as bleeding scores and not more reliable measures such as patient satisfaction, amenorrhoea rates, hysterectomy rate or quality of life measures. Not only that, but most authors are also reluctant to declare any financial interest or support from manufacturers.

Of the second-generation methods, only Therma-Choice™, MEA and Vestablate have published randomised trials and as Vestablate is no longer available, I will not discuss it further.

ThermaChoice™ is easy to use but has poor outcomes with only 15% becoming amenorrhoeic and poorer outcomes than rollerball ablation (REA), in a study where the results of REA were not as good as could be expected.[16] It can be performed under local anaesthetic but its relatively long treatment times, with uterine distension giving pain, may limit this. Perhaps the major disadvantage of this method is the inability to deal with large uterine cavities or irregular cavities due to fibroids. This will exclude around 30% of women currently dealt with in our practice.

MEA has perhaps the most evidence behind it. In our randomised study of 260 women comparing MEA to TCRE, we used our standard inclusion criteria of a uterus up to, and including, the size of a 10-week pregnancy and did not exclude fibroids or irregular cavities. MEA was faster than TCRE with fewer complications. The amenorrhoea rate following MEA was identical to TCRE 40% at 1 year[1] but had risen to 48% at 2 years.[2]

Satisfaction at 2 years was 90% (80% totally and 10% fairly satisfied) which was higher than for TCRE and the hysterectomy rate was 11% at 2 years.[2] TCRE and MEA gave identical results for the restoration of quality of life to normal as measured by Short Form 36. MEA, under local anaesthetic in a small-randomised trial, has also been studied.[17] This has shown that MEA is possible under local anaesthetic in the majority of unselected women and has given us the data to carry out a large randomised trial comparing both local and general anaesthetic.

Safety is an issue with the second-generation methods. All manufacturers claim their methods are safe and that there have never been any complications which seem to be at odds with the 'rumour factory'. There has been no formalised reporting system for most methods and indeed most manufacturers can only give accurate data for the number of pieces of equipment that have left the distributor. This is not the same as saying that all disposables have in fact been used.

There is only data for MEA on complications with a published prospective series of 1400 cases.[18] In this series, there was one major complication, a small bowel damage, secondary to a uterine false passage, which gives a complication less but similar to TCRE, in the MISTLETOE study. This study of MEA is better than nothing but is still too small, 5000 would be needed to give reliable figures.

Of the other methods there is, as yet, no good evidence to support their use. Personally speaking as a hysteroscopist, hydrothermablation (HTA) seems to me to be the most appealing of these methods. It is done under direct vision so hopefully preventing perforation or false passage formation in the uterus. This, however, is only true if the surgeon can recognise what he is seeing, which, unfortunately, is not always the case. There seems to be at least a theoretical risk of burns, if there is a sudden leak of the hot saline. The other advantage of this method is that it will treat irregular cavities.

My personal choice is between TCRE and MEA. TCRE has been proven to be effective and has given me good results over the years. It is inexpensive and gives material for histological assessment. MEA gives as good or better results than TCRE even in our hands. It is safer as it removes the risk of bleeding or fluid absorption. Its major advantage, to me, is that it is proven to be possible under local anaesthetic. Whether it is better under local or general anaesthetic and what patient perception and recovery differences there are, will be determined by a randomised trial currently being analysed. MEA is more expensive than TCRE but this may be reduced by local anaesthetic treatment and only if it can be removed from the operating theatre setting.

If you are able to do either TCRE or ELA well, with audited, reliably good results, then I would not advise any change unless you plan to move to a local anaesthetic regime outside the operating theatre. If, however, like the majority of gynaecologists, you have not taken up TCRE or found it difficult or disappointing, then based on the trial evidence at the time of writing this chapter in December 2001, MEA appears to offer the best alternative.

Declaration of interest

I have no financial connection with any manufacturer. Microsulis PLC have part funded some research activity in Aberdeen and provided travel support. The views are my own and not either those of Microsulis or The Chief Scientist's Office of the Scottish Executive who have funded most of the Aberdeen endometrial ablation research. I would like to thank all my research fellows from 1991 to 2001, Sheena Pinion, Siladitya Bhattacharya, Kevin Cooper, Christine Bain and Sarah Wallage.

References

1. Cooper KG, Bain C, Parkin DE. Comparison of microwave endometrial ablation with transcervical resection of the endometrium for the treatment of heavy menstrual loss. *Lancet* 1999; 354: 1859–1863.

2. Bain C, Cooper KG, Parkin DE. Two year follow up of a randomised controlled trial comparing microwave endometrial ablation to trans cervical resection of the endometrium in women complaining of excessive menstrual bleeding. *Obstet Gynecol* 2002 (in press).

3. Cooper KG, Jack S, Parkin DE, Grant AM. Five year follow-up of women randomised to medical management or transcervical resection of the endometrium for heavy menstrual loss: clinical and quality of life outcomes. *Br J Obstet Gynaecol* 2001 (in press).

4. Aberdeen Endometrial Ablation Trials Group. A randomised trial of endometrial ablation versus hysterectomy for the treatment of dysfunctional uterine bleeding: outcome at four years. *Br J Obstet Gynaecol* 1999; 106: 360–366.

5. Pinion SB, Parkin DE, Abramovich DR, Naji A, Alexander DA, Russell IT, Kitchener HC. Randomised trial of hysterectomy, endometrial laser ablation and transcervical endometrial resection for dysfunctional uterine bleeding. *Br Med J* 1994; 309: 979–983.

6. Parkin DE. Fatal toxic shock syndrome following endometrial resection. *Br J Obstet Gynaecol* 1995; 102: 163–164.

7. Scottish Hysteroscopic Audit Group. A Scottish audit of hysteroscopic surgery. *Br J Obstet Gynaecol* 1994; 102: 249–254.

8. Overton C, Hargreaves H, Maresh M. A national survey of the complications of endometrial destruction for menstrual disorders: the MISTLETOE study. *Br J Obstet Gynaecol* 1997; 104: 1351–1359.

9. Dwyer N, Hutton J, Stirrat GM. Randomised controlled trial comparing endometrial resection with abdominal hysterectomy for the surgical treatment of menorrhagia. *Br J Obstet Gynaecol* 1993; 100: 237–243.

10. O'Connor H, Broadbent J, Magos A et al. Medical research council randomised trial of endometrial resection versus hysterectomy in the management of menorrhagia. *Lancet* 1997; 349: 891–901.

11. Bhattacharya S, Cameron I, Parkin DE et al. A pragmatic randomised comparison of transcervical resection of the endometrium with endometrial laser ablation for the treatment of menorrhagia. *Br J Obstet Gynaecol* 1997; 104: 601–607.

12. Cooper KG, Parkin DE, Garret AM, Grant AM. Two year follow-up of women randomised to medical management or transcervical resection of the endometrium for heavy menstrual loss; clinical and quality of life outcomes. *Br J Obstet Gynaecol* 1999; 106: 258–265.

13. Lethaby AE, Shepperd S, Cooke I, Farquhar C. Endometrial resection and ablation versus hysterectomy for heavy menstrual bleeding (Cochrane review). Cochrane Library, Issue 2, 2000. Oxford: Update Software.

14. Parkin DE et al. Hysteroscopic Surgery: A national Clinical Guideline. Scottish Intercollegiate Guidelines Network. Guideline no 37. SIGN Edinburgh, 1999.

15. Dunkley MP, Brown LH, Robinson JM, Parkin DE. Initial training model for endometrial ablation. *Gynaecol Endosc* 2002 (in press).

16. Mayer WR, Walsh BW, Grainger DA, Peacock LM, Loffer FD, Steege JF. Thermal balloon and rollerball ablation to treat menorrhagia: a multicenter comparison. *Obstet Gynecol* 1998; 92: 98–103.

17. Bain C, Cooper KG, Parkin DE. A partially randomised patient preference trial of microwave endometrial ablation using local anaesthesia and intravenous sedation or general anaesthesia: a pilot study. *Gynaecol Endosc* 2001; 10: 223–228.

18. Parkin DE. Microwave endometrial ablation: a safe technique. Complication data from a prospective series of 1400 cases. *Gynaecol Endosc* 2000; 9: 385–388.

28

Future research on menorrhagia

Khalid S. Khan and T. Justin Clark

Introduction

In this book, the practical implications of the results of health research, as well as the personal views of experts in various aspects of conservative surgery for menorrhagia, have been provided. This chapter will look at the implications for future research in this field.

A recent postal questionnaire survey of 100 members of a gynaecological endoscopy society showed that 99% respondents believed that their society should play a proactive role in directing future research.[1] There was a substantial commitment to research with 47% respondents actively involved in research projects at the time of the survey, but there was no consensus about the topics suitable for health technology assessment in menorrhagia. This is not surprising, as the choice of research areas is usually a subjective judgement. However, one can attempt to determine future research topics by examining the following areas:

- the clinical process,
- current research findings and deficiencies in research,
- current patterns of practice and uncertainty in practice,
- views of practitioners, consumers, and grant giving bodies.

Considering these factors, we have chosen three aspects of menorrhagia research for more detailed discussion in this chapter. These include quality of life assessment, diagnostic strategies and therapeutic effectiveness.

Quality of life assessment in menorrhagia

The clinical process involves making a diagnosis and providing an appropriate therapy, usually in that sequence. Following institution of therapy, one needs to find ways of monitoring its success. Menorrhagia and its conservative surgery pose special research issues in all these aspects of clinical care.

Menorrhagia may be defined as excessive menstrual loss. Objectively, this means measured menstrual loss in excess of 80 ml per menstrual cycle. In clinical practice, it is not possible to routinely perform an objective assessment of menstrual loss and menorrhagia is, therefore, taken to be a subjective complaint of excessive menstrual loss. This causes problems from the outset. Many research studies employ objective measurements

as eligibility criteria for recruitment but what will be the generalisability of studies that include and exclude subjects without regard for clinical practice? Moreover, how would one assess the outcomes of conservative surgery if the disease symptoms were subjective?

One crucial area for menorrhagia research is development of disease specific 'quality of life' instruments. The overall aim of management of chronic, benign conditions, such as menorrhagia, is to reduce the adverse health impact of the condition in order to improve the patient's quality of life. Thus, it should be immediately apparent that use of instruments to measure life quality will be critical to diagnosis, as well as to evaluating success of therapy, in menorrhagia. The use of life quality instruments in menorrhagia research will allow more objective assessment of the clinical condition. Although generic instruments have been available for many years, quality of life measurement cannot ignore aspects that are unique to menorrhagia. Thus, disease specific instruments are required to obtain patient focussed measurements. In this way, research in menorrhagia can benefit both from generic as well as disease specific instruments.

Numerous definitions of quality of life exist, each with slightly different underlying theoretical emphasis. In simple terms, quality of life is a unique personal perception of both health related and non-health related factors. A quality of life instrument collects information about these factors (or domains) by using a questionnaire. Examples of domains include physical and cognitive function, psychological and social well-being, role activities (e.g. jobs, family, friends, finance) and personal factors (e.g. spirituality). Some instruments focus only on aspects of life more closely related to health status (e.g. physical and psychological well-being). Sometimes a single all-inclusive question is used to assess quality of life, e.g. 'How would you rate your quality of life?'

Quality of life instruments can be either generic or disease specific as indicated earlier. Generic instruments attempt to capture a broad range of aspects of life quality that are important to all patients. They allow comparison across different diseases. Disease specific instruments, on the other hand, are expected to capture how specific aspects of the disorder interfere with life quality, thereby providing specific information and ensuring sensitivity to change over time. However, the two most important aspects of any type of quality of life instrument are clinical appropriateness (or face validity) and measurement properties. In order for an instrument to have clinical face validity, it must include items that are of importance to patients and adequately reflect their experiences and concerns. Instruments with sound measurement properties are those instruments that have demonstrated reliability, validity, responsiveness, etc.

Evaluation of recent research on menorrhagia shows that, in studies where quality of life instruments are employed, there is good compliance with the criteria for measurement properties but not with those for clinical face validity.[2] Therefore, the appropriateness of the life quality measures used in menorrhagia research is questionable. The SF36 health survey questionnaire, the most commonly used instrument in menorrhagia, is seemingly reliable, valid and responsive. However, several of its questions are inappropriate or difficult to answer for women with menorrhagia. This results from the fact that symptoms are not generally constant but cyclical, they are distressing but non-life threatening and they do not last indefinitely.[3] Therefore, used on its own, the SF36 is inappropriate as a patient based outcome measure in menorrhagia. The available disease specific instruments have poor face validity because they do not use a more flexible questionnaire format incorporating global patient ratings, ratings of importance of constituents of quality of life and allowing supplemental patient comments.[4] It is disappointing that even recently developed disease specific instruments do not show compliance with criteria for face validity.[5,6] Thus, there is a need to develop methodologically sound disease specific quality of life instruments in menorrhagia focussing both on face validity and measurement properties.

Diagnostic strategies for menorrhagia

Accurate diagnosis is a critical part of the clinical process because it allows optimal management strategies to be employed. Incorrect diagnoses may put patients at risk and waste limited resources. Available diagnostic methods for the evaluation of women with menorrhagia include traditional dilatation and curettage under anaesthesia, outpatient blind endometrial biopsy, inpatient and outpatient hysteroscopy, transvaginal ultrasonography with or without colour flow doppler, 3-dimensional ultrasonography, sonohysterography, computerised tomography (CT) and magnetic resonance imaging (MRI). These have been used alone or in combination to assess the uterine cavity. The clinical process dictates that a detailed history should be

obtained and examination including general, abdominal and pelvic examination should be carried out, prior to any investigations.

Many of the tests for endometrial assessment are yet to undergo rigorous clinical evaluation but those event in routine use (e.g. hysteroscopy and ultrasonography) have been poorly evaluated. In a recent survey[1] of areas for the direction of future research in hysteroscopic diagnosis, 36/100 (36%) responders felt that this was important. Not all respondents supporting this research area specified particular research topics.[1] However, those that did, identified studies to determine the diagnostic accuracy of hysteroscopy in endometrial cancer and its diagnostic performance compared to ultrasonography (with or without saline contrast) to be of importance. However, when enquired about their current research activity, relatively few respondents indicated conducting diagnostic accuracy studies in gynaecological endoscopy. This may reflect a perceived lack of importance compared to developing new therapies or a lack of experience in designing diagnostic test studies.

One has to start evaluation of test accuracy with the premise that diagnosis will be based on information acquired from a variety of sources, i.e. history, examination and tests. The need to rigorously assess the accuracy of the clinical history and examination has been highlighted,[7] but it has seldom been integrated in the evaluation of diagnostic tests.[7,8] The whole clinical process should be borne in mind when conducting research to evaluate a diagnostic strategy because test accuracy studies in isolation from the rest of the clinical context do not necessarily indicate how useful the test will be in practice. Estimates of diagnostic accuracy derived in this way can lead to erroneous inferences and may artificially inflate the value of diagnostic tests.[9]

To determine the real value of the tests listed above, evaluation within the context of contemporary clinical practice is essential. The clinical value of tests lies in the added information over and above what was already known from the history and examination. Recent evaluation of literature addressing the diagnostic accuracy of ultrasound,[10,11] hysteroscopy[12] and endometrial biopsy[13,14] shows that only a limited number of existing studies consider the value of test in light of the clinical context, otherwise most of the literature evaluates tests in isolation. Multivariable analysis should be used to delineate the significance of diagnostic variables and it is important in facilitating meaningful clinical interpretation of tests. This is because it allows the added value of tests to be determined in light of information already available to the clinician from the history and examination, thereby reflecting the real contribution of the test in a clinical situation. Future diagnostic research should be done in a way as to allow one to determine how the tests add value to the overall diagnostic process.

Therapeutic effectiveness in menorrhagia

Traditionally, medical treatment with drugs is used as a first line intervention prior to surgery in benign menorrhagia. The treatment, hysteroscopically, ranges from resection of polyps[15] and submucous myoma[16] to resection or ablative procedures of the endometrium.[17,18] These procedures may be carried out in the outpatient setting.[15] More recently levenorgestrel-releasing intrauterine systems have been used as an alternative to surgery.[19] The definitive cure for menorrhagia is believed to be a hysterectomy, but this major surgery is associated with morbidity and rarely mortality.[20] Endometrial surgery with ablative and resection techniques has the potential benefits of less post-operative morbidity, shorter recovery time and lower cost. There is still debate on the role of endometrial surgery in the management of dysfunctional uterine bleeding. There is sufficient evidence to suggest that such surgery is no longer an experimental procedure, but there is still uncertainty about its role in clinical practice.[21] Should it be offered to women with dysfunctional uterine bleeding as an intermediate procedure after failed medical treatment and prior to hysterectomy or should it be used as a first line treatment in place of medical treatment? The concern for patients, consumer groups, third party payers and government agencies has been that approximately 35% of women with menorrhagia end up having a hysterectomy. However, the uptake of alternatives to hysterectomy like endometrial resection and ablation have been limited. The indications, effectiveness, operative risks and economic consequences of these techniques are all issues that need to be resolved with high quality research.

In a recent survey[1] of areas for the direction of future research in hysteroscopic therapy, 62/100 (62%) responders felt that this was important. Not all respondents supporting this research area specified particular research topics. However, those who did, identified studies into first and second-generation endometrial ablative techniques and their comparison with each other and the levenorgestrel-releasing intrauterine device to be important. Other studies included determining the feasibility and effectiveness of treatment of intrauterine lesions (polyps, fibroids and septae) and hysteroscopic sterilisation.

The majority of existing randomised trials in menorrhagia treatment, particularly those on medical treatment, have utilised reduction in measured menstrual blood loss prior to and after treatment as the outcome measure to assess efficacy. While such an outcome measure has the advantage in requiring a relatively small sample size to conduct the trial, it has no clinical relevance at all as an objective reduction in menstrual blood loss, does not necessarily correlate with the patient's perception of the clinical effectiveness of the treatment administered.[2] It has been previously indicated that there is a need to develop and use quality of life instruments for assessing effectiveness of menorrhagia treatments.

The research assessment of endometrial surgery has mainly been performed with observational studies over a moderate follow-up period. Almost all of these studies have enrolled women from the gynaecological outpatient clinic after failure with some form of medical intervention administered prior to surgery. Such studies may be biased as the study population is recruited exclusively from a hospital setting. Future studies may be targeted on a mix of women recruited from the general practitioners as well as from hospital outpatient clinics. Another problem with published observational cohort studies on the outcome of endometrial surgery is the use of simple proportions to quantify the rates of outcome events such as hysterectomy, patient satisfaction or amenorrhoea. Since these outcomes are time-dependent, i.e. the likelihood of being able to observe the outcome event is higher with those women with longer follow-up than those with shorter follow-up times, the use of simple proportions will tend to underestimate the true event rates.[21] On the other hand, use of survival analyses will allow the outcome of the entire cohort with variable follow-up times to be described without bias. In this way, a more realistic estimation of the likelihood of failure of endometrial surgery can be obtained. In this analysis, the outcome measure used should be an irreversible once-in-a-lifetime event since the cumulative probability of a woman experiencing that outcome, up to and including any particular time interval, assumes that she has not experienced it previously. The presence or absence of a subsequent hysterectomy or repeat endometrial surgery would satisfy this requirement. However, amenorrhoea (except when menopause is achieved) and patient satisfaction are reversible outcomes and hence, are not appropriate outcomes to be used with this method of analysis.

There is obviously a need to generate experimental (i.e. randomised) evidence to compare the effectiveness of the various treatment modalities for menorrhagia. The study populations should be followed-up for a long period of time in order for complications and hysterectomy rates in the various comparison groups to be ascertained in a more meaningful fashion. These trials should be robust and their design may take account of variation in current practice and views of practitioners and consumers. Without them, the effectiveness and the place of endometrial surgical modalities will remain uncertain.

Conclusion

Rigorous, relevant and timely research is essential for improvement in the quality of care we provide to our patients with menorrhagia. The conduct of such research requires an appraisal of the existing evidence, an examination of current medical practice and an appreciation of the whole clinical process. In addition, a multidisciplinary collaborative approach should be encouraged, incorporating the views of all stakeholders. In this way, increasingly effective diagnostic and therapeutic strategies, in such a common condition as menorrhagia, can be implemented in clinical practice in the future.

References

1. Clark TJ, Mahajan D, Sunder P, Bingham T, Khan KS, Gupta JK. What research should be done in gynaecological endoscopy: a national questionnaire survey of members of the British Society of Gynaecological Endoscopy. *Gynaecol Endosc* 2001 (in press).

2. Clark TJ, Khan KS, Foon R, Pattison H, Bryan S, Gupta JK. Quality of life instruments in studies of menorrhagia: a systematic review. *Eur J Obstet Gynecol Reprod* 2001 (submitted).

3. Jenkinson C, Peto V, Coulter A. Making sense of ambiguity: evaluation of internal reliability and face validity of the SF 36 questionnaire in women presenting with menorrhagia. *Qual Health Care* 1996; 5: 9–12.

4. Guyatt GH, Cook DJ. Health status, quality of life, and the individual. *JAMA* 1994; 272: 630–631.

5. Lamping DL, Rowe P, Clarke A, Black N, Lessof L. Development and validation of the menorrhagia outcomes questionnaire. *Br J Obstet Gynecol* 1998; 105: 766–779.

6. Shaw RW, Brickley MR, Evans L, Edwards MJ. Perceptions of women on the impact of menorrhagia on their health using multi-attribute utility assessment. *Br J Obstet Gynecol* 1998; 105: 1155–1159.

7. McAlister F, Straus S, Sackett D. Why we need large, simple studies of the clinical examination: the problem and a proposed solution. *Lancet* 1999; 354: 1721–1724.

8. Clark TJ, Bakour S, Gupta JK, Khan KS. Evaluation of outpatient hysteroscopy and ultrasonography in the diagnosis of endometrial disease. *Obstet Gynecol* 2001 (in press).

9. Bachmann LM, ter Riet G, Clark TJ, Gupta JK, Khan KS. Probability analysis for diagnosis of endometrial disease in postmenopausal bleeding: an approach for a rational diagnostic workup. *Gynecol Oncol* 2001 (submitted).

10. Smith-Bindman R, Kerlikowske K, Feldstein VA, Subak L, Scheidler J, Segal M et al. Endovaginal ultrasound to exclude endometrial cancer and other endometrial abnormalities. *JAMA* 1998; 280: 1510–1517.

11. Chien PFW, Voit D, Clark TJ, Khan KS, Gupta JK. Ultrasonographic endometrial thickness for diagnosing endometrial pathology in women with postmenopausal bleeding: a meta-analysis. *Acta Obstet Gynecol Scand* 2002 (in press).

12. Clark TJ, Voit D, Gupta JK, Hyde C, Song F, Khan KS. Accuracy of hysteroscopy in the diagnosis of endometrial cancer and hyperplasia: a systematic quantitative review. *JAMA* 2001 (submitted).

13. Clark TJ, Mann CH, Shah N, Song F, Khan KS, Gupta JK. Accuracy of outpatient endometrial biopsy in the diagnosis of endometrial cancer: a systematic quantitative review. *Br J Obstet Gynaecol* 2001; 109: 313–21.

14. Clark TJ, Mann CH, Shah N, Song F, Khan KS, Gupta JK. Accuracy of outpatient endometrial biopsy in the diagnosis of endometrial hyperplasia: a systematic quantitative review. *Acta Obstet Gynecol Scand* 2001; 80: 784–793.

15. Clark TJ, Godwin J, Khan KS, Gupta JK. Ambulatory endoscopic treatment of symptomatic benign endometrial polyps: a feasibility study. *Gynaecol Endosc* 2001 (in press).

16. Clark TJ, Mahajan D, Sunder P, Gupta JK. Hysteroscopic treatment of symptomatic submucous fibroids using a bipolar intrauterine system: a feasibility study. *Eur J Obstet, Gynecol and Reprod Biol* 2001 (in press).

17. Kremer C, Duffy S. Endometrial ablation: the next generation. *Br J Obstet Gynaecol* 2000; 107: 1443–1452.

18. O'Connor H, Magos A. Endometrial resection for the treatment of menorrhagia. *N Engl J Med* 1996; 335: 151–156.

19. Barrington JW, Bowen-Simpkins P. The levenorgestrel intrauterine system in the management of menorrhagia. *Br J Obstet Gynaecol* 1997; 104: 614–616.

20. Wingo PA, Huezo CM, Rubin GL, Ory HW, Peterson HB. The mortality risk associated with hysterectomy. *Am J Obstet Gynecol* 1985; 152: 803–808.

21. Chien PF, Khan KS, Garry R. Medical treatment or endometrial surgery for dysfunctional uterine bleeding? *Acta Obstet Gynecol Scand* 1998; 77(6): 587–590.

Index

Abbreviations: RCT, randomsied controlled trial; TCRE, transcervical resection of endometrium.